Concussion
Diagnosis and Management
Second Edition

SPORTS-RELATED

Concussion
Diagnosis and Management
Second Edition

Brian Sindelar
MD

Neurosurgery Chief Resident
University of Florida
Department of Neurosurgery
Gainesville, Florida

Julian E. Bailes
MD

Bennett Tarkington Chairman
Department of Neurosurgery
NorthShore Univ HealthSystem
Co-director, NorthShore Neurological Institute
Clinical Professor of Neurosurgery
University of Chicago Pritzker School of Medicine
Evanston, Illinois

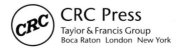

CRC Press
Taylor & Francis Group
Boca Raton London New York

CRC Press is an imprint of the
Taylor & Francis Group, an **informa** business

CRC Press
Taylor & Francis Group
6000 Broken Sound Parkway NW, Suite 300
Boca Raton, FL 33487-2742

© 2018 by Taylor & Francis Group, LLC
CRC Press is an imprint of Taylor & Francis Group, an Informa business

No claim to original U.S. Government works

Printed and bound in India by Replika Press Pvt. Ltd.

Printed on acid-free paper

International Standard Book Number-13: 978-1-4987-6457-5 (Paperback)

Contents

CHAPTER 5

Postconcussive syndrome   99

CHAPTER 6

Outpatient care of the concussed athlete: Gauging recovery to tailor rehabilitative needs   131

With Elizabeth M. Pieroth, Psy.D.

CHAPTER 7

Return to activity following concussion   161

CHAPTER 8

Neuroimaging in concussion   181

With Matthew T. Walker, M.D. and Monther Qandeel, M.D.

CHAPTER 9
The advent of subconcussion and chronic traumatic encephalopathy   195

With John Lee, M.D. Ph.D.

CHAPTER 10
Promising advances in concussion diagnosis and treatment   225

Preface

SINCE THE RELEASE OF THE FIRST EDITION almost two decades ago, sports-related concussion has been brought to the public's attention due the extreme popularity of sports, the wide participation, and extensive media coverage. This has led to an explosion in the science of concussion with efforts to better understand the true injury that occurs and therefore enable proper diagnosis, treatment, and reveal potential long-term effects. This book is intended to provide the reader with an understanding of concussion and its management through a review of extensive preclinical and clinical research, as well as best practices experience.

With the vast number of youth, high school, collegiate, and professional athletes, sports-related concussion is a significantly prevalent affliction. Therefore, a wide variety of people, whether medically trained or not, have the potential to interact with a concussed athlete, and play a role in the short-term and/or long-term care of the athlete. For this reason, this book has been written as a general foundation into sports-related concussion and management for anyone that is involved in the care of a concussed athlete: from medical professionals (physicians, therapists, psychologists, athletic trainers), to school and sporting staff (administrators, coaches, nurses), and also family members.

Starting from the coach, athletic trainers, school nurses, and parents, increased knowledge in concussion management can improve timely evaluation, diagnosis, and coordinated care focused towards the recovery of the athlete. Similarly, a better understanding of concussion literature by medical professionals will equip them to more thoroughly manage the process of recovery of a concussed athlete and his/her return to activity. There is more emphasis now being placed on concussion education for all those who come in contact with athletes.

This book is also written for the athlete. Since concussion care is individually tailored, a comprehensive understanding by the athlete of their injury is essential in providing them with the tools to be proactive in their care and hasten recovery. This notably enables the athlete to make an informed decision about concussion recognition as well as activity progression, therapeutic remedies, return to sport, and/or even retirement from sport. Additionally, it is imperative to understand that the consequences of a concussion may not be only limited to the immediate days to weeks following an injury. Strong evidence has demonstrated a correlation between cumulative concussive injuries, and even subconcussive injuries, to the potential development of a progressive neurodegenerative disease, chronic traumatic encephalopathy. Therefore, concussion education is imperative so that the athlete understands the risks of hazardous play in efforts to reduce concussion incidence, stress the importance of return to activity protocols, and potentially decrease any long-term sequelae.

As will be further illustrated in this book, care for the concussed athlete is a multidisciplinary effort; only through a unified understanding of the injury among all of these individuals can the athlete be best positioned for a timely recovery and return to their given sport. We hope that this text will provide such knowledge to the reader, and also stimulate intellectual thought and discussion to further progress research into the field of sports-related concussion.

Acknowledgments

- The senior author, Dr. Julian Bailes, for his invaluable mentorship, support, and guidance in my career.
- Our contributing authors, Dr. John Lee, Dr. Matthew Walker, Dr. Monther Qandeel, and Dr. Elizabeth Pieroth, for offering their expertise in their chosen fields.
- Dr. Vimal Patel, who was vital to the completion of this text through obtaining publication copyright permissions.
- Randal McKenzie, for animating the written words of complex concussion topics into incredible figures and also envisioning and producing the book cover.
- My mother, for leading by example. All that I am is because of you.
- Lastly, and most importantly, my wife Adriana, for not only enthusiastically editing chapters but providing endless love, support, encouragement, and laughter during the process.

CHAPTER I

Introduction to sports related concussion

Introduction

Prior to diving into the complex physiology, presentation, and treatment of concussion, an initial introduction of the historical definition is required followed by its evolution into its current designation. Though our knowledge of concussion has deepened through advanced neuroimaging and preclinical animal research, there still remains shortcomings regarding our understanding of this topic which has led to challenges in providing a stable definition. We will present these changes in the definition of concussion, and how this has influenced the ability to accurately provide a concussion incidence in sports. Lastly, we will review how the epidemiology of various sports-specific concussive injuries has influenced game-play alterations in order to make the sport safer for athletes.

"What's in a name?"

Concussion or mild traumatic brain injury?

Concussion comes from the Latin word "concutere" which means to shake violently. In the 1300s, Lanfrancus became the first modern physician to define concussion as a transient alteration in cerebral functioning.[1] Since that time, numerous terminologies have been used in order to describe this injury: "mild traumatic brain injury (mTBI)," "mild brain injury," "mild head injury," and "ding."[2] Even within the medical community, mTBI and concussion is used synonymously to denote a similar injury, which is actually erroneous.[3]

The Glasgow Coma Scale, GCS, was originally developed as a clinical classification scheme to rapidly describe traumatically injured patients by evaluating their alertness, mentation, and functional abilities. This crude but easily communicated system is determined by the following patient characteristics—eye opening, verbal response, and motor activity—with a total score ranging from 3 to 15 (Table 1.1). Scores between 13 and 15 denote a mild traumatic brain injury, or "mTBI." After a concussion, athletes are typically alert, communicative, and following commands. Therefore, in the majority of concussed athletes, the GCS scale would assign this player as having a "mTBI."

The use of the term mTBI to describe concussion, however, clusters patients that have similar clinical exams based on this rudimentary scale, yet may have vastly different intracranial pathologies. Clinical scales such as the GCS can therefore place a patient with a more structural lesions like intracranial hemorrhage in the same category as a patient with a concussion that typically has absent radiological findings on cranial imaging. Relying solely on this scale to evaluate a patient can either seriously overestimate or underestimate the time severity of their injury. For this reason, it is important to recognize that concussion is on the spectrum of traumatic brain injuries and is one of many types of mTBI, but not all mTBIs are concussions. Therefore, these terms should not be used synomously.[3–6]

Historical classification

Though most concussive symptoms are self-limited, resolving within 7–10 days, there are a minority of athletes that develop a protracted course following injury.[7,8] For this reason, historical grading scales were devised in efforts to further classify the severity of concussion based upon initial symptomatology, specifically duration of loss of consciousness

Table 1.1 Glasgow Coma Scale

	Eye Response	Verbal	Motor
1	Does not open	Non verbal	No movement
2	Opens to painful stimuli	Incomprehensible	Decerebrate posturing
3	Opens to voice	Uses inappropriate words	Decorticate posturing
4	Opens spontaneously	Confused	Withdraws to painful stimuli
5		Oriented	Localizes to painful stimuli
6			Follows commands

Note: A score of 3–8 denotes a severe TBI, 9–12 a moderate TBI, and 13–15 mild TBI.

(LOC) and/or post traumatic amnesia (PTA), with the hope that this would correlate and predict long-term outcomes.[9–16] The classification schemes were based on LOC because it was previously thought that LOC was associated/required for diagnosis of a concussion.[9,10]

To date, there have been a total of 25 different concussion-grading scales.[17] Three of the most common concussion scales were published by Cantu et al., the Colorado Medical Society Consortium, and the American Academy of Neurology (Table 1.2).[12,13,18,19] It is clearly evident that though these grading scales are simple and easy to use, there exists great variability between each concussion grade determined by the athlete's presence or absence of LOC and PTA. This lack of standardization consequently brought confusion to clinicians and made it difficult to compare results of clinical studies.[14]

Moreover, every one of these concussion-grading scales was dependent on the manifestation and duration of LOC following injury. With time, it was observed that only 5%–10% of concussions actually had a period of LOC and even the presence itself did not correlate with injury severity.[8,14,20–25] Analogously, Brown et al. demonstrated in a preclinical concussion model that extensive and diffuse axonal injury can occur without the presence of LOC.[26] For these reasons, currently most clinicians rely on presence or absence of concussion symptoms, and their duration, rather than a grading system that relief on LOC. Therefore, these concussion grading scales have only historical importance, but do not have any clinical application.

Current definition of concussion

With the understanding and acceptance that a concussive injury can occur without LOC, the Concussion in Sport Group released the Zurich Guidelines in 2012 defining concussion as:

1. "Caused by a *direct blow* to the head, face, neck, or *elsewhere on the body* with an 'impulsive' force transmitted to the head.
2. Typically results in the rapid onset of *short-lived impairment of neurological function* that resolves spontaneously. However, in some cases, symptoms and signs may evolve over a number of minutes to hours.
3. May result in neuropathological changes, but the acute clinical symptoms largely reflect a *functional disturbance rather than a structural injury*, and as such, *no abnormality* is seen on standard structural neuroimaging studies.

Table 1.2 Historical Concussion Grading Scales

Concussion Scale	Concussion Grade	LOC	PTA	Symptoms
Cantu Grading System[12]	1	None	<30 mins	
	2	<5 mins	>30 mins	
	3	>5 mins	>24 hours	
1999 Colorado Medical Society[19]	1	None	None	Confusion
	2	None	Present	None
	3	Present		
1999 American Academy of Neurology[18]	1	None		Transient (<15 mins) confusion, symptoms, or mental status changes
	2	None		Confusion, symptoms, or mental status changes (>15 mins)
	3	Present		

4. Results in a graded set of clinical symptoms that may or *may not involve loss of consciousness.* Resolution of the clinical and cognitive symptoms typically follows a sequential course. However, it is important to note that in some cases symptoms may be prolonged."[8]

Along with the importance of not requiring LOC to diagnose concussion, this definition of concussion was the first to emphasize that concussions occur from 1. direct and indirect impacts, 2. lead to a functional neuronal alteration, 3. have no radiographical correlate (lack of intracranial macrostructural lesions), and 4. that the path of recovery is just as important as the initial injury (to be further discussed in Chapters 2 and 3).[8,10,14–16,27–37] These points accentuated by the Zurich Guidelines have become adopted into the standardized definition of concussion, and have been presented in recent years by various medical professional societies like the American Academy of Neurology, the American Medical Society, the Institute of Medicine, and the National Athletic Trainers Association.[32,33,38,39]

The glaring inaccuracy regarding the definition of concussion by the Zurich guidelines is that they propose a concussion is "a *functional* disturbance rather than a *structural* injury."[8,40] To be further discussed throughout this book, it is now apparent that the functional disturbance that occurs in the neuron following a concussive blow, though unlikely to cause a macrostructural injury, can in fact result in microstructural damage.[41–70] This revelation has only been recently understood through the remarkable improvements in neuroimaging, such as diffusion tensor imaging. This concept will likely be addressed in the 5th International Consensus Conference on Concussion in Sport.

Concussion modifiers

For completeness in discussion, modifiers have also been attached to the definition of concussion in literature, but have been used to describe different criteria. "Simple versus complex concussion" or "uncomplicated versus complicated" modifiers have been inconsistently applied to patients with either the presence of intracranial blood products, those either with worse acute presentations (LOC, PTA, or lowered GCS), and if a patient is found

to develop a prolonged recovery upon retrospective review.[15,71–73] Until scientific validation of these modifiers is proven to predict recovery and functional outcome, use of them only brings perplexity and confusion to the definition without any clear benefit. Potentially, in the near future, will there be validation of a graded scale of concussive injuries based on outpatient recovery assessment tools (like neuropsychological testing, oculomotor/balance testing, or symptom checklists), serum/CSF biomarkers, or neuroimaging outcomes.[43,74–90]

Epidemiology

It has been published that 3.8 million sports and recreation concussions are reported annually in the U.S., but this incidence is likely an enormous underestimate.[10,39] First, as discussed above, there has been an evolution in the definition of concussion over the past decade therefore making epidemiological studies throughout the years difficult to compare in parallel. Second, athletes may present for evaluation in different settings (emergency department, primary care provider, or athletic trainer), potentially eluding a database that collects from only one specific location. Third, some athletes may have prompt resolution of symptoms, thereby precluding them from ever seeking medical attention. Lastly, it has been well studied that there exists a large body of athletes that do not report their injury to medical professionals.[16] In anonymous surveys, 90% of athletes expressed understanding of the potential serious consequences of playing while concussed or partaking in a premature return to play, yet roughly only 50%–60% of high school, collegiate, and professional athletes would report a concussion and seek medical attention.[39,91–98] Even more concerning, is that some players acknowledged they would knowingly hide symptoms in order to influence the diagnosis.[91,95] The reasons for nondisclosure of a concussive injury are numerous: internal pressures, lack of knowledge of serious consequences, underplaying symptoms/injury, stigma/stereotype of "being weak," external pressures from teammates/coaches/parents, importance of a specific match or game, not wanting to be removed from play/sport, and financial reasons like income and scholarships.[16,99–105] In a survey of 8–18 year old student athletes, the "worst part about a concussion" was the removal from participation and lack of activity.[105]

Therefore, taking only into account underreporting, the annual concussion rate can be re-estimated to be doubled in the range of 7–8 million people.[10,39,91–96] Interestingly, this number only continues to grow as demonstrated by studies analyzing the annual concussion incidence in high school, college, and patients presenting to the emergency department (Figure 1.1).[106–109] There are a multitude of factors attributed to this growing concussion incidence: litigation/legislation, increased concussion education to players, media coverage, improved detection, and also ever growing size and speed of athletes as sports continue to evolve.[106,110–112] Therefore, it is unknown whether we are observing a true increase in the incidence of concussion, or, if we are observing an increase in the reporting of concussion.

Across all sports, the risk of concussion has been projected to be in the range of 0.025–21.5 concussions per 1000 athletic exposures (1 athletic exposure is a single practice or game).[113–115] Depending on the specific study, either men's football, men's wrestling, men's rugby, men's baseball, women's softball, women's soccer, and women's lacrosse have been reported to have the highest incidence of concussions in either high school or collegiate sports.[32,109,115–119] Please refer to Table 1.3 for a summary of concussions per athletic exposures observed for each specific sport.[113,120–125]

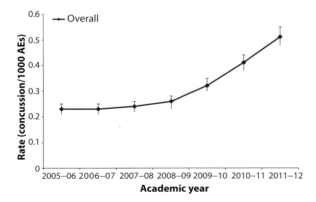

Figure 1.1 Annual concussion incidence has doubled in collegiate sports from 2005 to 2011. (From Rosenthal et al., *The American Journal of Sports Medicine* 42, 1710–1715, 2014. With permission from American Orthopaedic Society for Sports Medicine.)

Table 1.3 Concussion Rates per Athletic Exposures

Sport	Level of Play	Concussion Rate per 1000 Athletic Exposures (AE)[a]
Football	High school	0.48–1.03
	Collegiate	0.52–0.81
	Professional	4.56
Lacrosse	High School	Female: 0.21
		Male: 0.28
	Collegiate	Female: 0.32–0.64
		Male: 0.87–1.25
Hockey	High School	Male: 0.54
	Collegiate	Female: 0.71–1.11
		Male: 0.37–0.72
	Professional	Male: 1.45
Soccer	High School	Female: 0–0.27
		Male: 0.17
	Collegiate	Female: 0.38–0.44
		Male: 0.49–0.6
	Professional	Male: 1.2
Rugby		0.2–14.7

Sources: Clay MB et al., *Journal of Chiropractic Medicine*, 12(4), 230–251, 2013; Izraelski J., *The Journal of the Canadian Chiropractic Association*, 58(4), 346–352, 2014; Kirkwood G et al., *British Journal of Sports Medicine*, 49(8), 506–510, 2015; Gardner A et al., *British Journal of Sports Medicine*, 49(8), 495–498, 2015; Gardner AJ et al., *Sports Medicine (Auckland, NZ)*, 44(12), 1717–1731, 2014; Boden BP et al., *The American Journal of Sports Medicine*, 26(2), 238–241, 1998; O'Kane JW et al., *The Journal of the American Medical Association Pediatrics*, 168(3), 258–264, 2014.

[a] Athletic Exposure (AE) is equal to one practice or game participation.

Though the table document published incidences mostly for contact sports, noncollision sport athletes are also at risk. Noncontact sports like gymnastics, cheerleading/dancing, swimming, track and field, equestrian riding, cricket, volleyball, etc. also have the potential for a concussive injury.[126–133] Therefore, it is essential for all medical professionals to educate all athletes about concussion. Likewise, medical professionals should be ready to perform diagnostic assessment and evaluation for concussion in any sport, if the symptoms and mechanism of injury suggest potential concussive exposure.

Sport specific concussion details

Football

American football has the greatest volume of literature published regarding concussive injury in players for a specific sport. It has been estimated that 40% of all football players have experienced at least one concussion during their playing career.[97] Given there are over 1.2 million high school and collegiate players annually, 40% of this number is a staggeringly high number of exposed players.[134] Even within the National Football League (NFL), there is between 0.38 and 0.41 concussions per game; therefore it takes Any Given Sunday to witness at least five televised concussions.[23,135]

The specific positions in football that are most vulnerable to concussion are the lineman, wide receivers, defensive secondary, quarterbacks, and linebackers.[23,32,104] Studies have demonstrated that offensive and defensive linemen experience the highest frequency of impacts and therefore total cumulative G forces;[97,136] while running backs and quarterbacks, on average, are exposed to the greatest peak intensities.[137,138] Players that receive one concussion have also been demonstrated to be at an increased risk of repeat concussion within acute (within 10 days from first concussion)[139] and chronic time points (within 6 years)[140] along with an increased risk for musculoskeletal injuries.[125] Player positions that are at the highest risk of repeat concussions include quarterbacks, special team members, offensive linemen, wide receivers/tight-ends, and linebackers.[140,141] Therefore, being mindful of this risk per position, coaches could alter practice drills in order to reduce impact exposures.

It has also been demonstrated that players receive greater impacts during practice, and in some studies, of greater magnitude than game play, but this has been contested by further studies.[142–146] Daniel et al. found in a cohort of 7–8 year old football players that 76% of all impacts in the 95th percentile (>40 G forces) and all 8 impacts above 80 G linear acceleration occurred during practice.[142] Beckwith et al. also established that players were exposed to more impacts above the 50th and 95th percentile of peak linear and rotational acceleration on the day leading up to a concussive injury.[146] For this reason, youth (Pop-Warner Football), high school, collegiate, and professional sports teams have implemented a number of strict nonpadded, noncontact practices during the week in order to reduce collision exposures and hopefully the number of concussions.[112] Aside from practice participation, concussions were found to occur most frequently during kickoff returns. This evidence prompted the NFL to move the kickoff line to the 35 yard line to reduce the number of returned plays.[135]

Through analysis of concussive injuries in all levels of play, three fourths of football concussions were found to be due to direct player contact, where 45%–68% of them occur with helmet-to-helmet collisions.[7,23,145] Players fitted with helmet accelerometers have shown that head to head contact and hits to the top of the head are the cause of the greatest G force exposures during play.[136,137,143,147–150] Through head down tackling, or "spearing," a player increases his/her overall striking mass by 67% by coupling the head with the rest of the body and therefore increasing the overall blunt force delivered to the opposing player.[151,152] These conclusions have led youth, high school, collegiate, and professional football leagues to ban helmet-to-helmet contact, even resulting in ejections from play and hefty fines at the professional level.

Hockey

Another contact sport, 2%–14% of all hockey related injuries are attributed specifically to concussion.[120] Athletes playing the forward position are at the greatest risk of concussion, and it has also been demonstrated that these concussions are more likely to occur during the first period of play.[120,153] Similar to football, 88% of concussions are due to player-to-player contact where the head is struck by an opposing player's shoulder (44%), elbow (15%), or glove (5%).[154]

The National Hockey League has made strides in order to protect players by penalizing athletes for checking from behind, "boarding" (if an opposing player violently hits the player into the boards of the hockey rink), and "crosschecking" (when an opposing player uses his stick to strike the torso or back of a player). A study in youth ice hockey players by Mihalik et al. showed that 17% of all body collisions involved penalized plays. These infraction-associated impacts were also accompanied with the highest head accelerations to the opposing player.[155] Similar studies in other sports, like rugby, have also demonstrated a higher association of concussions due to greater head linear acceleration occurring during plays that involved illegal or aggressive play.[122,155,156] Therefore, simple measures at the coaching and referee level involving instruction in proper play and aggressive penalty calls will establish a culture of safe play among athletes, and ultimately reduce concussions.[157]

Soccer

In soccer, 8.6% of all injuries are due to concussion.[158] Players at greatest risk are the defenders and goalkeepers, with an increased incidence during game play versus practice (69%).[124,158] Similarly to the previous sports mentioned, 60%–78% of concussions are due to player contact with the opposing player's head (30%)/elbow (14%)/knee (3%), ball (24%), ground (10%), or goalpost (3%).[124,125,158,159] Due to the high risk of concussions from head-to-head contact, "heading" has been banned in youth leagues, and limited heading for teenagers during practice has been recommended.

Conclusion

The study of concussion has led to an evolving definition over the past decade. This definition will continue to change as further knowledge is gained through preclinical and clinical research of concussion. We invite the reader to continue through the chapters in order to gain knowledge regarding the different aspects of concussion, and how this influences clinical management. Before further discussion of concussion management in the following chapters, we will attempt to simplify the biomechanical properties that initiate the pathophysiological response of the neurons, vasculature, and even inflammatory cells. This knowledge will provide a comprehensive understanding of the injury of concussion and how this has guided our process of diagnosis, concerns with other associated features (like intracranial blood products, seizures, and second impact syndrome), evaluation of their recovery (through symptom assessment, various clinical tools, and neuropsychological testing), mitigation of prolonged symptom recovery, and proper return to activity. We will also explore current and potential therapeutic remedies for concussion along with advances in neuroimaging of the concussed athlete. We will conclude the text with a collective review of the research and understanding of the effects of chronic cumulative head trauma and the development of Chronic Traumatic Encephalopathy. We hope that this overview will not only improve the care of the concussed athlete,

but will also spark further discussion and interest into advancing the preclinical and clinical research in sports related concussion.

References

1. McCrory PR, Berkovic SF. Concussion: the history of clinical and pathophysiological concepts and misconceptions. *Neurology.* 2001; 57(12): 2283–2289.

2. Guskiewicz KM, Bruce SL, Cantu RC et al. National Athletic Trainers' Association Position Statement: Management of Sport-Related Concussion. *Journal of Athletic Training.* 2004; 39(3): 280–297.

3. Giza CC, Kutcher JS. An introduction to sports concussions. Continuum (Minneapolis, Minn). 2014; *Sports Neurology.* 20(6): 1545–1551.

4. Harmon KG, Drezner JA, Gammons M et al. American Medical Society for Sports Medicine position statement: concussion in sport. *British Journal of Sports Medicine.* 2013; 47(1): 15–26.

5. Stone JL, Patel V, Bailes JE. The history of neurosurgical treatment of sports concussion. *Neurosurgery.* 2014; 75 Suppl. 4: S3–S23.

6. Murray IR, Murray AD, Robson J. Sports concussion: time for a culture change. *Clinical Journal of Sport Medicine.* 2015; 25(2): 75–77.

7. Meehan WP, 3rd, d'Hemecourt P, Comstock RD. High school concussions in the 2008–2009 academic year: mechanism, symptoms, and management. *The American Journal of Sports Medicine.* 2010; 38(12): 2405–2409.

8. McCrory P, Meeuwisse W, Aubry M et al. Consensus statement on Concussion in Sport–The 4th International Conference on Concussion in Sport held in Zurich, November 2012. *Physical Therapy in Sport.* 2013; 14(2): e1–e13.

9. Denny-Brown DE, Russell WR. Experimental Concussion: (Section of Neurology). *Proceedings of the Royal Society of Medicine.* 1941; 34(11): 691–692.

10. Ropper AH, Gorson KC. Clinical practice. Concussion. *The New England Journal of Medicine*. 2007; 356(2): 166–172.

11. Warren WL, Jr., Bailes JE. On the field evaluation of athletic head injuries. *Clinics in Sports Medicine*. 1998; 17(1): 13–26.

12. Cantu RC. Return to play guidelines after a head injury. *Clinics in Sports Medicine*. 1998; 17(1): 45–60.

13. Collins MW, Lovell MR, McKeag DB. Current issues in managing sports-related concussion. *The Journal of the American Medical Association* 1999; 282(24): 2283–2285.

14. Echemendia RJ, Giza CC, Kutcher JS. Developing guidelines for return to play: consensus and evidence-based approaches. *Brain Injury* 2015; 29(2): 185–194.

15. Choe MC, Giza CC. Diagnosis and management of acute concussion. *Seminars in Neurology*. 2015; 35(1): 29–41.

16. McKee AC, Daneshvar DH. The neuropathology of traumatic brain injury. *Handbook of Clinical Neurology*. 2015; 127: 45–66.

17. Johnston KM, McCrory P, Mohtadi NG, Meeuwisse W. Evidence-based review of sport-related concussion: clinical science. *Clinical Journal of Sport Medicine*. 2001; 11(3): 150–159.

18. Quality Standards Subcommittee, American Academy of Neurology. Practice parameter. *Neurology*. 1997; 48: 581–585.

19. Colorado Medical Society. Report of the Sports Medicine Committee: Guidelines for the Management of Concussion in Sports. Denver: Colorado Medical Society. 1991.

20. Carney N, Ghajar J, Jagoda A et al. Concussion guidelines step 1: systematic review of prevalent indicators. *Neurosurgery*. 2014; 75 Suppl 1: S3–15.

21. Purcell L, Kissick J, Rizos J. Concussion. *CMAJ: Canadian Medical Association Journal*. 2013; 185(11): 981.

22. Guskiewicz KM, Weaver NL, Padua DA, Garrett WE, Jr. Epidemiology of concussion in collegiate and high school football players. *The American Journal of Sports Medicine*. 2000; 28(5): 643–650.

23. Pellman EJ, Powell JW, Viano DC et al. Concussion in professional football: epidemiological features of game injuries and review of the literature—part 3. *Neurosurgery*. 2004; 54(1): 81–94.

24. Concussion (mild traumatic brain injury) and the team physician: a consensus statement. *Medicine and Science in Sports and Exercise*. 2006; 38(2): 395–399.

25. Lovell MR, Iverson GL, Collins MW, McKeag D, Maroon JC. Does loss of consciousness predict neuropsychological decrements after concussion? *Clinical Journal of Sport Medicine*. 1999; 9(4): 193–198.

26. Browne KD, Chen XH, Meaney DF, Smith DH. Mild traumatic brain injury and diffuse axonal injury in swine. *Journal of Neurotrauma*. 2011; 28(9): 1747–1755.

27. McCrory P, Meeuwisse WH, Aubry M et al. Consensus statement on concussion in sport: the 4th International Conference on Concussion in Sport, Zurich, November 2012. *Journal of Athletic Training*. 2013; 48(4): 554–575.

28. Stein SC, Ross SE. Mild head injury: a plea for routine early CT scanning. *The Journal of Trauma*. 1992; 33(1): 11–13.

29. Zyluk A, Mazur A, Piotuch B, Safranow K. Analysis of the reliability of clinical examination in predicting traumatic cerebral lesions and skull fractures in patients with mild and moderate head trauma. *Polski Przeglad Chirurgiczny*. 2013; 85(12): 699–705.

30. Albers CE, von Allmen M, Evangelopoulos DS, Zisakis AK, Zimmermann H, Exadaktylos AK. What is the incidence of intracranial bleeding in patients with mild traumatic brain injury? A retrospective study in 3088 Canadian CT head rule patients. *BioMed Research International*. 2013; 2013: 453978.

31. Borg J, Holm L, Cassidy JD et al. Diagnostic procedures in mild traumatic brain injury: results of the WHO Collaborating Centre Task Force on Mild Traumatic Brain Injury. *Journal of Rehabilitation Medicine.* 2004(43 Suppl): 61–75.

32. Giza CC, Kutcher JS, Ashwal S et al. Summary of evidence-based guideline update: evaluation and management of concussion in sports: report of the Guideline Development Subcommittee of the American Academy of Neurology. *Neurology.* 2013; 80(24): 2250–2257.

33. Institute of Medicine (IOM) and National Research Council (NRC). In: Graham R, Rivara FP, Ford MA, Spicer CM, eds. *Sports-Related Concussions in Youth: Improving the Science, Changing the Culture.* Washington DC: The National Academics Press. 2014.

34. Caskey RC, Nance ML. Management of pediatric mild traumatic brain injury. *Advances in Pediatrics.* 2014; 61(1): 271–286.

35. Hovda DA. The neurophysiology of concussion. *Progress in Neurological Surgery.* 2014; 28: 28–37.

36. Giza CC, Hovda DA. The Neurometabolic Cascade of Concussion. *Journal of Athletic Training.* 2001; 36(3): 228–235.

37. Giza CC, Hovda DA. The new neurometabolic cascade of concussion. *Neurosurgery.* 2014; 75 Suppl 4: S24–33.

38. Broglio SP, Cantu RC, Gioia GA et al. National Athletic Trainers' Association position statement: management of sport concussion. *Journal of Athletic Training.* 2014; 49(2): 245–265.

39. Harmon KG, Drezner J, Gammons M et al. American Medical Society for Sports Medicine position statement: concussion in sport. *Clinical Journal of Sport Medicine.* 2013; 23(1): 1–18.

40. Bigler ED, Deibert E, Filley CM. When is a concussion no longer a concussion? *Neurology.* 2013; 81(1): 14–15.

41. Carman AJ, Ferguson R, Cantu R et al. Expert consensus document: Mind the gaps-advancing research into short-term and long-term neuropsychological outcomes of youth sports-related concussions. *Nature Reviews Neurology.* 2015; 11(4): 230–244.

42. Chamard E, Lefebvre G, Lassonde M, Theoret H. Long-term abnormalities in the corpus callosum of female concussed athletes. *Journal of Neurotrauma.* 2016; 33(13): 1220–1226.

43. Dean PJ, Sato JR, Vieira G, McNamara A, Sterr A. Long-term structural changes after mTBI and their relation to post-concussion symptoms. *Brain Injury.* 2015: 1–8.

44. Orr CA, Albaugh MD, Watts R et al. Neuroimaging biomarkers of a history of concussion observed in asymptomatic young athletes. *Journal of Neurotrauma.* 2015.

45. Waljas M, Lange RT, Hakulinen U et al. Biopsychosocial outcome after uncomplicated mild traumatic brain injury. *Journal of Neurotrauma.* 2014; 31(1): 108–124.

46. Henry LC, Tremblay J, Tremblay S et al. Acute and chronic changes in diffusivity measures after sports concussion. *Journal of Neurotrauma.* 2011; 28(10): 2049–2059.

47. Helmer KG, Pasternak O, Fredman E et al. Hockey Concussion Education Project, Part 1. Susceptibility-weighted imaging study in male and female ice hockey players over a single season. *Journal of Neurosurgery.* 2014; 120(4): 864–872.

48. Mayer AR, Ling J, Mannell MV et al. A prospective diffusion tensor imaging study in mild traumatic brain injury. *Neurology.* 2010; 74(8): 643–650.

49. Miles L, Grossman RI, Johnson G, Babb JS, Diller L, Inglese M. Short-term DTI predictors of cognitive dysfunction in mild traumatic brain injury. *Brain Injury.* 2008; 22(2): 115–122.

50. Messe A, Caplain S, Paradot G et al. Diffusion tensor imaging and white matter lesions at the subacute stage in mild traumatic brain injury with persistent neurobehavioral impairment. *Human Brain Mapping*. 2011; 32(6): 999–1011.

51. Murugavel M, Cubon V, Putukian M et al. A longitudinal diffusion tensor imaging study assessing white matter fiber tracts after sports-related concussion. *Journal of Neurotrauma*. 2014; 31(22): 1860–1871.

52. Rutgers DR, Toulgoat F, Cazejust J, Fillard P, Lasjaunias P, Ducreux D. White matter abnormalities in mild traumatic brain injury: a diffusion tensor imaging study. *AJNR American Journal of Neuroradiology*. 2008; 29(3): 514–519.

53. Rutgers DR, Fillard P, Paradot G, Tadie M, Lasjaunias P, Ducreux D. Diffusion tensor imaging characteristics of the corpus callosum in mild, moderate, and severe traumatic brain injury. *AJNR American Journal of Neuroradiology*. 2008; 29(9): 1730–1735.

54. Pasternak O, Koerte IK, Bouix S et al. Hockey Concussion Education Project, Part 2. Microstructural white matter alterations in acutely concussed ice hockey players: a longitudinal free-water MRI study. *Journal of Neurosurgery*. 2014; 120(4): 873–881.

55. Sasaki T, Pasternak O, Mayinger M et al. Hockey Concussion Education Project, Part 3. White matter microstructure in ice hockey players with a history of concussion: a diffusion tensor imaging study. *Journal of Neurosurgery*. 2014; 120(4): 882–890.

56. Chong CD, Schwedt TJ. White matter damage and brain network alterations in concussed patients: a review of recent diffusion tensor imaging and resting-state functional connectivity data. *Current Pain and Headache Reports*. 2015; 19(5): 485.

57. Shin SS, Pathak S, Presson N et al. Detection of white matter injury in concussion using high-definition fiber tractography. *Progress in Neurological Surgery*. 2014; 28: 86–93.

58. Wozniak JR, Krach L, Ward E et al. Neurocognitive and neuroimaging correlates of pediatric traumatic brain injury: a diffusion tensor imaging (DTI) study. *Archives of Clinical Neuropsychology*. 2007; 22(5): 555–568.

59. Wilde EA, McCauley SR, Hunter JV et al. Diffusion tensor imaging of acute mild traumatic brain injury in adolescents. *Neurology*. 2008; 70(12): 948–955.

60. Toth A, Kovacs N, Perlaki G et al. Multimodal magnetic resonance imaging in the acute and sub-acute phase of mild traumatic brain injury: can we see the difference? *Journal of Neurotrauma*. 2013; 30(1): 2–10.

61. Virji-Babul N, Borich MR, Makan N et al. Diffusion tensor imaging of sports-related concussion in adolescents. *Pediatric Neurology*. 2013; 48(1): 24–29.

62. Metting Z, Cerliani L, Rodiger LA, van der Naalt J. Pathophysiological concepts in mild traumatic brain injury: diffusion tensor imaging related to acute perfusion CT imaging. *PLoS One*. 2013; 8(5): e64461.

63. Goswami R, Dufort P, Tartaglia MC et al. Frontotemporal correlates of impulsivity and machine learning in retired professional athletes with a history of multiple concussions. *Brain Structure and Function*. 2015.

64. Bazarian JJ, Zhu T, Zhong J et al. Persistent, long-term cerebral white matter changes after sports-related repetitive head impacts. *PLoS One*. 2014; 9(4): e94734.

65. Bazarian JJ, Zhu T, Blyth B, Borrino A, Zhong J. Subject-specific changes in brain white matter on diffusion tensor imaging after sports-related concussion. *Magnetic Resonance Imaging*. 2012; 30(2): 171–180.

66. McAllister TW, Ford JC, Flashman LA et al. Effect of head impacts on diffusivity measures in a cohort of collegiate contact sport athletes. *Neurology*. 2014; 82(1): 63–69.

103. Kroshus E, Garnett B, Hawrilenko M, Baugh CM, Calzo JP. Concussion under-reporting and pressure from coaches, teammates, fans, and parents. *Social Science and Medicine (1982)*. 2015; 134: 66–75.

104. Kumar NS, Chin M, O'Neill C, Jakoi AM, Tabb L, Wolf M. On-field performance of national football league players after return from concussion. *The American Journal of Sports Medicine*. 2014; 42(9): 2050–2055.

105. Stein CJ, MacDougall R, Quatman-Yates CC et al. Young athletes' concerns about sport-related concussion: the patient's perspective. *Clinical Journal of Sport Medicine*. 2015.

106. Kilcoyne KG, Dickens JF, Svoboda SJ et al. Reported concussion rates for three division i football programs: an evaluation of the new ncaa concussion policy. *Sports Health*. 2014; 6(5): 402–405.

107. Zonfrillo MR, Kim KH, Arbogast KB. Emergency department visits and head computed tomography utilization for concussion patients from 2006 to 2011. *Academic Emergency Medicine*. 2015; 22(7): 872–877.

108. Macpherson A, Fridman L, Scolnik M, Corallo A, Guttmann A. A population-based study of paediatric emergency department and office visits for concussions from 2003 to 2010. *Paediatrics and Child Health*. 2014; 19(10): 543–546.

109. Rosenthal JA, Foraker RE, Collins CL, Comstock RD. national high school athlete concussion rates from 2005–2006 to 2011–2012. *The American Journal of Sports Medicine*. 2014; 42(7): 1710–1715.

110. LaRoche AA, Nelson LD, Connelly PK, Walter KD, McCrea MA. Sport-related concussion reporting and state legislative effects. *Clinical Journal of Sport Medicine*. 2015.

111. Mackenzie B, Vivier P, Reinert S, Machan J, Kelley C, Jacobs E. Impact of a state concussion law on pediatric emergency department visits. *Pediatric Emergency Care*. 2015; 31(1): 25–30.

112. Daneshvar DH, Nowinski CJ, McKee AC, Cantu RC. The epidemiology of sport-related concussion. *Clinics in Sports Medicine*. 2011; 30(1): 1–17, vii.

113. Clay MB et al., *Journal of Chiropractic Medicine*, 12(4), 230–251, 2013.

114. Guerriero RM, Proctor MR, Mannix R, Meehan WP, 3rd. Epidemiology, trends, assessment and management of sport-related concussion in United States high schools. *Current Opinion in Pediatrics*. 2012; 24(6): 696–701.

115. Zuckerman SL, Kerr ZY, Yengo-Kahn A, Wasserman E, Covassin T, Solomon GS. Epidemiology of sports-related concussion in ncaa athletes from 2009–2010 to 2013–2014: incidence, recurrence, and mechanisms. *The American Journal of Sports Medicine*. 2015; 43(11): 2654–2662.

116. Gessel LM, Fields SK, Collins CL, Dick RW, Comstock RD. Concussions among United States high school and collegiate athletes. *Journal of Athletic Training*. 2007; 42(4): 495–503.

117. Lam KC, Snyder Valier AR, Valovich McLeod TC. Injury and treatment characteristics of sport-specific injuries sustained in interscholastic athletics: a report from the athletic training practice-based research network. *Sports Health*. 2015; 7(1): 67–74.

118. Marar M, McIlvain NM, Fields SK, Comstock RD. Epidemiology of concussions among United States high school athletes in 20 sports. *The American Journal of Sports Medicine*. 2012; 40(4): 747–755.

119. Covassin T, Swanik CB, Sachs ML. Epidemiological considerations of concussions among intercollegiate athletes. *Applied Neuropsychology*. 2003; 10(1): 12–22.

120. Izraelski J., *The Journal of the Canadian Chiropractic Association*, 58(4), 346–352, 2014.

121. Kirkwood G, et al, *British Journal of Sports Medicine*, 49(8), 506–510, 2015.

122. Gardner A, et al., *British Journal of Sports Medicine*, 49(8), 495–498, 2015.

123. Gardner AJ et al., *Sports Medicine (Auckland, NZ)*, 44(12), 1717–1731, 2014.

124. Boden BP et al., *The American Journal of Sports Medicine*, 26(2), 238–241, 1998.

125. O'Kane JW et al., *The Journal of the American Medical Association Pediatrics*, 168(3), 258–264, 2014.

126. Covassin T, Swanik CB, Sachs ML. Sex differences and the incidence of concussions among collegiate athletes. *Journal of Athletic Training*. 2003; 38(3): 238–244.

127. Pieter W, Zemper ED. Incidence of reported cerebral concussion in adult taekwondo athletes. *The Journal of the Royal Society for the Promotion of Health*. 1998; 118(5): 272–279.

128. Heath CJ, Callahan JL. Self-reported concussion symptoms and training routines in mixed martial arts athletes. *Research in Sports Medicine* (Print). 2013; 21(3): 195–203.

129. Cantu RC, Mueller FO. The prevention of catastrophic head and spine injuries in high school and college sports. *British Journal of Sports Medicine*. 2009; 43(13): 981–986.

130. Kuhl HN, Ritchie D, Taveira-Dick AC, Hoefling KA, Russo SA. Concussion history and knowledge base in competitive equestrian athletes. *Sports Health*. 2014; 6(2): 136–138.

131. Ranson C, Peirce N, Young M. Batting head injury in professional cricket: a systematic video analysis of helmet safety characteristics. *British Journal of Sports Medicine*. 2013; 47(10): 644–648.

132. Petraglia AL, Walker CT, Bailes JE, Callerame KJ, Thompson KE, Burnham JM. Concussion in the absence of head impact: a case in a collegiate hammer thrower. *Current Sports Medicine Reports*. 2015; 14(1): 11–15.

133. Stein CJ, Kinney SA, McCrystal T et al. Dance-related concussion: a case series. *Journal of Dance Medicine and Science*. 2014; 18(2): 53–61.

134. Cuellar TA, Lottenberg L, Moore FA. Blunt cerebrovascular injury in rugby and other contact sports: case report and review of the literature. *World Journal of Emergency Surgery*. 2014; 9: 36.

135. Yengo-Kahn AM, Johnson DJ, Zuckerman SL, Solomon GS. Concussions in the National Football League: A Current Concepts Review. *The American Journal of Sports Medicine*. 2015.

136. Mihalik JP, Bell DR, Marshall SW, Guskiewicz KM. Measurement of head impacts in collegiate football players: an investigation of positional and event-type differences. *Neurosurgery*. 2007; 61(6): 1229–1235.

137. Crisco JJ, Wilcox BJ, Machan JT et al. Magnitude of head impact exposures in individual collegiate football players. *Journal of Applied Biomechanics*. 2012; 28(2): 174–183.

138. Funk JR, Rowson S, Daniel RW, Duma SM. Validation of concussion risk curves for collegiate football players derived from HITS data. *Annals of Biomedical Engineering*. 2012; 40(1): 79–89.

139. McCrea M, Guskiewicz K, Randolph C et al. Effects of a symptom-free waiting period on clinical outcome and risk of reinjury after sport-related concussion. *Neurosurgery*. 2009; 65(5): 876–882.

140. Pellman EJ, Viano DC, Casson IR et al. Concussion in professional football: repeat injuries—part 4. *Neurosurgery*. 2004; 55(4): 860–873.

141. Casson IR, Viano DC, Powell JW, Pellman EJ. Repeat concussions in the national football league. *Sports Health*. 2011; 3(1): 11–24.

142. Daniel RW, Rowson S, Duma SM. Head impact exposure in youth football. *Annals of Biomedical Engineering*. 2012; 40(4): 976–981.

143. Mihalik JP, Guskiewicz KM, Marshall SW, Blackburn JT, Cantu RC, Greenwald RM. Head impact biomechanics in youth hockey: comparisons across playing position, event types, and impact locations. *Annals of Biomedical Engineering*. 2012; 40(1): 141–149.

144. Dompier TP, Kerr ZY, Marshall SW et al. Incidence of concussion during practice and games in youth, high school, and collegiate american football players. *The Journal of the American Medical Association Pediatrics*. 2015; 169(7): 659–665.

145. Kontos AP, Elbin RJ, Fazio-Sumrock VC et al. Incidence of sports-related concussion among youth football players aged 8–12 years. *Journal of Pediatrics*. 2013; 163(3): 717–720.

146. Beckwith JG, Greenwald RM, Chu JJ et al. Head impact exposure sustained by football players on days of diagnosed concussion. *Medicine and Science in Sports and Exercise*. 2013; 45(4): 737–746.

147. Guskiewicz KM, Mihalik JP, Shankar V et al. Measurement of head impacts in collegiate football players: relationship between head impact biomechanics and acute clinical outcome after concussion. *Neurosurgery*. 2007; 61(6): 1244–1252.

148. Guskiewicz KM, Mihalik JP. Biomechanics of sport concussion: quest for the elusive injury threshold. *Exercise and Sport Sciences Reviews*. 2011; 39(1): 4–11.

149. Withnall C, Shewchenko N, Gittens R, Dvorak J. Biomechanical investigation of head impacts in football. *British Journal of Sports Medicine*. 2005; 39 Suppl 1: i49–57.

150. Zhang L, Yang KH, King AI. A proposed injury threshold for mild traumatic brain injury. *Journal of Biomechanical Engineering*. 2004; 126(2): 226–236.

151. Viano DC, Casson IR, Pellman EJ et al. Concussion in professional football: comparison with boxing head impacts–part 10. *Neurosurgery*. 2005; 57(6): 1154–1172.

152. Casson IR, Pellman EJ, Viano DC. Concussion in the National Football League: an overview for neurologists. *Physical Medicine and Rehabilitation Clinics of North America*. 2009; 20(1): 195–214, x.

153. Hutchison MG, Comper P, Meeuwisse WH, Echemendia RJ. A systematic video analysis of National Hockey League (NHL) concussions, part I: who, when, where and what? *British Journal of Sports Medicine*. 2015; 49(8): 547–551.

154. Hutchison MG, Comper P, Meeuwisse WH, Echemendia RJ. A systematic video analysis of National Hockey League (NHL) concussions, part II: how concussions occur in the NHL. *British Journal of Sports Medicine*. 2015; 49(8): 552–555.

155. Mihalik JP, Greenwald RM, Blackburn JT, Cantu RC, Marshall SW, Guskiewicz KM. Effect of infraction type on head impact severity in youth ice hockey. *Medicine and Science in Sports and Exercise*. 2010; 42(8): 1431–1438.

156. Gardner AJ, Iverson GL, Quinn TN et al. A preliminary video analysis of concussion in the National Rugby League. *Brain Injury*. 2015: 1–4.

157. Ruhe A, Gansslen A, Klein W. The incidence of concussion in professional and collegiate ice hockey: are we making progress? A systematic review of the literature. *British Journal of Sports Medicine*. 2014; 48(2): 102–106.

158. Maher ME, Hutchison M, Cusimano M, Comper P, Schweizer TA. Concussions and heading in soccer: a review of the evidence of incidence, mechanisms, biomarkers and neurocognitive outcomes. *Brain Injury*. 2014; 28(3): 271–285.

159. Comstock RD, Currie DW, Pierpoint LA, Grubenhoff JA, Fields SK. An evidence-based discussion of heading the ball and concussions in high school soccer. *The Journal of the American Medical Association Pediatrics*. 2015; 169(9): 830–837.

CHAPTER 2

Biomechanics and pathophysiology of concussion

Introduction

In order to appreciate the injury of concussion, it is imperative to obtain a basic understanding of the types of impacts and biomechanical forces that are transmitted through the skull that act upon the cerebrum causing concussion. The physics of concussive forces initiate neurometabolic changes at a cellular level leading to clinical symptomatology. Established by preclinical and clinical models, we will discuss our current understanding of the complex metabolic, chemical, inflammatory, and vascular responses following concussive injury that produce *functional* alterations perpetuating clinical symptomatology but can also induce *microstructural* damage. Most importantly, attention should be focused on the window period of injury to recovery seen in studies in order to appreciate why cognitive and physical exertion during this period has been hypothesized and shown to cause further detriment.[1]

Biomechanics of concussion

Direct and indirect impacts

Direct or impact loading collisions involve direct head trauma from the head striking against a fixed surface or object (ground, shoulder, head, goal post, etc.) (Figure 2.1a,b). Conversely another cause of a concussive injury, an indirect impact, also known as inertial, "whiplash," or impulsive loading, occurs when the head of a player is forcefully set in motion due to an impact involving the body (Figure 2.1c).[2,3] Indirect impacts are commonly seen with tackling on the football field, where the momentum of the player's body is abruptly stopped and redirected.

Direct and indirect impact mechanisms cause a concussive injury due to the anatomical and physiological properties of the brain and intracranial space. When a blow occurs to a stationary head or there is a forceful redirection of a moving head, the global acceleration–deceleration of the head is propagated to the brain causing microscopic shear stress on the neurons, erythrocytes and their axons.[4] Early preclinical models by Holbourn and Ommaya highlighted that this inertial strain, and not the direct head impact, is what causes a head injury, most notably illustrated when neuronal damage did not occur when striking a fixed cranium.[5,6] Important to this concept is that not only does the brain behave in a viscoelastic manner, but it is also floating within the cerebrospinal fluid (CSF) surrounded by the rigid skull.[7,8] Therefore, the brain's intrinsic properties allow a decoupled movement within the skull, causing strain at a cellular level (similar to shaking gelatin), but also more globally the brain can have degrees of movement where it can tear bridging blood vessels or strike against the fixed skull causing cerebral contusions (not common in concussive injury, but likely in more severe TBIs). The macroscopic and microscopic fluid-like property of the brain, its vasculature, and CSF, in reaction to a force, has been termed "slosh" (slosh is the dynamics of fluids within moving containers).[9,10] See Figure 2.2.

In the 1950s, Schneider first confirmed that movement of the cerebral hemispheres occurs in response to an impact within a thinned rhesus monkey skull, which was then further described in cadaveric studies.[6,8] More recently, groups have been able to demonstrate in vivo "slosh" or brain deformation and strain through the application of mild rapid translational forces to the heads of

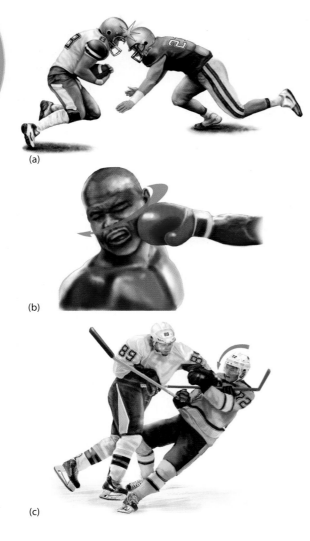

Figure 2.1 Illustration of a direct linear (a), direct rotational (b), and indirect contact (c) in sports.

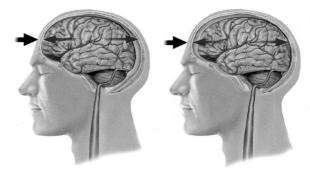

Figure 2.2 Movement of the brain within the cranium creating the slosh like effect.

patients during MRI acquisition.[11,12] This strain, specifically upon the white matter, initiates a complex cascade that leads to an alteration in neuronal functioning that can either recover with time or end in cell death depending on the degree of injury.[13]

Besides the more popular theory of brain "slosh" directly causing white matter strain and injury; a less known, previously theorized mechanism of TBI has been through cavitation. Cavitation is the formation of bubbles within a liquid following a perturbed state that release high levels of energy when colliding with and bursting upon an object.[14,15] Therefore, when a player's head is struck, cavitation bubbles are presumed to form within the cerebrospinal fluid, travel through this space at high velocities, and cause injury to the brain parenchyma and blood vessels, like a projectile of shotgun pellets. This theory has been exhibited in scientific (hitting a water filled glass vial with a hammer)[14,15] and ex vivo animal models[16] and therefore hypothesized with a potential application to explain concussive TBI. Without any true clinical evidence or even direct animal models, this theory, though intriguing, is only in its infancy. More recently, this premise has been further reevaluated as a possible mechanism in blast TBI.[17–19]

Linear and rotational acceleration

Besides direct and indirect impacts, the specific vector of force and its relation to the object's center of gravity is important in determining concussive injury. First described by Ommaya and Gennarelli, the two main types of acceleration are linear and rotational.[21] Linear, or translational, acceleration occurs when the force points towards the object's center of gravity (Figure 2.3).

Through the use of helmet accelerometers, linear acceleration has been shown to be greatest when the player is struck at the top of their head along the sagittal plane.[21–23] With significant impact, the brain collides with the fixed skull causing focal injuries like parenchymal and intracerebral hemorrhages/contusions and skull fractures. See Figure 2.4.[5,23,24] These lesions can appear directly adjacent to where the hit occurred (coup injury) or at the opposite side of impact (contra-coup).[23,25]

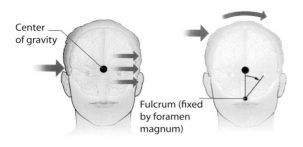

Center of gravity

Fulcrum (fixed by foramen magnum)

Linear acceleration   **Rotational acceleration**

Figure 2.3 Direction of force in relation to the head to cause either linear or rotational acceleration. (Reprinted from Petraglia AL et al., *Handbook of neurological sports medicine: Concussion and other nervous system injuries in the athlete*, 2015. Champaign, IL: Human Kinetics. With permission.)

Rotational, or angular, acceleration is where the force is directed around or tangential to the object's center (Figure 2.3). This most commonly occurs in players that are struck to the back, front, or side of the head, with temporal side impacts being the cause of greatest rotational acceleration.[21,22] This force, directed in the coronal plane, leads to excessive strain within the deep brain parenchyma often causing diffuse white matter injury and petechial hemorrhages

(Figure 2.4).[8,23,25] First noted by Oppenheimer pathologically, it was presumed that significant rotational injury, with the brainstem acting as a fulcrum, produced brainstem microhemorrhages and shearing of white matter tracts in a cohort of severe TBI patients.[26] To a lesser degree, this same mechanism has been postulated as the cause of loss of consciousness in concussive injury[27] (Figure 2.5). In concert with this is the "centripetal theory" proposed by Ommaya.[5,28] It was noted in preclinical models that shear strain increased directly in relation to distance from an object's center. Therefore, the cortical surface receives the greatest strain with an acceleration–deceleration injury and only with significant forces does the brainstem become involved.

It has been held that angular acceleration is the principal element of concussive injury because it has been shown experimentally to produce diffuse neuronal strain and not focal injury, has a lower injurious threshold than translational acceleration, is not reproducible in models where the head was suspended, and there is a higher incidence of concussion occurring with temporal side impacts in preclinical models.[5,6,28–30] More recently, with the advent of head accelerometers, this theory has been further validated in clinical studies in that the degree of head rotation

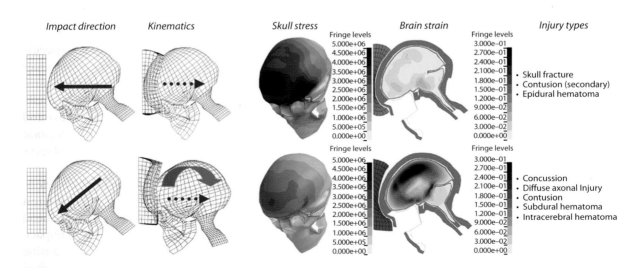

Figure 2.4 Illustration of the biomechanics of an oblique impact (lower), compared to a corresponding perpendicular one, when impacted against the same padding using an identical initial velocity of **6.7 m/s.** The perpendicular impact would create a true linear acceleration while the oblique impact would cause a rotational acceleration. (From Kleiven S. *Frontiers in Bioengineering and Biotechnology*. 1:15, 2013.)

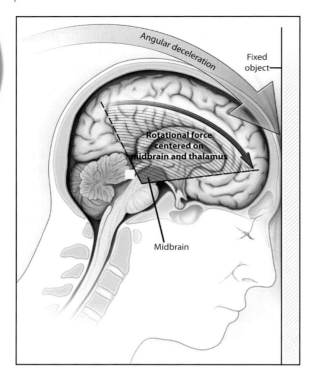

Figure 2.5 Rotational acceleration/deceleration force with the brainstem and thalamus acting as a fulcrum. With escalating forces, loss of consciousness or comatose state ensues.

was more predictive of developing a concussion than translational acceleration.[31,32] In an Australian football cohort, McIntosh described that angular acceleration of 1747 rad/s^2 and 2296 rad/s^2 were 50% and 75% likely to cause a concussion and was more predictive of concussive injury than linear acceleration.[32] But counterintuitively, temporal side impacts occur the least in football, where hits to the top of the head cause the greatest linear acceleration, and impacts to the crown of the head have also shown more correlation with causing a concussion in clinical studies.[13,21,22,30,33–36] Most likely the discrepancy in these findings is that pure angular or translational forces in preclinical models are not replicated in vivo. Most concussive injuries on the playing field are a combination of angular and translational acceleration dictating the extent of both diffuse and focal injury. Bayley et al. performed MRI imaging in human subjects where a purely translational force was applied to

the patient's head.[11] Though no angular acceleration was applied, rotational brain deformation and strain was seen with the linear force presumably created due to an alteration in the force vector from the brain being tethered to the skull base.

Magnitude of force

The biomechanical components of a concussion including acceleration and magnitude have been evaluated by finite element modeling and helmet accelerometers.[8] Finite element modeling applies mathematical computations with video analysis or collision of mannequins and helmets to calculate and classify the various involving forces.[37] Helmet accelerometers were originally only used in experimental situations, but advanced technology has allowed real-time practice and game acquisition through the use of such devices as the Head Impact Telemetry System.[13,38] A challenging feature to studying concussions through the use of helmet accelerometers is the difficulty in properly mounting them within a form fitting helmet, poor accuracy and error of measurements, and the lack of concussion reporting leaving many collisions to not be correctly evaluated as a concussion causing event.[39]

Though these measures have many limitations, they have provided researchers with an understanding of the G-force exposures in different sports and the variations that occur within age groups. Refer to Table 2.1 for the published linear acceleration G forces for each sport. In general, the average translational G force among all sports is between 20 and 50 G, with one study showing a maximum of 191 G during a sparing practice.[40]

Through multiple seasons of data collection, specifically in tandem with a concussive injury, researchers have attempted to determine

Table 2.1 Linear Acceleration G Forces for Each Sport

Soccer	15–20: Head to ball collision 80–90: Head to head collision (most common, 40% of all soccer concussions)[49–51]
Rugby	3.8–36.2[52]
Hockey	10–45 (average 18–35)[21,53,88]
Lacrosse (stick check)	50–60[54,55]
Football (youth)	10–100 (average 18)[56]
Football (college–pro)	30–144 (20, 50th percentile; 62, 95th percentile)[56,59]
Boxing	10–191 (average 30–71)[40,57,58]

a concussion threshold value based on linear and angular acceleration.[41–46] Presumably, it was believed that this cutoff for linear acceleration causing concussion was roughly 80–100 G.[42–47] But multiple groups have published that of those diagnosed with a concussion only a small percentage, <0.4%, were actually exposed to an impact greater than 80–100 G.[33,44,48] Similarly, Funk et al. noted that 1 in every 1000 plays would expose a player to a 100 G hit in their cohort of 64 Virginia Tech collegiate football players. Therefore, based on a 100 G threshold, concussive injuries would presumably occur more frequently than what was actually seen.

Further attempts at obtaining a specific concussion threshold only brought more inconsistent results, ranging from as low as 60 G to as high as 168 G of linear acceleration.[22,33,42,44,45,48,59,60] In a review of 88 players during 2 years of collegiate football play with a total of 13 analyzed concussions, Guskiewics et al. concluded that there was no correlation with impact location or magnitude, and due to the large variation (60–168 G), stated that a specific threshold value was not attainable.[34] This data illustrates the fact that no two collisions are alike. Players have different body and brain anatomy, neck strength, prior environmental exposures (previous concussions, exposure to neurotoxic agents, etc.), genetic susceptibility, permutation of biomechanical properties for each collision (blend of linear and angular acceleration, magnitude, duration, location, distribution, etc.), and an unknown likely variable extent of propagation of these forces intracranially to the brain.[13,61–63] At this time, a threshold value that is applicable to all athletes is not available as a diagnostic marker of concussion and appears to be an unrealistic goal even in the future.[8,48] A different approach that has been taken statistically, rather than obtaining a definite cutoff, has been in formulating a concussion risk curve based on both linear and angular accelerations.[59,64] Zhang et al. published that linear accelerations at 66, 82, and 106 G along with angular accelerations of 4600, 5900, and 7900 rad/s² were 25%, 50%, and 80% likely to cause concussion in their collegiate football cohort.[59]

Force mitigators

As mentioned, there are nonmodifiable factors (anatomy, sex, genetics, etc.), and more importantly, modifiable factors that have been shown to influence G force and therefore concussion risk. Mitigation of injury exposure has become the cornerstone to concussion management. Greater scrutiny and evidence-based proof of force mitigation has become emphasized for protective equipment in different sports, specifically helmets. This has led to the development of the star rating for both hockey and football helmets based on their ability to reduce linear acceleration following blunt impact.[65–67] Researchers have studied and proposed changes to current helmet designs in many different sports through the addition of external foam pieces to reduce peak intensities, specifically in both football and baseball pitcher's helmets[68,69] (Figure 2.6). Though this technology is shown

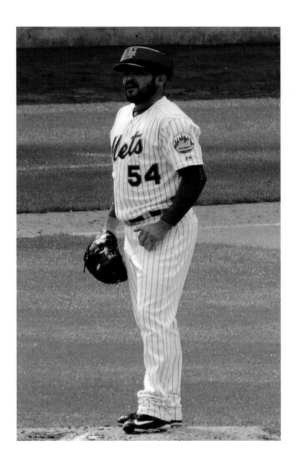

Figure 2.6 Protective cap worn by MLB pitcher. (Courtesy of slgckgc on Flickr [original version] UCinternational [Crop]. Originally posted to Flickr as "Alex Torres" Cropped by UCinternational, CC BY 2.0. Available at https://commons .wikimedia.org/w/index.php?curid=39785714.)

to reduce the peak G force experienced, Tong et al. demonstrated, through a forensic head model, that external protective layers just increased the duration and therefore did not change the overall total energy that the brain is exposed to.[70,71] By reducing peak force applied focally to the skull but not total intracranial strain, helmets reduce impact injuries like skull fractures, but have limitations in concussion prevention.[1,72–74] This concept has been echoed in the many studies that have published conflicting data in support and against helmets, even specific models, in their ability, or lack thereof, at reducing concussion incidence.[2,75–78]

A novel approach to intracranial slosh mitigation has been proposed through the application of internal jugular vein compression (IJV). Prophylactic mild IJV compression restricts cerebral venous outflow, enlarging the brain and increasing brain turgor (making it stiffer).[79,80] Therefore, this causes a reduction in relative motion between the brain and skull and deformation/strain through decreasing brain compliance (Figure 2.7). This mechanism has been used in preclinical models, revealing dramatic reductions in markers of traumatic brain injury.[10,11]

Recently, development of a collar for clinical use and application in high school hockey and football players has also shown a dramatic decrease in diffusion tensor image findings of white matter pathology in the athletes who wore the collar during a season of play (Figure 2.8).[81,82] Due to concerns of worsening hemorrhagic lesions at greater injury severities, the authors have investigated IJV

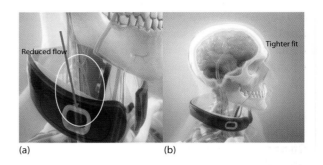

Figure 2.8 Q-collar designed to reduce venous blood outflow of the brain (a) and produce a tighter fit of the brain within the cranium (b). (From Myer GD et al. *Front Neurol.* Jun 6;7:74, 2016.)

compression in a porcine cortical impact model with remarkable evidence suggestive of a protective effect of IJV compression in preventing intracranial hemorrhagic lesions.[83]

Another greatly researched topic of debate is the effect of neck mass/strength on concussions. It has been postulated that anticipation of a collision results in constriction of the neck muscles, presumably reducing acceleration–deceleration of the athlete's head; and therefore, reducing the biomechanical forces acting on the brain.[47,84–88] Studies have shown that anticipatory contraction of the neck prior to injury does reduce head acceleration during impacts, but counterintuitively, there is conflicting results regarding the correlation of cervical muscle strength and size and their effects on concussion reduction.[84,85,87,89–91] This theory of neck muscle strength has been speculated as the reason why children and female athletes have repeatedly shown to have a reduced threshold for injury, higher incidence of concussion, and worse outcomes, but this has not been scientifically validated.[89,92] Due to the anticipatory effect of neck muscle contraction on concussion, all levels of competitive football and hockey have instituted penalties against aggressive play like hits to a "defenseless receiver" (when a defender strikes an offensive player to the upper chest, neck, or head as the receiver is looking at the ball and not the defender) or checking from behind.[93]

Lastly, mouth guards have long been believed to reduce concussion incidence by reducing cranial forces when blunt forces to the head occur. But, this

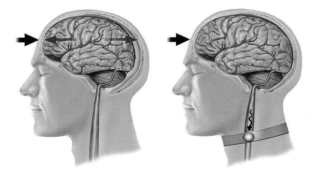

Figure 2.7 Reduction of brain slosh through mild internal jugular vein compression and increased cerebral volume and turgor.

is a great misconception. Mouth guards have consistently demonstrated their ability to only reduce dental trauma but not able to reduce the risk of concussion.[78,91,94]

Molecular pathophysiology of concussion

Shortcomings of preclinical and clinical models

The direct or indirect impact creating rotational acceleration and strain upon the neurons incites complex molecular changes at a cellular level within the neuron. These changes affect the functionality of the neuron, creating clinical symptomatology of concussion, and can lead to long term microstructural injury. The extent of our knowledge of the pathophysiology of concussion comes from extensive preclinical models and more recently clinical studies. A brief understanding of each model, specifically the force applied, aids the reader in analytically evaluating further concussion research by understanding the shortcomings of each. There are four main animal models to study traumatic brain injury/concussion and they are organized from least to greatest acceleration/deceleration injury (Figures 2.9 and 2.10, Table 2.2)[95,97]:

◆ Controlled Cortical Impact (CCI).[98]
   ◇ Through a craniectomy, a piston is placed over the dura of the brain and a specific

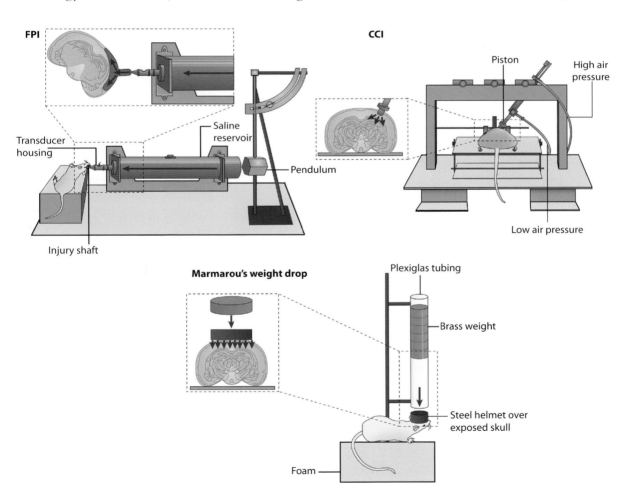

Figure 2.9 Traumatic brain injury models: fluid percussion injury (FPI), controlled cortical impact (CCI), and Marmarou drop weight model (MDW). (Reprinted by permission from Macmillan Publishers Ltd: Xiong Y et al. *Nature Reviews Neuroscience* 2013 Feb;14(2):128–42.)

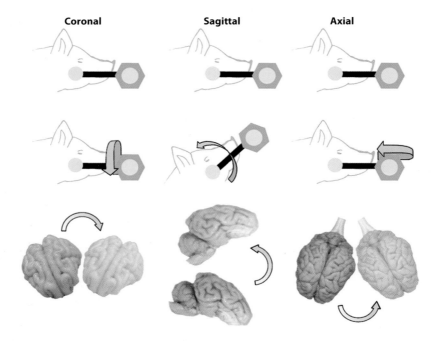

Coronal   **Sagittal**   **Axial**

Figure 2.10 **Depiction of a rotational acceleration animal model.** (With kind permission from Springer Science+Business Media: A Porcine Model of Traumatic Brain Injury via Head Rotational Acceleration, D. Kacy Cullen, PhD, 2016.)

impact force is mechanically applied directly to the brains surface.

◆ Lateral Fluid Percussion model (LFP).[99]
  ◇ Through a craniectomy, a fluid wave is used to strike the dura overlying the animal's brain.
◆ Marmarou Drop weight model (MDW).[100]
  ◇ A weight is dropped from a given height above the animal, striking a steel disk that is cemented to the animal's skull. The steel disk dissipates the force over a larger area to prevent fractures. The head is also suspended by a foam pad allowing

some head movement, specifically rotational acceleration.

◆ Rotational acceleration model.[101]
  ◇ Involves the use of a pneumatic piston device attached to the head to provide purely rotational motion without translational force.

Studies are designed so that the injury model is appropriately used to match the specific hypothesis being tested. For example, a purely rotational model is not appropriate to assess focal injuries. Through fine-tuning the various animal models,

Table 2.2 Extent of Focal and Diffuse Injury by Specific Animal Models

Model	Concussion	Contusion	Axonal Injury	ASDH	Skull Fracture
Weight drop	+++	+	+	−	+++
Fluid percussion	+++	+	+	−	−
Controlled cortical impact (CCI)	+++	++	++	−	−
Dynamic cortical deformation	−	−	−	−	−
Inertial	+++	±	+++	++	−
Impact acceleration	+++	+	++	−	±

Abbreviation: ASDH = acute subdural hematoma; ICH = intracerebral hematoma. − does not duplicate the condition; ± inconsistent; + duplicates to some degree; ++ greater fidelity; and +++ greatest fidelity.

Source: Reprinted from Pharmacology & Therapeutics, Vol. 130, O'Connor WT et al., Animal models of traumatic brain injury: A critical evaluation, Copyright 2011, with permission from Elsevier.

specific injury mechanisms have been developed that truly emulate a concussive injury, a functional and potentially microstructural injury, without macrostructural pathology. For example, Gurkoff et al. demonstrated with LFP model the ability to have rats that demonstrated deficits on behavioral testing but did not show neuronal loss on histological analysis.[99]

Also, understanding of concussion physiology has then been exposed through invasive monitoring, imaging, and pathology in patients with severe traumatic brain injury (TBI). This approach is assuming that there is a continuum and increasing extent of injury from concussion to more severe TBI. But, experimental results may be difficult to extrapolate from severe TBI to concussed patients due to the presence and possibly different influence of an intensive structural lesion more commonly seen with severe TBI.[102] Therefore, within this chapter, there is an attempt to mostly focus on concussive, specifically sports-related, or mild TBI studies and only present those with severe TBI when appropriate.

Primary and secondary injury

All forms of TBI are due to a force that is applied to the skull, causing brain deformation and strain. Depending on the magnitude of force, immediate, nonreversible neuronal or blood vessel damage may occur.[103] Examples of gross macrostructural injuries include coup and contra-coup parenchymal and intraparenchymal contusions occurring at the frontal and temporal poles,[104] large hemorrhages in the subdural, epidural, or subarachnoid spaces, and skull fractures.[104] All of these lesions require a significant amount of force and therefore may–but are not commonly–seen in concussive injuries.[105] At a microscopic level, primary injury can occur in the form of instant axonal stretching or tearing (axotomy), glial injury, and microhemorrhages. This microstructural white matter injury has been extensively characterized through MRI DTI imaging following concussion in adolescent, collegiate, and professional sports at both acute and chronic time points.[81,83,106,133] Therefore, as discussed in Chapter 1, concussion does cause structural injury, but occurs at a micro scale.

When an impact occurs, a cascade of events ensue that initiates changes in lipid membrane permeability, ion shifts, neurotransmitter release, mitochondrial dysfunction, changes in cerebral blood flow, hypoxia, impaired glucose metabolism, free radical formation, and activation of inflammatory cells.[134–140] This neurometabolic, chemical, vascular, and inflammatory cascade occurs hours to days in response to the injury, and is presumed to be the cause of post concussive symptoms. To be discussed in Chapter 7, extensive research has shown that there exists a sensitive window following concussion where additional cognitive or physical stress prior to complete recovery from this reactionary stage only further heightens this response, propagating further neuronal injury. This concept is the motivator for designing proper return to learn and play recommendations.

Neurometabolic cascade of concussion

For simplicity of discussion, the following description will be explained in a sequential manner but these molecular changes are occurring in tandem. An indirect or direct impact creates shear forces to the axon segment, damaging the membrane and forming small pores, termed "mechanoporation."[8] Ions are now permeable through the membrane, via these traumatically induced holes, causing electrochemical shifts as sodium travels into and potassium moves out of the neuron (Figure 2.11a).[141]

The change in neuronal electrochemical gradients causes the neuron, and nearby neurons, to depolarize (Figure 2.11b) and release excitatory neurotransmitters into the presynaptic space Figure 2.11c.[105,134,142–149] These neurotransmitters (dopamine, glutamate, aspartate, choline) are then able to affect downstream (postsynaptic) neurons through excitation or inhibition.[150,151]

The most important neurotransmitter within this cascade is glutamate.[152] It is presumably released from a depolarized presynaptic neuron, but it has also been proposed to be due to blood brain barrier breakdown.[153] Kierans et al. demonstrated in vivo through magnetic resonance spectrometry that following a concussive injury, patients had significant increases in glutamate.[154] Once released, glutamate binds to downstream postsynaptic neurons N-methyl-D-aspartate receptors (NMDAr) leading to further opening of sodium and potassium channels within the postsynaptic neuron.[155,156] Katayama et al. demonstrated in a rat LFP model that mild

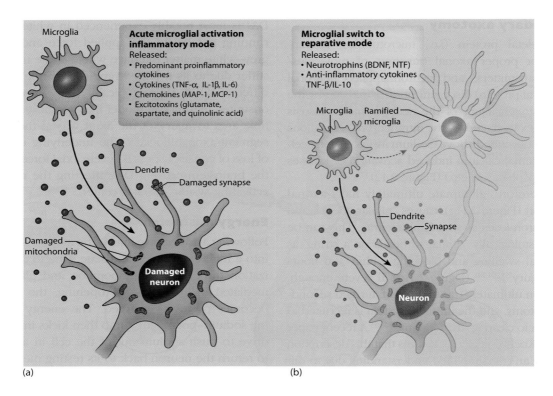

Figure 2.14 (a) Release of proinflammatory factors by microglia leading to further neuronal damage. (b) Microglia in reparative mode where they secrete anti-inflammatory and neurotrophic factors. (Reprinted from Petraglia AL et al., *Handbook of Neurological Sports Medicine: Concussion and Other Nervous System Injuries in the Athlete*, 2015. Champaign, IL: Human Kinetics. With permission.)

brain normally is able to maintain a steady state of oxygenation through sensing changes in carbon dioxide and constricting or dilating its vessels to increase or decrease blood flow.[181,182] Following injury, there is an immediate (within minutes) increase followed by a rebound reduction[193,194] in cerebral blood flow, up to 30%–40%,[190,195] with a loss of the mentioned cerebral vascular autoregulation.[196,197] This altered vascular physiology has been demonstrated to persist for weeks–months after injury (even after the normalization of neurocognitive testing), becomes exponentially worse following successive blows, is predictive of those with protracted recovery, and therefore is suggested as a possible diagnostic tool (Figures 2.13).[27,135] Along with the reduced cerebral blood flow, the intraneuronal alterations, specifically calcium influx, causes impairment in proper mitochondrial functioning and an inability for the neuron to perform aerobic respiration.[161,168] The energy mismatch (high energy demand with lack thereof) leads to intracellular

stress, neuronal hypoxia, free radical formation, lactate accumulation, and acidosis,[27,156,212] only further potentiating cell membrane damage and abnormal cellular functioning. Possibly attributable to this energy state, neurons have been shown to revert to a state of neuronal depression, termed as "spreading depression," that is seen greatest at areas closest to a focal lesion.[27,213–215] This alteration in neuronal activation has been demonstrated in clinical studies in athlete's postconcussion through advanced neuroimaging techniques.[216,217]

The taxing state that the neuron is placed into has also been even found to effect proper functioning of the endoplasmic reticulum (ER), a cellular structure responsible for proper protein folding. In diseased states, the cell is required to manufacture and package an increased level of proteins within the ER, but this high demand coupled with its poorly functioning state, leads to accumulation of misfolded proteins, termed ER stress.[218,219] If unable to reverse this process, the cell will increase reactive oxygen species and caspases ultimately leading to cell death.[220]

Neuroinflammation

Following a cerebral injury, microglia (the immune cell of the brain) proliferate and migrate to the site of injury.[221–228] Once the microglia arrive, there is a release of either proinflammatory or anti-inflammatory cytokines, chemokines, and prostaglandins to either promote repair or phagocytosis (remove the damaged cells), and measurement of gene expression of these inflammatory markers has been proposed for use as a diagnostic tool of concussion.[105,227,229–233] If this process remains unchecked and perpetuates into a continuous nature, secondary cellular damage occurs[234] (Figure 2.14). A preclinical study by Mierzwa et al. demonstrated pathological changes of diffuse axonal injury within the corpus callosum along with corresponding inflammatory cells (microglia) and diffuse cerebral injury/scarring (astrogliosis).[235] There have been multiple animal studies with the use of various immune modulating medications that resulted in limited secondary injury, reduced neuronal loss, and improved cognitive results on behavioral testing.[236–239] To be discussed in Chapter 9, preclinical research has proposed a theory that a perpetual inflammatory state prevents microglia from effectively clearing protein accumulations following microtubule dissociation, leading to aggregation, accumulation, and possible progression to Chronic Traumatic Encephalopathy, a neurodegenerative disease.[240–246]

Blood–brain barrier breakdown

The blood–brain barrier (BBB) is composed of endothelial tight junctions within the walls of blood vessels that separate the brain from the rest of the body.[237] This prevents plasma proteins, red blood cells, or immune cells from entering the brain. In preclinical models, it has been demonstrated that following a head injury, the BBB breaks down hours after injury, usually resolving after a week.[155,248–250] This leads to not only cerebral edema but also detrimental effects of exposing the brain to proteins and inflammatory cells it is normally naive to. The mechanism of BBB breakdown is likely multifactorial: direct injury, response to inflammatory cytokines, metabolic changes, and/or release of mediators following cell death.[155,248] Preclinical models have shown direct correlation between areas with BBB breakdown within the brain colocalized with inflammatory cells and glial scaring.[251,252] The role of matrix metalloproteinase-9, fibrinogen, aquaporin 4, and CD34+ inflammatory cells in BBB breakdown and resolution have been recently discovered, giving promise to possible therapeutic targets.[249,251,253]

Conclusion

Though the literature in concussion biomechanics and pathophysiology is growing, our understanding is still in its infancy. Our current knowledge is developed largely from preclinical animal research and clinical trials in severe traumatic brain injury and therefore has its limitations. Our lack of ability to successfully develop treatments for concussion is likely due to an incomplete understanding of the pathophysiology of a concussive injury. A better understanding of the neurometabolic, chemical, vascular, and inflammatory alterations after injury has taken shape, but with new information comes many more questions. Previously, it was thought that symptom resolution could solely guide return to play, but now it is known that symptoms, though usually resolved by 7–10 days, is not in parallel with the extensive metabolic changes that have been demonstrated on neuroimaging—even up to 1 month from injury.[254–258] At the present moment, the long-term consequences of cognitive or even physical exertion with persistent neurochemical alterations seen on neuroimaging is unknown. Only as we acquire greater information through translational research, can we potentially acquire better recommendations to properly instruct an athlete when it is safe to return to activity, possibly with the use of neuroimaging as a diagnostic and prognostic concussion biomarker.

References

1. Harmon KG, Drezner JA, Gammons M et al. American Medical Society for Sports Medicine position statement: concussion in sport. *British Journal of Sports Medicine*. 2013; 47(1): 15–26.

2. McCrory P, Meeuwisse W, Aubry M et al. Consensus statement on Concussion in Sport—The 4th International Conference on Concussion in Sport held in Zurich, November 2012. *Physical Therapy in Sport.* 2013; 14(2): e1–e13.

3. Giza CC, Kutcher JS, Ashwal S et al. Summary of evidence-based guideline update: evaluation and management of concussion in sports: report of the Guideline Development Subcommittee of the American Academy of Neurology. *Neurology.* 2013; 80(24): 2250–2257.

4. McCrory P, Johnston KM, Mohtadi NG, Meeuwisse W. Evidence-based review of sport-related concussion: basic science. *Clinical Journal of Sport Medicine.* 2001; 11(3): 160–165.

5. Ommaya AK. Head injury mechanisms and the concept of preventive management: a review and critical synthesis. *Journal of Neurotrauma.* 1995; 12(4): 527–546.

6. Stone JL, Patel V, Bailes JE. The history of neurosurgical treatment of sports concussion. *Neurosurgery.* 2014; 75 Suppl 4: S3–s23.

7. Ommaya AK, Goldsmith W, Thibault L. Biomechanics and neuropathology of adult and paediatric head injury. *British Journal of Neurosurgery.* 2002; 16(3): 220–242.

8. Meaney DF, Morrison B, Dale Bass C. The mechanics of traumatic brain injury: a review of what we know and what we need to know for reducing its societal burden. *Journal of Biomechemical Engineering.* 2014; 136(2): 021008.

9. Turner RC, Naser ZJ, Bailes JE, Smith DW, Fisher JA, Rosen CL. Effect of slosh mitigation on histologic markers of traumatic brain injury: laboratory investigation. *Journal of Neurosurgery.* 2012; 117(6): 1110–1118.

10. Smith DW, Bailes JE, Fisher JA, Robles J, Turner RC, Mills JD. Internal jugular vein compression mitigates traumatic axonal injury in a rat model by reducing the intracranial slosh effect. *Neurosurgery.* 2012; 70(3): 740–746.

11. Bayly PV, Cohen TS, Leister EP, Ajo D, Leuthardt EC, Genin GM. Deformation of the human brain induced by mild acceleration. *Journal of Neurotrauma.* 2005; 22(8): 845–856.

12. Knutsen AK, Magrath E, McEntee JE et al. Improved measurement of brain deformation during mild head acceleration using a novel tagged MRI sequence. *Journal of Biomechanics.* 2014; 47(14): 3475–3481.

13. Guskiewicz KM, Mihalik JP. Biomechanics of sport concussion: quest for the elusive injury threshold. *Exercise and Sport Sciences Reviews.* 2011; 39(1): 4–11.

14. Ward JW, Montgomery LH, Clark SL. A Mechanism of Concussion: A Theory. *Science (New York, NY).* 1948; 107(2779): 349–353.

15. Gross AG. A new theory on the dynamics of brain concussion and brain injury. *Journal Eurosurgery.* 1958; 15(5): 548–561.

16. Chen H, Brayman AA, Bailey MR, Matula TJ. Blood vessel rupture by cavitation. *Urological Research.* 2010; 38(4): 321–326.

17. Goeller J, Wardlaw A, Treichler D, O'Bruba J, Weiss G. Investigation of cavitation as a possible damage mechanism in blast-induced traumatic brain injury. *Journal of Neurotrauma.* 2012; 29(10): 1970–1981.

18. Panzer MB, Myers BS, Capehart BP, Bass CR. Development of a finite element model for blast brain injury and the effects of CSF cavitation. *Annals of Biomedical Engineering.* 2012; 40(7): 1530–1544.

19. Taylor PA, Ludwigsen JS, Ford CC. Investigation of blast-induced traumatic brain injury. *Brain Injury.* 2014; 28(7): 879–895.

20. Ommaya AK, Thibault L, Bandak F. Mechanisms of impact head injury. *International Journal of Impact Engineering.* 1994; 15(4): 535–560.

21. Mihalik JP, Guskiewicz KM, Marshall SW, Blackburn JT, Cantu RC, Greenwald RM. Head impact biomechanics in youth hockey: comparisons across playing position, event types, and impact locations. *Annals of Biomedical Engineering*. 2012; 40(1): 141–149.

22. Crisco JJ, Wilcox BJ, Machan JT et al. Magnitude of head impact exposures in individual collegiate football players. *Journal of Applied Biomechanics*. 2012; 28(2): 174–183.

23. Goldsmith W, Plunkett J. A biomechanical analysis of the causes of traumatic brain injury in infants and children. *The American Journal of Forensic Medicine and Pathology*. 2004; 25(2): 89–100.

24. Kleiven S. Why most traumatic brain injuries are not caused by linear acceleration but skull fractures are. *Frontiers Bioengineering Biotechnology*. 2013; 1: 15.

25. Morrison AL, King TM, Korell MA, Smialek JE, Troncoso JC. Acceleration–deceleration injuries to the brain in blunt force trauma. *The American Journal of Forensic Medicine and Pathology*. 1998; 19(2): 109–112.

26. Oppenheimer DR. Microscopic lesions in the brain following head injury. *Journal of Neurology, Neurosurgery, and Psychiatry*. 1968; 31(4): 299–306.

27. MacFarlane MP, Glenn TC. Neurochemical cascade of concussion. *Brain Injury*. 2015; 29(2): 139–153.

28. Ommaya AK, Thibault L, Bandak F Mechanisms of impact head injury. *International Journal of Impact Engineering*. 1994; 15(4): 535–660.

29. Patton DA, McIntosh AS, Kleiven S. The biomechanical determinants of concussion: finite element simulations to investigate brain tissue deformations during sporting impacts to the unprotected head. *Journal of Applied Biomechanics*. 2013; 29(6): 721–730.

30. Delaney JS, Al-Kashmiri A, Correa JA. Mechanisms of injury for concussions in university football, ice hockey, and soccer. *Clinical Journal of Sport Medicine*. 2014; 24(3): 233–237.

31. Hernandez F, Wu LC, Yip MC et al. Six degree-of-freedom measurements of human mild traumatic brain injury. *Annals of Biomedical Engineering*. 2015; 43(8): 1918–1934.

32. McIntosh AS, Patton DA, Frechede B, Pierre PA, Ferry E, Barthels T. The biomechanics of concussion in unhelmeted football players in Australia: a case-control study. *BMJ Open*. 2014; 4(5): e005078.

33. Guskiewicz KM, Mihalik JP, Shankar V et al. Measurement of head impacts in collegiate football players: relationship between head impact biomechanics and acute clinical outcome after concussion. *Neurosurgery*. 2007; 61(6): 1244–1252.

34. Mihalik JP, Bell DR, Marshall SW, Guskiewicz KM. Measurement of head impacts in collegiate football players: an investigation of positional and event-type differences. *Neurosurgery*. 2007; 61(6): 1229–1235.

35. Post A, Blaine Hoshizaki T. Rotational acceleration, brain tissue strain, and the relationship to concussion. *Journal of Biomechanical Engineering*. 2015; 137(3).

36. Kerr ZY, Collins CL, Mihalik JP, Marshall SW, Guskiewicz KM, Comstock RD. Impact locations and concussion outcomes in high school football player-to-player collisions. *Pediatrics*. 2014; 134(3): 489–496.

37. Patton DA, McIntosh AS, Kleiven S. The biomechanical determinants of concussion: finite element simulations to investigate tissue-level predictors of injury during sporting impacts to the unprotected head. *Journal of Applied Biomechanics*. 2015; 31(4): 264–268.

38. Allison MA, Kang YS, Maltese MR, Bolte JHt, Arbogast KB. Measurement of hybrid III head impact kinematics using an accelerometer and gyroscope system in ice hockey helmets. *Annals of Biomedical Engineering.* 2015; 43(8): 1896–1906.

39. Jadischke R, Viano DC, Dau N, King AI, McCarthy J. On the accuracy of the Head Impact Telemetry (HIT) System used in football helmets. *Journal of Biomechanics.* 2013; 46(13): 2310–2315.

40. Stojsih S, Boitano M, Wilhelm M, Bir C. A prospective study of punch biomechanics and cognitive function for amateur boxers. *British Journal of Sports Medicine.* 2010; 44(10): 725–730.

41. Rowson S, Duma SM, Beckwith JG et al. Rotational head kinematics in football impacts: an injury risk function for concussion. *Annals of Biomedical Engineering.* 2012; 40(1): 1–13.

42. Broglio SP, Schnebel B, Sosnoff JJ et al. Biomechanical properties of concussions in high school football. *Medicine and Science in Sports and Exercise.* 2010; 42(11): 2064–2071.

43. Beckwith JG, Greenwald RM, Chu JJ et al. Head impact exposure sustained by football players on days of diagnosed concussion. *Medicine and Science in Sports and Exercise.* 2013; 45(4): 737–746.

44. Funk JR, Duma SM, Manoogian SJ, Rowson S. Biomechanical risk estimates for mild traumatic brain injury. *Annual Proceedings/Association for the Advancement of Automotive Medicine Association for the Advancement of Automotive Medicine.* 2007; 51: 343–361.

45. Casson IR, Pellman EJ, Viano DC. Concussion in the National Football League: an overview for neurologists. *Physical Medicine and Rehabilitation Clinics of North America.* 2009; 20(1): 195–214, x.

46. Pellman EJ, Viano DC, Tucker AM, Casson IR, Waeckerle JF. Concussion in professional football: reconstruction of game impacts and injuries. *Neurosurgery.* 2003; 53(4): 799–812.

47. Pellman EJ, Viano DC, Tucker AM, Casson IR. Concussion in professional football: location and direction of helmet impacts-Part 2. *Neurosurgery.* 2003; 53(6): 1328–1340.

48. Greenwald RM, Gwin JT, Chu JJ, Crisco JJ. Head impact severity measures for evaluating mild traumatic brain injury risk exposure. *Neurosurgery.* 2008; 62(4): 789–798.

49. Withnall C, Shewchenko N, Gittens R, Dvorak J. Biomechanical investigation of head impacts in football. *British Journal of Sports Medicine.* 2005; 39 Suppl 1: i49–57.

50. Boden BP, Kirkendall DT, Garrett WE, Jr. Concussion incidence in elite college soccer players. *The American Journal of Sports Medicine.* 1998; 26(2): 238–241.

51. Naunheim RS, Bayly PV, Standeven J, Neubauer JS, Lewis LM, Genin GM. Linear and angular head accelerations during heading of a soccer ball. *Medicine and Science in Sports and Exercise.* 2003; 35(8): 1406–1412.

52. King D, Hume PA, Brughelli M, Gissane C. Instrumented mouthguard acceleration analyses for head impacts in amateur rugby union players over a season of matches. *The American Journal of Sports Medicine.* 2015; 43(3): 614–624.

53. Naunheim RS, Standeven J, Richter C, Lewis LM. Comparison of impact data in hockey, football, and soccer. *The Journal of Trauma.* 2000; 48(5): 938–941.

54. Crisco JJ, Costa L, Rich R, Schwartz JB, Wilcox B. Surrogate headform accelerations associated with stick checks in girls' lacrosse. *Journal of Applied Biomechanics.* 2015; 31(2): 122–127.

55. Morse JD, Franck JA, Wilcox BJ, Crisco JJ, Franck C. An experimental and numerical investigation of head dynamics due to stick impacts in girls' lacrosse. *Annals of Biomedical Engineering.* 2014; 42(12): 2501–2511.

56. Daniel RW, Rowson S, Duma SM. Head impact exposure in youth football. *Annals of Biomedical Engineering.* 2012; 40(4): 976–981.

57. Walilko TJ, Viano DC, Bir CA. Biomechanics of the head for Olympic boxer punches to the face. *British Journal of Sports Medicine.* 2005; 39(10): 710–719.

58. Viano DC, Casson IR, Pellman EJ et al. Concussion in professional football: comparison with boxing head impacts–part 10. *Neurosurgery.* 2005; 57(6): 1154–1172.

59. Zhang L, Yang KH, King AI. A proposed injury threshold for mild traumatic brain injury. *Journal of Biomechanical Engineering.* 2004; 126(2): 226–236.

60. McCaffrey MA, Mihalik JP, Crowell DH, Shields EW, Guskiewicz KM. Measurement of head impacts in collegiate football players: clinical measures of concussion after high- and low-magnitude impacts. *Neurosurgery.* 2007; 61(6): 1236–1243.

61. Morley WA, Seneff S. Diminished brain resilience syndrome: A modern day neurological pathology of increased susceptibility to mild brain trauma, concussion, and downstream neurodegeneration. *Surgical Neurology International.* 2014; 5: 97.

62. Weaver AA, Danelson KA, Stitzel JD. Modeling brain injury response for rotational velocities of varying directions and magnitudes. *Annals of Biomedical Engineering.* 2012; 40(9): 2005–2018.

63. Mihalik JP, Greenwald RM, Blackburn JT, Cantu RC, Marshall SW, Guskiewicz KM. Effect of infraction type on head impact severity in youth ice hockey. *Medicine and Science in Sports and Exercise.* 2010; 42(8): 1431–1438.

64. Rowson S, Duma SM. Brain injury prediction: assessing the combined probability of concussion using linear and rotational head acceleration. *Annals of Biomedical Engineering.* 2013; 41(5): 873–882.

65. Rowson S, Daniel RW, Duma SM. Biomechanical performance of leather and modern football helmets. *Journal of Neurosurgery.* 2013; 119(3): 805–809.

66. Rowson S, Duma SM. Development of the STAR evaluation system for football helmets: integrating player head impact exposure and risk of concussion. *Annals of Biomedical Engineering.* 2011; 39(8): 2130–2140.

67. Rowson B, Rowson S, Duma SM. Hockey STAR: A methodology for assessing the biomechanical performance of hockey helmets. *Annals of Biomedical Engineering.* 2015; 43(10): 2429–2443.

68. Nakatsuka AS, Yamamoto LG. External foam layers to football helmets reduce head impact severity. *Hawai'i Journal of Medicine and Public Health.* 2014; 73(8): 256–261.

69. Post A, Karton C, Hoshizaki TB, Gilchrist MD, Bailes J. Evaluation of the protective capacity of baseball helmets for concussive impacts. *Computer Methods in Biomechanics and Biomedical Engineering.* 2015: 1–10.

70. Tong DC, Winter TJ, Jin J, Bennett AC, Waddell JN. Quantification of subconcussive impact forces to the head using a forensic model. *Journal of Clinical Neuroscience.* 2015; 22(4): 747–751.

71. Bar-Kochba E, Scimone MT, Estrada JB, Franck C. Strain and rate-dependent neuronal injury in a 3D in vitro compression model of traumatic brain injury. *Scientific Report.* 2016; 6: 30550.

72. Bergmann KR, Flood A, Kreykes NS, Kharbanda AB. Concussion Among Youth Skiers and Snowboarders: A Review of the National Trauma Data Bank From 2009 to 2010. *Pediatric Emergency Care.* 2015.

73. Pellman EJ, Viano DC, Withnall C, Shewchenko N, Bir CA, Halstead PD. Concussion in professional football: helmet testing to assess impact performance–part 11. *Neurosurgery.* 2006; 58(1): 78–96.

74. Gammons MR. Helmets in sport: fact and fallacy. *Current Sports Medicine Reports.* 2013; 12(6): 377–380.

75. Rowson S, Duma SM, Greenwald RM et al. Can helmet design reduce the risk of concussion in football? *Journal of Neurosurgery.* 2014; 120(4): 919–922.

76. McGuine TA, Hetzel S, McCrea M, Brooks MA. Protective equipment and player characteristics associated with the incidence of sport-related concussion in high school football players: a multifactorial prospective study. *The American Journal of Sports Medicine.* 2014; 42(10): 2470–2478.

77. Zuckerman SL, Lee YM, Odom MJ, Forbes JA, Solomon GS, Sills AK. Sports-related concussion in helmeted vs. unhelmeted athletes: who fares worse? *International Journal of Sports Medicine.* 2015; 36(5): 419–425.

78. Armstrong C. Evaluation and management of concussion in athletes: recommendations from the AAN. *American Family Physician.* 2014; 89(7): 585–587.

79. Rakate H. Brain turgor (Kb): Intrinsic property of the brain to resist distortion. *Pediatric Neurosurgery.* 1992; 18: 257–262.

80. Hatt A, Cheng S, Tan K, Sinkus R, Bilston LE. MR elastography can be used to measure brain stiffness changes as a result of altered cranial venous drainage during jugular compression. *AJNR American Journal of Neuroradiology.* 2015; 36(10): 1971–1977.

81. Myer GD, Yuan W, Barber Foss KD et al. The effects of external jugular compression applied during head impact exposure on longitudinal changes in brain neuroanatomical and neurophysiological biomarkers: a preliminary investigation. *Frontiers Neurology.* 2016; 7: 74.

82. Myer GD, Yuan W, Barber Foss KD et al. Analysis of head impact exposure and brain microstructure response in a season-long application of a jugular vein compression collar: a prospective, neuroimaging investigation in American football. *British Journal of Sports Medicine.* 2016.

83. Sindelar B, Bailes JE, Sherman SA et al. Effect of internal jugular vein compression on intracranial hemorrhage in a porcine controlled cortical impact model. *Journal of Neurotrauma.* 2016.

84. Mihalik JP, Guskiewicz KM, Marshall SW, Greenwald RM, Blackburn JT, Cantu RC. Does cervical muscle strength in youth ice hockey players affect head impact biomechanics? *Clinical Journal of Sport Medicine.* 2011; 21(5): 416–421.

85. Schmidt JD, Guskiewicz KM, Blackburn JT, Mihalik JP, Siegmund GP, Marshall SW. The influence of cervical muscle characteristics on head impact biomechanics in football. *The American Journal of Sports Medicine.* 2014; 42(9): 2056–2066.

86. Hasegawa K, Takeda T, Nakajima K et al. Does clenching reduce indirect head acceleration during rugby contact? *Dental Traumatology.* 2014; 30(4): 259–264.

87. Eckner JT, Oh YK, Joshi MS, Richardson JK, Ashton-Miller JA. Effect of neck muscle strength and anticipatory cervical muscle activation on the kinematic response of the head to impulsive loads. *The American Journal of Sports Medicine.* 2014; 42(3): 566–576.

88. Mihalik JP, Blackburn JT, Greenwald RM, Cantu RC, Marshall SW, Guskiewicz KM. Collision type and player anticipation affect head impact severity among youth ice hockey players. *Pediatrics.* 2010; 125(6): e1394–1401.

89. Viano DC, Casson IR, Pellman EJ. Concussion in professional football: biomechanics of the struck player—part 14. *Neurosurgery.* 2007; 61(2): 313–327.

90. Collins CL, Fletcher EN, Fields SK et al. Neck strength: a protective factor reducing risk for concussion in high school sports. *The Journal of Primary Prevention*. 2014; 35(5): 309–319.

91. Benson BW, McIntosh AS, Maddocks D, Herring SA, Raftery M, Dvorak J. What are the most effective risk-reduction strategies in sport concussion? *British Journal of Sports Medicine*. 2013; 47(5): 321–326.

92. Viano DC, Pellman EJ. Concussion in professional football: biomechanics of the striking player–part 8. *Neurosurgery*. 2005; 56(2): 266–280.

93. Fuller CW, Taylor A, Raftery M. Epidemiology of concussion in men's elite Rugby-7s (Sevens World Series) and Rugby-15s (Rugby World Cup, Junior World Championship and Rugby Trophy, Pacific Nations Cup and English Premiership). *British Journal of Sports Medicine*. 2015; 49(7): 478–483.

94. Viano DC, Withnall C, Wonnacott M. Effect of mouthguards on head responses and mandible forces in football helmet impacts. *Annals of Biomedical Engineering*. 2012; 40(1): 47–69.

95. Bolouri H, Zetterberg H. Frontiers in Neuroengineering Animal Models for Concussion: Molecular and Cognitive Assessments–Relevance to Sport and Military Concussions. In: Kobeissy FH, ed. *Brain Neurotrauma: Molecular, Neuropsychological, and Rehabilitation Aspects*. 2015. Boca Raton (FL): CRC Press.

96. Bondi CO, Semple BD, Noble-Haeusslein LJ et al. Found in translation: understanding the biology and behavior of experimental traumatic brain injury. *Neuroscience and Biobehavioral Reviews*. 2014.

97. O'Connor WT, Smyth A, Gilchrist MD. Animal models of traumatic brain injury: a critical evaluation. *Pharmacology & Therapeutics*. 2011: 130.

98. Chen JQ, Zhang CC, Lu H, Wang W. Assessment of traumatic brain injury degree in animal model. *Asian Pacific Journal of Tropical Medicine*. 2014; 7(12): 991–995.

99. Gurkoff GG, Giza CC, Hovda DA. Lateral fluid percussion injury in the developing rat causes an acute, mild behavioral dysfunction in the absence of significant cell death. *Brain Research*. 2006; 1077(1): 24–36.

100. Marmarou A, Foda MA, van den Brink W, Campbell J, Kita H, Demetriadou K. A new model of diffuse brain injury in rats. Part I: Pathophysiology and biomechanics. *Journal of Neurosurgery*. 1994; 80(2): 291–300.

101. Gutierrez E, Huang Y, Haglid K et al. A new model for diffuse brain injury by rotational acceleration: I model, gross appearance, and astrocytosis. *Journal of Neurotrauma*. 2001; 18(3): 247–257.

102. McCrory PR, Berkovic SF. Concussion: the history of clinical and pathophysiological concepts and misconceptions. *Neurology*. 2001; 57(12): 2283–2289.

103. McKee AC, Stein TD, Kiernan PT, Alvarez VE. The neuropathology of chronic traumatic encephalopathy. *Brain Pathology (Zurich, Switzerland)*. 2015; 25(3): 350–364.

104. Gurdjian ES. Cerebral contusions: reevaluation of the mechanism of their development. *The Journal of Trauma*. 1976; 16(1): 35–51.

105. McKee AC, Daneshvar DH. The neuropathology of traumatic brain injury. *Handbook Clinical Neurology*. 2015; 127: 45–66.

106. Carman AJ, Ferguson R, Cantu R et al. Expert consensus document: Mind the gaps-advancing research into short-term and long-term neuropsychological outcomes of youth sports-related concussions. *Nature Reviews Neurology*. 2015; 11(4): 230–244.

107. Chamard E, Lefebvre G, Lassonde M, Theoret H. Long-term abnormalities in the corpus callosum of female concussed athletes. *Journal of Neurotrauma*. 2016; 33(13): 1220–1226.

108. Dean PJ, Sato JR, Vieira G, McNamara A, Sterr A. Long-term structural changes after mTBI and their relation to post-concussion symptoms. *Brain Injury*. 2015: 1–8.

109. Orr CA, Albaugh MD, Watts R et al. Neuroimaging Biomarkers of a history of concussion observed in asymptomatic young athletes. *Journal of Neurotrauma*. 2015.

110. Waljas M, Lange RT, Hakulinen U et al. Biopsychosocial outcome after uncomplicated mild traumatic brain injury. *Journal of Neurotrauma*. 2014; 31(1): 108–124.

111. Henry LC, Tremblay J, Tremblay S et al. Acute and chronic changes in diffusivity measures after sports concussion. *Journal of Neurotrauma*. 2011; 28(10): 2049–2059.

112. Helmer KG, Pasternak O, Fredman E et al. Hockey Concussion Education Project, Part 1. Susceptibility-weighted imaging study in male and female ice hockey players over a single season. *Journal of Neurosurgery*. 2014; 120(4): 864–872.

113. Mayer AR, Ling J, Mannell MV et al. A prospective diffusion tensor imaging study in mild traumatic brain injury. *Neurology*. 2010; 74(8): 643–650.

114. Miles L, Grossman RI, Johnson G, Babb JS, Diller L, Inglese M. Short-term DTI predictors of cognitive dysfunction in mild traumatic brain injury. *Brain Injury*. 2008; 22(2): 115–122.

115. Messe A, Caplain S, Paradot G et al. Diffusion tensor imaging and white matter lesions at the subacute stage in mild traumatic brain injury with persistent neurobehavioral impairment. *Human Brain Mapping*. 2011; 32(6): 999–1011.

116. Murugavel M, Cubon V, Putukian M et al. A longitudinal diffusion tensor imaging study assessing white matter fiber tracts after sports-related concussion. *Journal of Neurotrauma*. 2014; 31(22): 1860–1871.

117. Rutgers DR, Toulgoat F, Cazejust J, Fillard A, Lasjaunias P, Ducreux D. White matter abnormalities in mild traumatic brain injury: a diffusion tensor imaging study. *AJNR American Journal of Neuroradiology*. 2008; 29(3): 514–519.

118. Rutgers DR, Fillard P, Paradot G, Tadie M, Lasjaunias P, Ducreux D. Diffusion tensor imaging characteristics of the corpus callosum in mild, moderate, and severe traumatic brain injury. *AJNR American Journal of Neuroradiology*. 2008; 29(9): 1730–1735.

119. Pasternak O, Koerte IK, Bouix S et al. Hockey Concussion Education Project, Part 2. Microstructural white matter alterations in acutely concussed ice hockey players: a longitudinal free-water MRI study. *Journal of Neurosurgery*. 2014; 120(4): 873–881.

120. Sasaki T, Pasternak O, Mayinger M et al. Hockey Concussion Education Project, Part 3. White matter microstructure in ice hockey players with a history of concussion: a diffusion tensor imaging study. *Journal of Neurosurgery*. 2014; 120(4): 882–890.

121. Chong CD, Schwedt TJ. White matter damage and brain network alterations in concussed patients: a review of recent diffusion tensor imaging and resting-state functional connectivity data. *Current Pain and Headache Reports*. 2015; 19(5): 485.

122. Shin SS, Pathak S, Presson N et al. Detection of white matter injury in concussion using high–definition fiber tractography. *Progress in Neurological Surgery*. 2014; 28: 86–93.

123. Wozniak JR, Krach L, Ward E et al. Neurocognitive and neuroimaging correlates of pediatric traumatic brain injury: a diffusion tensor imaging (DTI) study. *Archives of Clinical Neuropsychology*. 2007; 22(5): 555–568.

124. Wilde EA, McCauley SR, Hunter JV et al. Diffusion tensor imaging of acute mild traumatic brain injury in adolescents. *Neurology*. 2008; 70(12): 948–955.

125. Toth A, Kovacs N, Perlaki G et al. Multimodal magnetic resonance imaging in the acute and sub-acute phase of mild traumatic brain injury: can we see the difference? *Journal of Neurotrauma*. 2013; 30(1): 2–10.

126. Virji-Babul N, Borich MR, Makan N et al. Diffusion tensor imaging of sports-related concussion in adolescents. *Pediatric Neurology*. 2013; 48(1): 24–29.

127. Metting Z, Cerliani L, Rodiger LA, van der Naalt J. Pathophysiological concepts in mild traumatic brain injury: diffusion tensor imaging related to acute perfusion CT imaging. *PLoS One*. 2013; 8(5): e64461.

128. Goswami R, Dufort P, Tartaglia MC et al. Frontotemporal correlates of impulsivity and machine learning in retired professional athletes with a history of multiple concussions. *Brain Structure and Function*. 2015.

129. Bazarian JJ, Zhu T, Zhong J et al. Persistent, long-term cerebral white matter changes after sports-related repetitive head impacts. *PLoS One*. 2014; 9(4): e94734.

130. Bazarian JJ, Zhu T, Blyth B, Borrino A, Zhong J. Subject-specific changes in brain white matter on diffusion tensor imaging after sports-related concussion. *Magnetic Resonance Imaging*. 2012; 30(2): 171–180.

131. McAllister TW, Ford JC, Flashman LA et al. Effect of head impacts on diffusivity measures in a cohort of collegiate contact sport athletes. *Neurology*. 2014; 82(1): 63–69.

132. Davenport EM, Whitlow CT, Urban JE et al. Abnormal white matter integrity related to head impact exposure in a season of high school varsity football. *Journal of Neurotrauma*. 2014; 31(19): 1617–1624.

133. Koerte IK, Ertl-Wagner B, Reiser M, Zafonte R, Shenton ME. White matter integrity in the brains of professional soccer players without a symptomatic concussion. *The Journal of the American Medical Association*. 2012; 308(18): 1859–1861.

134. Choe MC, Giza CC. Diagnosis and management of acute concussion. *Seminar in Neurology*. 2015; 35(1): 29–41.

135. Caskey RC, Nance ML. Management of pediatric mild traumatic brain injury. *Advances in Pediatrics*. 2014; 61(1): 271–286.

136. Hovda DA. The neurophysiology of concussion. *Progress in Neurological Surgery*. 2014; 28: 28–37.

137. Giza CC, Hovda DA. The neurometabolic cascade of concussion. *Journal of Athletic Training*. 2001; 36(3): 228–235.

138. Giza CC, Hovda DA. The new neurometabolic cascade of concussion. *Neurosurgery*. 2014; 75 Suppl 4: S24–33.

139. Nariai T, Inaji M, Tanaka Y et al. PET molecular imaging to investigate higher brain dysfunction in patients with neurotrauma. *Acta Neuro chirurgica Supplement*. 2013; 118: 251–254.

140. Selwyn R, Hockenbury N, Jaiswal S, Mathur S, Armstrong RC, Byrnes KR. Mild traumatic brain injury results in depressed cerebral glucose uptake: An (18)FDG PET study. *Journal of Neurotrauma*. 2013; 30(23): 1943–1953.

141. Rishal I, Fainzilber M. Axon-soma communication in neuronal injury. *Nature Reviews Neuroscience*. 2014; 15(1): 32–42.

142. Smith DH, Meaney DF, Shull WH. Diffuse axonal injury in head trauma. *The Journal of Head Trauma Rehabilitation*. 2003; 18(4): 307–316.

143. Siedler DG, Chuah MI, Kirkcaldie MT, Vickers JC, King AE. Diffuse axonal injury in brain trauma: insights from alterations in neurofilaments. *Frontiers in Cellular Neuroscience*. 2014; 8: 429.

144. Povlishock JT, Pettus EH. Traumatically induced axonal damage: evidence for enduring changes in axolemmal permeability with associated cytoskeletal change. *Acta Neurochirurgica Supplement.* 1996; 66: 81–86.

145. Pettus EH, Povlishock JT. Characterization of a distinct set of intra-axonal ultrastructural changes associated with traumatically induced alteration in axolemmal permeability. *Brain Research.* 1996; 722(1–2): 1–11.

146. Maxwell WL, McCreath BJ, Graham DI, Gennarelli TA. Cytochemical evidence for redistribution of membrane pump calcium-ATPase and ecto-Ca-ATPase activity, and calcium influx in myelinated nerve fibres of the optic nerve after stretch injury. *Journal of Neurocytology.* 1995; 24(12): 925–942.

147. Maxwell WL, Graham DI. Loss of axonal microtubules and neurofilaments after stretch-injury to guinea pig optic nerve fibers. *Journal of Neurotrauma.* 1997; 14(9): 603–614.

148. Farkas O, Lifshitz J, Povlishock JT. Mechanoporation induced by diffuse traumatic brain injury: an irreversible or reversible response to injury? *Journal of Neuroscience.* 2006; 26(12): 3130–3140.

149. Seifert T, Shipman V. The pathophysiology of sports concussion. *Current Pain and Headache Reports.* 2015; 19(8): 36.

150. Huang EY, Tsai TH, Kuo TT et al. Remote effects on the striatal dopamine system after fluid percussion injury. *Behavioural Brain Research.* 2014; 267: 156–172.

151. Patt S, Brodhun M. Neuropathological sequelae of traumatic injury in the brain. An overview. *Experimental and Toxicologic Pathology.* 1999; 51(2): 119–123.

152. Guerriero RM, Giza CC, Rotenberg A. Glutamate and GABA imbalance following traumatic brain injury. *Current Neurology and Neuroscience Reports.* 2015; 15(5): 27.

153. van Landeghem FK, Stover JF, Bechmann I et al. Early expression of glutamate transporter proteins in ramified microglia after controlled cortical impact injury in the rat. *Glia.* 2001; 35(3): 167–179.

154. Kierans AS, Kirov, II, Gonen O et al. Myoinositol and glutamate complex neurometabolite abnormality after mild traumatic brain injury. *Neurology.* 2014; 82(6): 521–528.

155. Barkhoudarian G, Hovda DA, Giza CC. The molecular pathophysiology of concussive brain injury. *Clinics in Sports Medicine.* 2011; 30(1): 33–48, vii–iii.

156. Yi JH, Hazell AS. Excitotoxic mechanisms and the role of astrocytic glutamate transporters in traumatic brain injury. *Neurochemistry International.* 2006; 48(5): 394–403.

157. Katayama Y, Becker DP, Tamura T, Hovda DA. Massive increases in extracellular potassium and the indiscriminate release of glutamate following concussive brain injury. *Journal of Neurosurgery.* 1990; 73(6): 889–900.

158. Faden AI, Demediuk P, Panter SS, Vink R. The role of excitatory amino acids and NMDA receptors in traumatic brain injury. *Science (New York, NY).* 1989; 244(4906): 798–800.

159. Giza CC, Maria NS, Hovda DA. N-methyl-D-aspartate receptor subunit changes after traumatic injury to the developing brain. *Journal of Neurotrauma.* 2006; 23(6): 950–961.

160. McDevitt J, Tierney RT, Phillips J, Gaughan JP, Torg JS, Krynetskiy E. Association between GRIN2A promoter polymorphism and recovery from concussion. *Brain Injury.* 2015: 1–8.

161. McDonald JW, Johnston MV. Physiological and pathophysiological roles of excitatory amino acids during central nervous system development. *Brain Research Brain Research Reviews.* 1990; 15(1): 41–70.

162. Kim JY, Kim N, Yenari MA, Chang W. Hypothermia and pharmacological regimens that prevent overexpression and overactivity of the extracellular calcium-sensing receptor protect neurons against traumatic brain injury. *Journal of Neurotrauma*. 2013; 30(13): 1170–1176.

163. Kampfl A, Posmantur RM, Zhao X, Schmutzhard E, Clifton GL, Hayes RL. Mechanisms of calpain proteolysis following traumatic brain injury: implications for pathology and therapy: a review and update. *Journal of Neurotrauma*. 1997; 14(3): 121–134.

164. Saatman KE, Abai B, Grosvenor A, Vorwerk CK, Smith DH, Meaney DF. Traumatic axonal injury results in biphasic calpain activation and retrograde transport impairment in mice. *Journal Cerebral Blood Flow Metabolism*. 2003; 23(1): 34–42.

165. Morgan JI, Curran T. Role of ion flux in the control of c-fos expression. *Nature*. 1986; 322(6079): 552–555.

166. Inci S, Ozcan OE, Kilinc K. Time-level relationship for lipid peroxidation and the protective effect of alpha-tocopherol in experimental mild and severe brain injury. *Neurosurgery*. 1998; 43(2): 330–335.

167. Lifshitz J, Sullivan PG, Hovda DA, Wieloch T, McIntosh TK. Mitochondrial damage and dysfunction in traumatic brain injury. *Mitochondrion*. 2004; 4(5–6): 705–713.

168. Verity MA. Ca(2+)–dependent processes as mediators of neurotoxicity. *Neurotoxicology*. 1992; 13(1): 139–147.

169. Villapol S, Byrnes KR, Symes AJ. Temporal dynamics of cerebral blood flow, cortical damage, apoptosis, astrocyte-vasculature interaction and astrogliosis in the pericontusional region after traumatic brain injury. *Frontiers in Neurology*. 2014; 5: 82.

170. Dean PJ, Sterr A. Long-term effects of mild traumatic brain injury on cognitive performance. *Frontiers in Human Neuroscience*. 2013; 7: 30.

171. Hicks RR, Smith DH, Lowenstein DH, Saint Marie R, McIntosh TK. Mild experimental brain injury in the rat induces cognitive deficits associated with regional neuronal loss in the hippocampus. *Journal of Neurotrauma*. 1993; 10(4): 405–414.

172. Di Pietro V, Amorini AM, Tavazzi B et al. Potentially neuroprotective gene modulation in an in vitro model of mild traumatic brain injury. *Molecular and Cellular Biochemistry*. 2013; 375(1–2): 185–198.

173. Zetterberg H, Smith DH, Blennow K. Biomarkers of mild traumatic brain injury in cerebrospinal fluid and blood. *Nature Reviews Neurology*. 2013; 9(4): 201–210.

174. Robertson CL, Saraswati M, Fiskum G. Mitochondrial dysfunction early after traumatic brain injury in immature rats. *Journal of Neurochemistry*. 2007; 101(5): 1248–1257.

175. Xiong Y, Gu Q, Peterson PL, Muizelaar JP, Lee CP. Mitochondrial dysfunction and calcium perturbation induced by traumatic brain injury. *Journal of Neurotrauma*. 1997; 14(1): 23–34.

176. Fineman I, Hovda DA, Smith M, Yoshino A, Becker DP. Concussive brain injury is associated with a prolonged accumulation of calcium: a 45Ca autoradiographic study. *Brain Research*. 1993; 624(1–2): 94–102.

177. Verweij BH, Muizelaar JP, Vinas FC, Peterson PL, Xiong Y, Lee CP. Mitochondrial dysfunction after experimental and human brain injury and its possible reversal with a selective N-type calcium channel antagonist (SNX-111). *Neurological Research*. 1997; 19(3): 334–339.

178. Smith DH, Stewart W. Tackling concussion, beyond Hollywood. The *Lancet Neurology*. 2016; 15(7): 662–663.

179. Tang-Schomer MD, Patel AR, Baas PW, Smith DH. Mechanical breaking of microtubules in axons during dynamic stretch injury underlies delayed elasticity, microtubule disassembly, and axon degeneration. *FASEB Journal*. 2010; 24(5): 1401–1410.

180. Nakamura Y, Takeda M, Angelides KJ, Tanaka T, Tada K, Nishimura T. Effect of phosphorylation on 68 KDa neurofilament subunit protein assembly by the cyclic AMP dependent protein kinase in vitro. *Biochemical and Biophysical Research Communications*. 1990; 169(2): 744–750.

181. Povlishock JT, Becker DP, Cheng CL, Vaughan GW. Axonal change in minor head injury. *Journal of Neuropathology and Experimental Neurology*. 1983; 42(3): 225–242.

182. Johnson VE, Stewart W, Smith DH. Axonal pathology in traumatic brain injury. *Experimental Neurology*. 2013; 246: 35–43.

183. Hanell A, Greer JE, McGinn MJ, Povlishock JT. Traumatic brain injury-induced axonal phenotypes react differently to treatment. *Acta Neuropathologica*. 2015; 129(2): 317–332.

184. Mittl RL, Grossman RI, Hiehle JF et al. Prevalence of MR evidence of diffuse axonal injury in patients with mild head injury and normal head CT findings. *AJNR American Journal of Neuroradiology*. 1994; 15(8): 1583–1589.

185. Giordano C, Kleiven S. Evaluation of axonal strain as a predictor for mild traumatic brain injuries using finite element modeling. *Stapp Car Crash Journal*. 2014; 58: 29–61.

186. Greer JE, Hanell A, McGinn MJ, Povlishock JT. Mild traumatic brain injury in the mouse induces axotomy primarily within the axon initial segment. *Acta Neuropathologica*. 2013; 126(1): 59–74.

187. Browne KD, Chen XH, Meaney DF, Smith DH. Mild traumatic brain injury and diffuse axonal injury in swine. *Journal of Neurotrauma*. 2011; 28(9): 1747–1755.

188. Gennarelli TA, Thibault LE, Adams JH, Graham DI, Thompson CJ, Marcincin RP. Diffuse axonal injury and traumatic coma in the primate. *Annals of Neurology*. 1982; 12(6): 564–574.

189. Yoshino A, Hovda DA, Kawamata T, Katayama Y, Becker DP. Dynamic changes in local cerebral glucose utilization following cerebral conclusion in rats: evidence of a hyper- and subsequent hypometabolic state. *Brain Research*. 1991; 561(1): 106–119.

190. Ginsberg MD, Zhao W, Alonso OF, Loor-Estades JY, Dietrich WD, Busto R. Uncoupling of local cerebral glucose metabolism and blood flow after acute fluid-percussion injury in rats. *The American Journal of Physiology*. 1997; 272(6 Pt 2): H2859–2868.

191. Gardner AJ, Tan CO, Ainslie PN et al. Cerebrovascular reactivity assessed by transcranial Doppler ultrasound in sport-related concussion: a systematic review. *British Journal of Sports Medicine*. 2015; 49(16): 1050–1055.

192. Tan CO, Meehan WP, 3rd, Iverson GL, Taylor JA. Cerebrovascular regulation, exercise, and mild traumatic brain injury. *Neurology*. 2014; 83(18): 1665–1672.

193. Muir JK, Boerschel M, Ellis EF. Continuous monitoring of posttraumatic cerebral blood flow using laser–Doppler flowmetry. *Journal of Neurotrauma*. 1992; 9(4): 355–362.

194. Yamakami I, McIntosh TK. Effects of traumatic brain injury on regional cerebral blood flow in rats as measured with radiolabeled microspheres. *Journal of Cereb Blood Flow Metabolism*. 1989; 9(1): 117–124.

195. Buckley EM, Miller BF, Golinski JM et al. Decreased microvascular cerebral blood flow assessed by diffuse correlation spectroscopy after repetitive concussions in mice. *Journal of Cereb Blood Flow Metabolism*. 2015.

196. Chan ST, Evans KC, Rosen BR, Song TY, Kwong KK. A case study of magnetic resonance imaging of cerebrovascular reactivity: a powerful imaging marker for mild traumatic brain injury. *Brain Injury*. 2015; 29(3): 403–407.

197. Mutch WA, Ellis MJ, Graham MR et al. Brain MRI CO2 stress testing: a pilot study in patients with concussion. *PLoS One*. 2014; 9(7): e102181.

198. Wang Y, Nelson LD, LaRoche AA et al. Cerebral blood flow alterations in acute sport-related concussion. *Journal of Neurotrauma*. 2016; 33(13): 1227–1236.

199. Yu GX, Mueller M, Hawkins BE et al. Traumatic brain injury in vivo and in vitro contributes to cerebral vascular dysfunction through impaired gap junction communication between vascular smooth muscle cells. *Journal of Neurotrauma*. 2014; 31(8): 739–748.

200. Sword J, Masuda T, Croom D, Kirov SA. Evolution of neuronal and astroglial disruption in the peri-contusional cortex of mice revealed by in vivo two-photon imaging. *Brain*. 2013; 136(Pt 5): 1446–1461.

201. Len TK, Neary JP. Cerebrovascular pathophysiology following mild traumatic brain injury. *Clinical Physiology and Functional imaging*. 2011; 31(2): 85–93.

202. Auerbach PS, Baine JG, Schott ML, Greenhaw A, Acharya MG, Smith WS. Detection of concussion using cranial accelerometry. *Clinical Journal of Sport Medicine*. 2015; 25(2): 126–132.

203. Militana AR, Donahue MJ, Sills AK et al. Alterations in default-mode network connectivity may be influenced by cerebrovascular changes within 1 week of sports related concussion in college varsity athletes: a pilot study. *Brain Imaging and Behavior*. 2015.

204. Wang Y, Nelson LD, LaRoche AA et al. Cerebral Blood Flow Alterations in Acute Sport-Related Concussion. *Journal of Neurotrauma*. 2015.

205. Maugans TA, Farley C, Altaye M, Leach J, Cecil KM. Pediatric sports-related concussion produces cerebral blood flow alterations. *Pediatrics*. 2012; 129(1): 28–37.

206. Len TK, Neary JP, Asmundson GJ et al. Serial monitoring of CO2 reactivity following sport concussion using hypocapnia and hypercapnia. *Brain Injury*. 2013; 27(3): 346–353.

207. Junger EC, Newell DW, Grant GA et al. Cerebral autoregulation following minor head injury. *Journal of Neurosurgery*. 1997; 86(3): 425–432.

208. Strebel S, Lam AM, Matta BF, Newell DW. Impaired cerebral autoregulation after mild brain injury. *Surgical Neurology*. 1997; 47(2): 128–131.

209. Bartnik-Olson BL, Holshouser B, Wang H et al. Impaired neurovascular unit function contributes to persistent symptoms after concussion: a pilot study. *Journal of Neurotrauma*. 2014; 31(17): 1497–1506.

210. Meier TB, Bellgowan PS, Singh R, Kuplicki R, Polanski DW, Mayer AR. Recovery of cerebral blood flow following sports-related concussion. *The Journal of the American Medical Association Neurology*. 2015; 72(5): 530–538.

211. Wang Y, West JD, Bailey JN et al. Decreased cerebral blood flow in chronic pediatric mild TBI: an MRI perfusion study. *Developmental Neuropsychology*. 2015; 40(1): 40–44.

212. Kalimo H, Rehncrona S, Soderfeldt B. The role of lactic acidosis in the ischemic nerve cell injury. *Acta Neuropathologica Supplementum*. 1981; 7: 20–22.

213. Kubota M, Nakamura T, Sunami K et al. Changes of local cerebral glucose utilization, DC potential and extracellular potassium concentration in experimental head injury of varying severity. *Neurosurgical Review*. 1989; 12 Suppl 1: 393–399.

214. Johnstone VP, Shultz SR, Yan EB, O'Brien TJ, Rajan R. The acute phase of mild traumatic brain injury is characterized by a distance-dependent neuronal hypoactivity. *Journal of Neurotrauma*. 2014; 31(22): 1881–1895.

215. Signoretti S, Di Pietro V, Vagnozzi R et al. Transient alterations of creatine, creatine phosphate, N-acetylaspartate and high-energy phosphates after mild traumatic brain injury in the rat. *Molecular and Cellular Biochemistry*. 2010; 333(1–2): 269–277.

216. Saluja RS, Chen JK, Gagnon IJ, Keightley M, Ptito A. Navigational memory functional magnetic resonance imaging: a test for concussion in children. *Journal of Neurotrauma*. 2015; 32(10): 712–722.

217. Urban KJ, Barlow KM, Jimenez JJ, Goodyear BG, Dunn JF. Functional near-infrared spectroscopy reveals reduced interhemispheric cortical communication after pediatric concussion. *Journal of Neurotrauma*. 2015; 32(11): 833–840.

218. Lucke-Wold BP, Turner RC, Logsdon AF, Bailes JE, Huber JD, Rosen CL. Linking traumatic brain injury to chronic traumatic encephalopathy: identification of potential mechanisms leading to neurofibrillary tangle development. *Journal of Neurotrauma*. 2014; 31(13): 1129–1138.

219. Walter P, Ron D. The unfolded protein response: from stress pathway to homeostatic regulation. *Science (New York, NY)*. 2011; 334(6059): 1081–1086.

220. Zhang K, Kaufman RJ. From endoplasmic-reticulum stress to the inflammatory response. *Nature*. 2008; 454(7203): 455–462.

221. Susarla BT, Villapol S, Yi JH, Geller HM, Symes AJ. Temporal patterns of cortical proliferation of glial cell populations after traumatic brain injury in mice. *American Society Neurochemistry Neuro*. 2014; 6(3): 159–170.

222. Tsai YD, Liliang PC, Cho CL et al. Delayed neurovascular inflammation after mild traumatic brain injury in rats. *Brain Injury*. 2013; 27(3): 361–365.

223. Tang C, Xue HL, Bai CL, Fu R. Regulation of adhesion molecules expression in TNF-alpha-stimulated brain microvascular endothelial cells by tanshinone IIA: involvement of NF-kappaB and ROS generation. *Phytotherapy Research*. 2011; 25(3): 376–380.

224. Tang C, Xue H, Bai C, Fu R, Wu A. The effects of Tanshinone IIA on blood–brain barrier and brain edema after transient middle cerebral artery occlusion in rats. *Phytomedicine*. 2010; 17(14): 1145–1149.

225. Davalos D, Grutzendler J, Yang G et al. ATP mediates rapid microglial response to local brain injury in vivo. *Nature Neuroscience*. 2005; 8(6): 752–758.

226. Zhang WJ, Feng J, Zhou R et al. Tanshinone IIA protects the human blood–brain barrier model from leukocyte-associated hypoxia-reoxygenation injury. *European Journal of Pharmacology*. 2010; 648(1–3): 146–152.

227. Rhodes JK, Sharkey J, Andrews PJ. The temporal expression, cellular localization, and inhibition of the chemokines MIP-2 and MCP-1 after traumatic brain injury in the rat. *Journal of Neurotrauma*. 2009; 26(4): 507–525.

228. Blaylock RL, Maroon J. Immunoexcitotoxicity as a central mechanism in chronic traumatic encephalopathy—A unifying hypothesis. *Surgical Neurology International*. 2011; 2: 107.

229. Finnie JW. Neuroinflammation: beneficial and detrimental effects after traumatic brain injury. *Inflammopharmacology*. 2013; 21(4): 309–320.

230. Perez-Polo JR, Rea HC, Johnson KM et al. Inflammatory consequences in a rodent model of mild traumatic brain injury. *Journal of Neurotrauma*. 2013; 30(9): 727–740.

231. Rancan M, Otto VI, Hans VH et al. Upregulation of ICAM-1 and MCP-1 but not of MIP-2 and sensorimotor deficit in response to traumatic axonal injury in rats. *Journal of Neuroscience Research*. 2001; 63(5): 438–446.

232. Ghirnikar RS, Lee YL, Eng LF. Inflammation in traumatic brain injury: role of cytokines and chemokines. *Neurochemical Research*. 1998; 23(3): 329–340.

233. Gill J, Merchant-Borna K, Lee H et al. Sports-Related Concussion Results in Differential Expression of Nuclear Factor-kappaB Pathway Genes in Peripheral Blood During the Acute and Subacute Periods. *The Journal of Head Trauma Rehabilitation*. 2015.

234. Loane DJ, Byrnes KR. Role of microglia in neurotrauma. *Neurotherapeutics*. 2010; 7(4): 366–377.

235. Mierzwa AJ, Marion CM, Sullivan GM, McDaniel DP, Armstrong RC. Components of myelin damage and repair in the progression of white matter pathology after mild traumatic brain injury. *Journal of Neuropathology and Experimental Neurology*. 2015; 74(3): 218–232.

236. Perez-Polo JR, Rea HC, Johnson KM et al. Inflammatory cytokine receptor blockade in a rodent model of mild traumatic brain injury. *Journal of Neuroscience Research*. 2016; 94(1): 27–38.

237. Feuerstein GZ, Wang X, Barone FC. The role of cytokines in the neuropathology of stroke and neurotrauma. *Neuroimmunomodulation*. 1998; 5(3–4): 143–159.

238. Baratz R, Tweedie D, Wang JY et al. Transiently lowering tumor necrosis factor-alpha synthesis ameliorates neuronal cell loss and cognitive impairments induced by minimal traumatic brain injury in mice. *Journal of Neuroinflammation*. 2015; 12: 45.

239. Homsi S, Piaggio T, Croci N et al. Blockade of acute microglial activation by minocycline promotes neuroprotection and reduces locomotor hyperactivity after closed head injury in mice: a twelve-week follow-up study. *Journal of Neurotrauma*. 2010; 27(5): 911–921.

240. Baugh CM, Stamm JM, Riley DO et al. Chronic traumatic encephalopathy: neurodegeneration following repetitive concussive and subconcussive brain trauma. *Brain Imaging and Behavior*. 2012; 6(2): 244–254.

241. Gavett BE, Stern RA, McKee AC. Chronic traumatic encephalopathy: a potential late effect of sport-related concussive and subconcussive head trauma. *Clinics in Sports Medicine*. 2011; 30(1): 179–188, xi.

242. Stern RA, Riley DO, Daneshvar DH, Nowinski CJ, Cantu RC, McKee AC. Long-term consequences of repetitive brain trauma: chronic traumatic encephalopathy. *PM & R*. 2011; 3(10 Suppl 2): S460–467.

243. Kiernan PT, Montenigro PH, Solomon TM, McKee AC. Chronic traumatic encephalopathy: a neurodegenerative consequence of repetitive traumatic brain injury. *Seminars in Neurology*. 2015; 35(1): 20–28.

244. Smith DH, Chen XH, Pierce JE et al. Progressive atrophy and neuron death for one year following brain trauma in the rat. *Journal of Neurotrauma*. 1997; 14(10): 715–727.

245. Breunig JJ, Guillot-Sestier MV, Town T. Brain injury, neuroinflammation and Alzheimer's disease. *Frontiers in Aging Neuroscience*. 2013; 5: 26.

246. Sivanandam TM, Thakur MK. Traumatic brain injury: a risk factor for Alzheimer's disease. *Neuroscience and Biobehavioral Reviews*. 2012; 36(5): 1376–1381.

247. Zlokovic BV. The blood–brain barrier in health and chronic neurodegenerative disorders. *Neuron*. 2008; 57(2): 178–201.

248. Shlosberg D, Benifla M, Kaufer D, Friedman A. Blood–brain barrier breakdown as a therapeutic target in traumatic brain injury. *Nature Reviews Neurology*. 2010; 6(7): 393–403.

249. Ren Z, Iliff JJ, Yang L et al. 'Hit & Run' model of closed-skull traumatic brain injury (TBI) reveals complex patterns of post-traumatic AQP4 dysregulation. *Journal of Cerebral Blood Flow Metabolism*. 2013; 33(6): 834–845.

250. Shapira Y, Setton D, Artru AA, Shohami E. Blood–brain barrier permeability, cerebral edema, and neurologic function after closed head injury in rats. *Anesthesia and Analgesia*. 1993; 77(1): 141–148.

251. Jin X, Wang F, Liu X et al. Negative correlation of CD34+ cells with blood–brain barrier permeability following traumatic brain injury in a rat model. *Microcirculation (New York, NY: 1994)*. 2014; 21(8): 696–702.

252. Glushakova OY, Johnson D, Hayes RL. Delayed increases in microvascular pathology after experimental traumatic brain injury are associated with prolonged inflammation, blood–brain barrier disruption, and progressive white matter damage. *Journal of Neurotrauma.* 2014; 31(13): 1180–1193.

253. Muradashvili N, Benton RL, Saatman KE, Tyagi SC, Lominadze D. Ablation of matrix metalloproteinase-9 gene decreases cerebrovascular permeability and fibrinogen deposition post traumatic brain injury in mice. *Metabolic Brain Disease.* 2015; 30(2): 411–426.

254. Vagnozzi R, Signoretti S, Cristofori L et al. Assessment of metabolic brain damage and recovery following mild traumatic brain injury: a multicentre, proton magnetic resonance spectroscopic study in concussed patients. *Brain.* 2010; 133(11): 3232–3242.

255. Ramos-Zuniga R, Gonzalez-de la Torre M, Jimenez-Maldonado M et al. Postconcussion syndrome and mild head injury: the role of early diagnosis using neuropsychological tests and functional magnetic resonance/spectroscopy. *World Neurosurgery.* 2014; 82(5): 828–835.

256. Henry LC, Tremblay S, Boulanger Y, Ellemberg D, Lassonde M. Neurometabolic changes in the acute phase after sports concussions correlate with symptom severity. *Journal of Neurotrauma.* 2010; 27(1): 65–76.

257. Chamard E, Lassonde M, Henry L et al. Neurometabolic and microstructural alterations following a sports-related concussion in female athletes. *Brain Injury.* 2013; 27(9): 1038–1046.

258. Mondello S, Schmid K, Berger RP et al. The challenge of mild traumatic brain injury: role of biochemical markers in diagnosis of brain damage. *Medicinal Research Reviews.* 2014; 34(3): 503–531.

CHAPTER 3

Acute assessment, diagnosis, and management of the concussed athlete

Introduction

Due to the nonspecific, and at times, vague symptomatology of concussion, the initial diagnosis can be quite challenging. Only through a complete evaluation of the athlete including a history of the injury, neurological examination, symptomatology, and changes from baseline on sideline assessment tools, will the perceptive provider be able to make the early diagnosis of concussion.

Within this chapter, we will discuss these aspects of the acute evaluation that may occur either at the field of play, emergency department, or even outpatient clinic. Woven within this process of the initial diagnosis, further assessment, and repeated evaluation, the provider will also be required to make prompt decisions regarding when the player necessitates a higher level of care due to their clinical presentation (Figure 3.1).

The same basic principles of acute management overlap through each tier of care (onfield management, emergency department setting, inpatient hospital facility, and outpatient initial assessment); and therefore, emphasis will be placed on the unique and numerous decisions that need to be made at each specific level. These decisions encompass the following questions: can the player return to play, do they need to be evaluated at a hospital, is neuroimaging required, when should the outpatient follow-up occur, etc.? Further detailed outpatient management, like return to activity recommendations, postconcussive syndrome management, and various concussion measurement modalities, will be discussed in Chapters 4, 5, and 6 respectively.

Onfield preparedness

A critical failure regarding concussion recognition and care is a lack of preparation. A 1999 review showed that an athletic trainer would see roughly eight concussions per year, in which even this value is likely outdated and underestimated.[1] Therefore, due to this low but still very prevalent incidence, complacency can easily develop within the protocol of managing the concussed athlete. It is essential to establish an Emergency Action Plan (EAP) at each level of care that should be understood by all personnel involved, and practiced on a routine basis.[2] Depending on the level of competitive play, this should be a coordinated effort between the team physician and/or athletic trainer.[3,4] These protocols will provide a stepwise direction to the person providing care to the concussed athlete especially in life-threatening situations, for example, an expanding subdural/epidural hematoma or malignant cerebral edema. These previously determined algorithms are necessary in providing time-efficient care, therefore reducing long-term neurological deficits and mortality. For example, following an injurious event where a player is found to be neurologically compromised, questions that already need to be addressed are:

◆ Who is tasked with the initial assessment of the player to determine the need for notifying emergency medical services (EMS)?
◆ Who will be calling EMS, where does the ambulance enter the stadium, who will be directing the ambulance onto the field, or

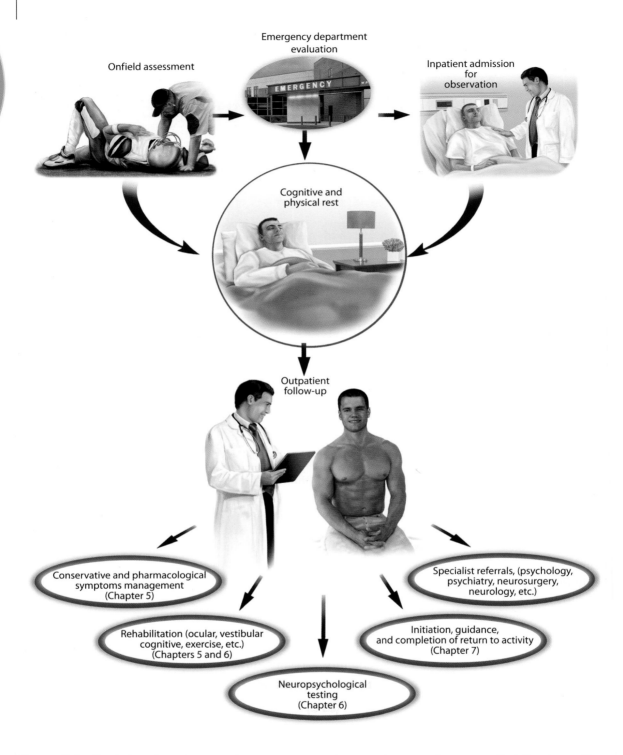

Figure 3.1 **Escalation of care in concussion management and progression towards recovery.** First, the player will receive a primary survey followed by the secondary survey that includes a multimodal approach to diagnosis of concussion. Depending on the severity of injury, the player may require further evaluation and possible admission to an inpatient hospital. All players, once diagnosed with a concussion, require a few days of complete rest followed by a return to activity escalation guided by the medical provider.

how will the spectators be guided to allow the ambulance access to the field?

◆ Where is the closest Level 1 trauma facility?
◆ Where are specific medical supplies located, for example the cervical collar and backboard to maintain spinal precautions, the cardiac defibrillator if cardiopulmonary resuscitation (CPR) needs to take place, or even personal protective equipment like surgical gloves to minimize exposures to bodily fluids?

This is just an example of a fraction of the specific tasks and responsibilities that can be predelegated to avoid any delay or confusion during a high-stress event.

Onfield evaluation and diagnosis

An obvious initial step to the diagnosis is to understand what type of impacts can cause a concussive injury. As detailed in Chapter 2, a concussion can be caused by not only a direct blow to the head, but also an impact to the neck or torso that creates an "impulsive force transmitted to the head (whiplash type mechanism)."[5–12] It is imperative to educate athletic trainers, coaches, and athletes on this crucial point because the media has engrained in popular thought that concussions are only possible through blunt head impacts. With this knowledge, the medical provider is able to identify potentially concussive-causing events prompting further investigation in those players that walk away immediately from the play but begin to have slight behavioral changes or symptoms (irritability, incoordination, mild confusion, forgetfulness of play or role on the field etc.).[6] It is easy to diagnose concussion in players with loss of consciousness or traumatic amnesia, but this occurrence is few in the majority of injuries. Other subtler signs may ensue following the incident where the player appears confused or forgetful of the next play, unsure of the score or his/her position role, appears unsteady or clumsy, walks to the wrong huddle or sidelines, and/or appears dazed. Any player with overt symptoms or even a concern for concussive injury should be immediately removed from play, evaluated by a physician or other licensed medical provider with a rapid primary assessment followed by a more formal

secondary evaluation in the locker room. This evaluation includes a history and physical, symptom checklist, and cognitive functioning with the aid of sideline assessment tools if immediate transport to the hospital is not indicated (Figure 3.1).[4,6–8,13–17]

Primary assessment

Especially in the players that remain down after the injury or subsequently fall down after reaching the sidelines, a prompt and focused assessment of the athlete's level of consciousness, respiratory, and cardiac function is made upon initially approaching the athlete.[2,18] In general, if the person is communicative without any signs of respiratory distress (use of accessory respiratory muscles, rapid or shallow breaths, discoloration of the lips, etc.) they are likely producing adequate respirations. If the patient is unresponsive, then EMS should be contacted and a trained individual should begin Basic Life Support (BLS) or Advanced Cardiac Life Support (ACLS), which may entail placement of an advanced airway, based on the technical expertise of personnel and equipment present.[19,20] A review article by Jung et al. evaluated the literature on airway management in patients with suspected cervical spine instability. It was emphasized that standard techniques of mask ventilation and even intubation with manual in-line stabilization does cause significant cervical motion. Relevant for the emergency department setting, it was felt that the use of a nasal fiber optic bronchoscope had the least cervical motion, but was very technically challenging and time consuming. Therefore, if possible, one should consider video laryngoscope intubation in the concussed athlete with cervical spine concerns.[21] Whether on the field, within the ambulance, or the emergency department, the available equipment and training of the handler will determine the specific type of airway that is employed.

Medical personnel must also determine if there is concern for cervical spine instability following an injury.[6] Any direct blow to the head or body can cause an aggressive flexion, extension, or rotational force that can lead to cervical spine injury. If the athlete is functionally altered, with neck pain, or neurological symptoms (weakness or numbness to part of their body), spinal immobilization must be applied and EMS notified.[22–24]

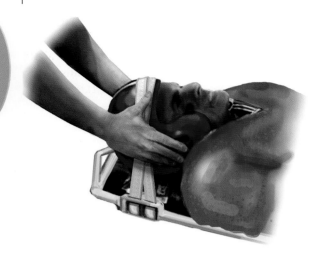

Figure 3.2 Spinal immobilization in an athlete where the helmet and shoulder pads are not able to be removed safely.

This may be initiated by manual in-line stabilization, cervical collar application, and followed by placement onto a hard backboard with the assistance of EMS personnel or athletic trainers. If there are sufficient personnel present to maintain manual cervical stabilization, the player's equipment, helmet and shoulder pads, should be removed.[25] In the scenario where there are not sufficient trained personnel present, cervical spine immobilization should be provided with the athletic gearing remaining in place, but the facemask should be removed to allow easy access to the athlete's airway (Figure 3.2).

Further need for immediate notification of EMS to transfer the patient to the nearest trauma facility should occur if the player has an abnormal neurological exam, seizure episode, or other pathological conditions that exceed the expertise of present personnel. If the player is neurologically intact without any of the above mentioned "red flags," requiring immediate transport to the hospital, the player should be moved to the locker room for the secondary assessment.[4,6,7,14,15,22,26]

Secondary assessment

Now that the athlete has been removed from the field of play, a more complex assessment for diagnosis including a history of the injury, thorough clinical exam, extent of subjective symptomatology, neurocognitive testing, and other adjunctive sideline tools such as postural assessment, reaction time, and oculomotor testing (King Devick occurs).[2,4,7,14,26–31] This detailed, multimodal, and systematic approach should be standardized for the initial assessment of all injured athletes and can be further used on follow-up appointments to measure recovery. Similarly, if the patient presents first to an outpatient clinic, this same thorough method of diagnosis and assessment should be undertaken.

History

A complete history should be obtained from the athlete including past medical/surgical history, current medications, the date of injury (if presenting first to outpatient clinic), specific mechanism of injury (head to head contact with other player, head striking against ground, etc.), amnesia/loss of consciousness, specific symptom onset/duration/type currently experiencing, and neurological issues. Specific attention should be directed towards demographics (age, gender), past medical history (ADHD, migraine, or psychiatric history), or concussion history (number, length of recovery, extent of symptoms, etc.) that allude to a potential prolonged recovery from concussion (to be further discussed in Chapter 5).[7,32–38] These details may be obtained from the athlete, but also from the assistance of the athletic trainer, coach, parent, or anyone else that witnessed the injury or was with the athlete following the injury.

Physical exam

A detailed neurological examination may cue the examiner in on specific clinical postconcussive findings but may also prompt further imaging to rule out a macroscopic injury, like intracranial hematoma.[4,5,7,14,26–29] It is imperative that the exam be repeated in a serial fashion in order to detect, early, any neurological deterioration, again prompting a more immediate escalation of care.[22] Please refer to Table 3.1 to provide a brief overview of the neurological clinical exam. Commonly, the general neurological exam is benign in a concussed patient. Lethargy, profound confusion, hemiparesis (weakness to one half of the body), or anisocoric pupils (unequal sizes) is due to a more serious condition of an expanding space occupying lesion and warrants emergency medical care (refer to Chapter 4).

Table 3.1 Basic Overview of the Neurological Exam Including Cranial Nerve, Motor Strength, and Sensory Examination Testing

Cranial Nerve Testing	Olfactory (1)	• Provides sense of smell • May test with coffee beans (clinic setting)
	Optic (2)	• Provides sight • Test with the Snellen chart (clinic setting) or have patient count fingers at a distance • Also use of fingers to test medial, lateral, superior, and inferior visual fields
	Oculomotor (3)	• Controls inferior oblique, superior rectus, and inferior rectus muscle of the eye • Test eye by instructing patient to look medially (Figure 3.3) • Carries parasympathetic nerves to ciliary ganglion in eye that causes constriction of pupil (pupillary sphincter). Look for equal and bilateral pupillary response to light • Also innervates the levator palpebrae superioris (raises eye brow)
	Trochlear (4)	• Controls superior oblique muscle of the eye • Test by instructing patient to look medially and downward (Figure 3.3)
	Trigeminal (5)	• Provides sensation (light touch, pain, temperature, and proprioception) to face in a forehead, midface, and mandibular distribution • Test by touching specific distribution on athlete's face (Figure 3.4) • Provides control of muscles of mastication • Test by instructing the patient to bite down and palpate contraction of masseter muscles • Also provides sensation to the intracranial dura mater
	Abducens (6)	• Controls lateral rectus muscle of the eye • Test by instructing the patient to look laterally Figure 3.3
	Facial (7)	• Controls muscles of facial expression • Observe symmetry of face at rest then instruct patient to close eyes and also smile (Figure 3.5) • Also provides sense of taste to anterior 2/3 of tongue and carries parasympathetic fibers to innervate the sublingual, submandibular, and lacrimal glands
	Vestibulocochlear (8)	• Provides balance and hearing • Evaluate by dedicated audiology testing (clinic setting) or by producing sound (rubbing fingers together) next to athlete's ear and asking to localize sound
	Glossopharyngeal (9) and vagus (10)	• Motor control of soft palate, pharynx, larynx • Test by inspecting posterior pharynx for a deviated uvula • Sense of taste over posterior portion of tongue and pharynx • Also carries parasympathetic fibers to innervate parotid gland (9) and thoracic and abdominal viscera (10) • Regulates blood pressure/heart rate through aortic and carotid receptors (9&10)
	Accessory (11)	• Motor control of trapezius and sternocleidomastoid muscle • Test muscle groups by having athlete shrug shoulders and turn head against resistance (Figure 3.6)
	Hypoglossal (12)	• Provides motor control to tongue • Tongue should be midline and not deviated when protruded by athlete

Motor		• In clinical practice, graded as:
		  • 0: no movement
		  • 1: twitch/contractility of muscle without movement of extremity
		  • 2: able to move extremity with gravity eliminated
		  • 3: able to move against gravity but not against any resistance
		  • 4: provides movement against some resistance, not full strength
		  • 5: full strength

(Continued)

Table 3.1 (Continued) Basic Overview of the Neurological Exam Including Cranial Nerve, Motor Strength, and Sensory Examination Testing

	• Commonly, an expanding intracranial mass causes contralateral hemiparesis (weakness in one's arm and leg), but this is very dependent on the location of the lesion
	• Details of specific myotomes for the spinal nerves will be deferred due to the nature of this book addressing concussive injuries only
Sensory	• All athletes should be tested for specific deficits in sensation especially in the presence of neck/back trauma, pain, or extremity weakness
	• Dermatomes and peripheral nerve sensory deficits will also be deferred as noted above

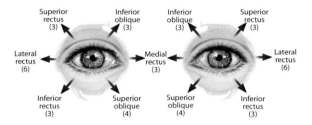

Figure 3.3 Ocular muscle motor testing of the Oculomotor (3), Trochlear (4), and Abducens (6) Nerve. Also, perform simple back and forth saccadic eye movements, the oculocephalic reflex (briefly turning the player's head with eyes maintaining fixed position), single and bilateral eye convergence, and monitor for nystagmus on lateral gaze.

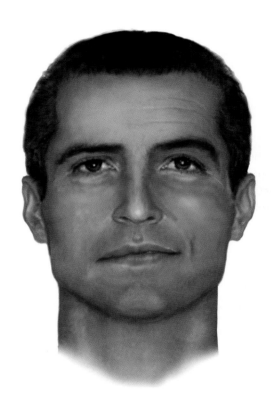

Figure 3.5 Facial Nerve (7) controls the muscles of facial expression. Complete or partial involvement of the face helps to identify the location of nerve injury one can appreciate right facial asymmetry of the mouth denoting a facial nerve injury.

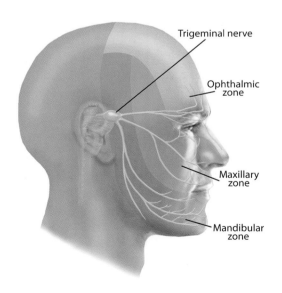

Figure 3.4 Main role of the Trigeminal Nerve (5) is to provide facial sensation to the forehead, maxillae, and mandible.

Symptoms

Following injury, medical personnel should assess the athlete for postconcussive symptoms and also what factors mitigate or exacerbate these symptoms. The symptoms of concussion are numerous and with low sensitivity and specificity, but particularly need to occur in relation to trauma

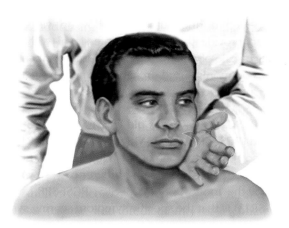
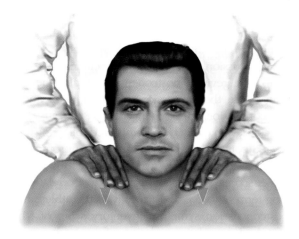

Figure 3.6 Testing of the Accessory Nerve (11) involves having the patient shrug their shoulders and turn their head against resistance (only perform if spinal cord injury has been ruled out).

(see Table 3.2 for a detailed listing).[5,23,26,39–46] Due to the heterogeneous nature of concussion, symptoms can be variable, vague, and overlap other medical issues making the diagnosis more challenging.[24] For example, an athlete may complain of headache, nausea, and vertigo, but this may be due to exertion or dehydration and not a concussive injury.[47] Therefore, careful assessment of traumatic exposure is required. Lastly, symptoms may not always present immediately following a concussion making the diagnosis more difficult and potentially delayed.[12,26] In a review of 48 concussions within a collegiate football and hockey cohort, only half had immediate symptoms following injury.[12]

The most common symptom of concussion is headache (in 60%–90% of athletes, more common in females), with the symptoms of headache, fatigue, lethargy, and sleep disturbance lasting the longest after injury.[45,48–56] On average, these symptoms typically resolve between 7 and 10 days, and only in a small minority do symptoms last longer than 1 month.[57]

Also, the extent and presence of specific symptoms acutely after injury have also been related to protracted recovery.[58] Post-traumatic migraine and the complaint of dizziness following a concussive injury have been related to a two- and sixfold risk, respectively, of protracted recovery and reduced performance on neurocognitive testing 1–2 weeks from injury.[59–62]

Symptom checklists

Symptom checklists are a written list of subjective complaints that require the athlete to select which symptoms they are currently experiencing. The initial symptom checklist developed was the Pittsburgh

Table 3.2 The Many Symptoms of Concussion

Somatic	• Headache
	• Balance difficulties/dizziness/vertigo/ataxia
	• Nausea/vomiting
	• Light and sound sensitivity
	• Tinnitus
	• Double or blurred vision
	• Seizures
	• Loss of consciousness
Cognitive	• Slowed reaction time and mentation
	• Amnesia of event or surrounding event
	• Feeling "in a fog"/groggy/sluggish
	• Concentration difficulties
	• Memory difficulties
	• Anterograde/retrograde amnesia (usually improves within hours)
	• Disorientation/confusion
Affective	• Irritability
	• Emotional lability
	• Personality changes
	• Anxiety
	• Depression
	• Eating disturbances
Sleep-related	• Sleep difficulties
	• Insomnia
	• Fatigue/drowsiness

◆ Neck examination:
  ◇ Flags examiner to potential cervical spine pathology through extremity strength/sensory examination, range of motion, and evaluation of neck pain upon palpation.
◆ Balance Error Scoring System (BESS):
  ◇ A total score is determined by the number of errors performed by the athlete while attempting to balance on a flat surface or foam pad with both legs, one leg, and then tandem stance.[82]
  ◇ Added to the SCAT score because early balance deficits seen immediately following injury that may persist up to 1 week, even in the absence of neuropsychological testing abnormalities.[83,84]
  ◇ 24%–37% of concussed athletes have balance deficits at 24 h and 20%–24% by 48 h.[45]
  ◇ It is important to be aware that the BESS has been found to have mild practice effects (where improved test performance occurs simply by learning from repetitive testing) and therefore, results should be scrutinized if repeated use has been employed (Figure 3.9).[81,85]
◆ Upper extremity coordination:
  ◇ This is tested by having the athlete touch their nose with their index finger and then touching your index finger repeatedly back and forth for five times.
  ◇ It is important to always use the same arm in baseline and post concussive testing due to effects of hand dominance within the athlete.[86]
  See Figure 3.8.

Acute concussion evaluation (ACE): The ACE was released by the Centers for Disease Control and Prevention (Figure 3.10).[87,88] This is a more limited assessment in comparison to the SCAT, that encompasses a description of the event of the concussion, a symptom checklist, recognition of possible red flags to seek further evaluation, and also potential risk factors for prolonged recovery. The ACE questions can be asked of the athlete or parent, and also has the ability to be delivered in an interview format over the phone.

Military acute concussion evaluation (MACE): For completeness of discussion, the MACE has also been used in the acute evaluation of concussion, but as the name implies, strictly within the military population.[68,89] This assessment modality is composed of obtaining a history of the event including important features of loss of consciousness and amnesia, the SAC, and a "yes/no" symptom checklist.

Adjunctive sideline tools

Due to the ease of administration, reproducibility, and low cost of equipment, these tests have already made an appearance on the sidelines/locker room and outpatient clinic in high school, collegiate, and professional levels. Due to the more recent development, there is limited but strong evidence for the addition of reaction time and ocular testing (King Devick) in the acute assessment of the concussed athlete that was even recognized by the Zurich Guidelines in 2012.[6] These adjunctive tools will likely appear as a standard in further editions of the SCAT.

Reaction time   The testing of an athlete's reaction time is a very efficient and inexpensive acute assessment tool that can be repeated to measure player recovery after injury. Reaction time can be evaluated by simple bedside measures (see Figure 3.11)[90] but also through the use of computerized testing. This validated measure has not only shown strong sensitivity early after injury <24 h in 40%–70% of athletes, it also has good testing reliability, and was not affected by exercise.[45,66,90–94] Moreover, this testing identified athletes with persistent delayed reaction time even after resolution of concussion symptoms.[45,66,90–95] Similar to all sideline assessment tools, baseline testing is important to obtain and also the specific test should always be repeated and not changed in order for comparison.[96]

King Devick   The King Devick tool (KD) is a sideline tool that can also be used in the outpatient/rehabilitation phase to assess saccadic eye movements. This test requires the athlete to read a series of single digit numbers from multiple cards in the span of 2 min. A score is obtained based on the number of errors and time to completion (Figure 3.12).[97] Changes in the KD have been associated with reduced scores in neuropsychological testing and sideline tests, but the reliability and validity have demonstrated a range of results.[97–102]

SCAT3™

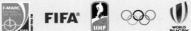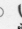

Sport Concussion Assessment Tool – 3rd edition

For use by medical professionals only

Name: _____   Date / Time of Injury: _____   Examiner: _____

Date of Assessment: _____

What is the SCAT3?[1]

The SCAT3 is a standardized tool for evaluating injured athletes for concussion and can be used in athletes aged from 13 years and older. It supersedes the original SCAT and the SCAT2 published in 2005 and 2009, respectively[2]. For younger persons, ages 12 and under, please use the Child SCAT3. The SCAT3 is designed for use by medical professionals. If you are not qualified, please use the Sport Concussion Recognition Tool[1]. Preseason baseline testing with the SCAT3 can be helpful for interpreting post-injury test scores.

Specific instructions for use of the SCAT3 are provided on page 3. If you are not familiar with the SCAT3, please read through these instructions carefully. This tool may be freely copied in its current form for distribution to individuals, teams, groups and organizations. Any revision or any reproduction in a digital form requires approval by the Concussion in Sport Group.
NOTE: The diagnosis of a concussion is a clinical judgment, ideally made by a medical professional. The SCAT3 should not be used solely to make, or exclude, the diagnosis of concussion in the absence of clinical judgement. An athlete may have a concussion even if their SCAT3 is "normal".

What is a concussion?

A concussion is a disturbance in brain function caused by a direct or indirect force to the head. It results in a variety of non-specific signs and / or symptoms (some examples listed below) and most often does not involve loss of consciousness. Concussion should be suspected in the presence of any one or more of the following:

- Symptoms (e.g., headache), or
- Physical signs (e.g., unsteadiness), or
- Impaired brain function (e.g. confusion) or
- Abnormal behaviour (e.g., change in personality).

SIDELINE ASSESSMENT

Indications for Emergency Management

NOTE: A hit to the head can sometimes be associated with a more serious brain injury. Any of the following warrants consideration of activating emergency procedures and urgent transportation to the nearest hospital:

- Glasgow Coma score less than 15
- Deteriorating mental status
- Potential spinal injury
- Progressive, worsening symptoms or new neurologic signs

Potential signs of concussion?

If any of the following signs are observed after a direct or indirect blow to the head, the athlete should stop participation, be evaluated by a medical professional and **should not be permitted to return to sport the same day** if a concussion is suspected.

Any loss of consciousness?	Y	N
"If so, how long?"		
Balance or motor incoordination (stumbles, slow / laboured movements, etc.)?	Y	N
Disorientation or confusion (inability to respond appropriately to questions)?	Y	N
Loss of memory:	Y	N
"If so, how long?"		
"Before or after the injury?"		
Blank or vacant look:	Y	N
Visible facial injury in combination with any of the above:	Y	N

1 Glasgow Coma Scale (GCS)

Best eye response (E)

No eye opening	1
Eye opening in response to pain	2
Eye opening to speech	3
Eyes opening spontaneously	4

Best verbal response (V)

No verbal response	1
Incomprehensible sounds	2
Inappropriate words	3
Confused	4
Oriented	5

Best motor response (M)

No motor response	1
Extension to pain	2
Abnormal flexion to pain	3
Flexion / Withdrawal to pain	4
Localizes to pain	5
Obeys commands	6

Glasgow Coma score (E + V + M) — of 15

GCS should be recorded for all athletes in case of subsequent deterioration.

2 Maddocks Score[3]

"I am going to ask you a few questions, please listen carefully and give your best effort."

Modified Maddocks questions (1 point for each correct answer)

What venue are we at today?	0	1
Which half is it now?	0	1
Who scored last in this match?	0	1
What team did you play last week / game?	0	1
Did your team win the last game?	0	1

Maddocks Score — of 5

Maddocks score is validated for sideline diagnosis of concussion only and is not used for serial testing.

Notes: Mechanism of injury ("Tell me what happened"?):

Any athlete with a suspected concussion should be REMOVED FROM PLAY, medically assessed, monitored for deterioration (i.e., should not be left alone) and should not drive a motor vehicle until cleared to do so by a medical professional. No athlete diagnosed with concussion should be returned to sports participation on the day of injury.

(a)

Figure 3.8   Sideline Concussion Assessment Tool.   *(Continued)*

BACKGROUND

Name: _____   Date: _____

Examiner: _____

Sport / team / school: _____   Date / time of injury: _____

Age: _____   Gender: ☐ M   ☐ F

Years of education completed: _____

Dominant hand: ☐ right   ☐ left   ☐ neither

How many concussions do you think you have had in the past? _____

When was the most recent concussion? _____

How long was your recovery from the most recent concussion? _____

Have you ever been hospitalized or had medical imaging done for a head injury?   ☐ Y   ☐ N

Have you ever been diagnosed with headaches or migraines?   ☐ Y   ☐ N

Do you have a learning disability, dyslexia, ADD / ADHD?   ☐ Y   ☐ N

Have you ever been diagnosed with depression, anxiety or other psychiatric disorder?   ☐ Y   ☐ N

Has anyone in your family ever been diagnosed with any of these problems?   ☐ Y   ☐ N

Are you on any medications? If yes, please list: ☐ Y   ☐ N

SCAT3 to be done in resting state. Best done 10 or more minutes post exercise.

3 How do you feel?

"You should score yourself on the following symptoms, based on how you feel now".

	none	mild		moderate		severe	
Headache	0	1	2	3	4	5	6
"Pressure in head"	0	1	2	3	4	5	6
Neck pain	0	1	2	3	4	5	6
Nausea or vomiting	0	1	2	3	4	5	6
Dizziness	0	1	2	3	4	5	6
Blurred vision	0	1	2	3	4	5	6
Balance problems	0	1	2	3	4	5	6
Sensitivity to light	0	1	2	3	4	5	6
Sensitivity to noise	0	1	2	3	4	5	6
Feeling slowed down	0	1	2	3	4	5	6
Feeling like "in a fog"	0	1	2	3	4	5	6
"Don't feel right"	0	1	2	3	4	5	6
Difficulty concentrating	0	1	2	3	4	5	6
Difficulty remembering	0	1	2	3	4	5	6
Fatigue or low energy	0	1	2	3	4	5	6
Confusion	0	1	2	3	4	5	6
Drowsiness	0	1	2	3	4	5	6
Trouble falling asleep	0	1	2	3	4	5	6
More emotional	0	1	2	3	4	5	6
Irritability	0	1	2	3	4	5	6
Sadness	0	1	2	3	4	5	6
Nervous or anxious	0	1	2	3	4	5	6

Total number of symptoms (Maximum possible 22) ☐

Symptom severity score (Maximum possible 132) ☐

Do the symptoms get worse with physical activity?   ☐ Y   ☐ N

Do the symptoms get worse with mental activity?   ☐ Y   ☐ N

☐ self rated   ☐ self rated and clinician monitored

☐ clinician interview   ☐ self rated with parent input

Overall rating: If you know the athlete well prior to the injury, how different is the athlete acting compared to his / her usual self? Please circle one response:

no different   very different   unsure   N/A

Scoring on the SCAT3 should not be used as a stand-alone method to diagnose concussion, measure recovery or make decisions about an athlete's readiness to return to competition after concussion. Since signs and symptoms may evolve over time, it is important to consider repeat evaluation in the acute assessment of concussion.

4 Cognitive assessment

Standardized Assessment of Concussion (SAC)[4]

Orientation (1 point for each correct answer)

What month is it?	0	1
What is the date today?	0	1
What is the day of the week?	0	1
What year is it?	0	1
What time is it right now? (within 1 hour)	0	1

Orientation score   of 5

Immediate memory

List	Trial 1		Trial 2		Trial 3		Alternative word list		
elbow	0	1	0	1	0	1	candle	baby	finger
apple	0	1	0	1	0	1	paper	monkey	penny
carpet	0	1	0	1	0	1	sugar	perfume	blanket
saddle	0	1	0	1	0	1	sandwich	sunset	lemon
bubble	0	1	0	1	0	1	wagon	iron	insect
Total									

Immediate memory score total   of 15

Concentration: Digits Backward

List	Trial 1		Alternative digit list		
4-9-3	0	1	6-2-9	5-2-6	4-1-5
3-8-1-4	0	1	3-2-7-9	1-7-9-5	4-9-6-8
6-2-9-7-1	0	1	1-5-2-8-6	3-8-5-2-7	6-1-8-4-3
7-1-8-4-6-2	0	1	5-3-9-1-4-8	8-3-1-9-6-4	7-2-4-8-5-6
Total					

Concentration: **Month in Reverse Order** (1 pt. for entire sequence correct)

Dec-Nov-Oct-Sept-Aug-Jul-Jun-May-Apr-Mar-Feb-Jan   0   1

Concentration score   of 5

5 Neck examination

Range of motion   Tenderness   Upper and lower limb sensation & strength

Findings:

6 Balance examination

Do one or both of the following tests.
Footwear (shoes, barefoot, braces, tape, etc.)

Modified Balance Error Scoring System (BESS) testing[5]
Which foot was tested (i.e. which is the non-dominant foot)   ☐ L   ☐ R
Testing surface (hard floor, field, etc.)
Condition

Double leg stance:	Errors
Single leg stance (non-dominant foot):	Errors
Tandem stance (non-dominant foot at back):	Errors

And / Or

Tandem gait[6,7]
Time (best of 4 trials):

7 Coordination examination

Upper limb coordination
Which arm was tested: ☐ L   ☐ R

Coordination score   of 1

8 SAC Delayed Recall[4]

Delayed recall score   of 5

(b)

Figure 3.8 (Continued) Sideline Concussion Assessment Tool. (*From Br J Sports Med.* Apr;47(5):259, 2013. With permission of BMJ Publishing Group Limited.)

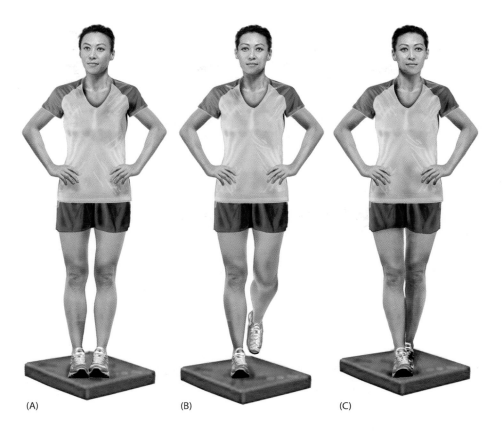

Figure 3.9 **Balance Error Scoring System (BESS).** The athlete is instructed to stand with (A) both legs together, (B) with one leg, and (C) in tandem. This may be performed on the flat ground or foam pad. Keep the footwear similar (cleats, tennis shoes, etc.) consistent between baseline and post concussive balance testing.[85]

Incorporation of this short, easy to administer test of ocular motility may improve the accuracy of concussion diagnostic sideline tests.[97,103]

Testing accuracy

Diagnostic accuracy of a disease is only as good as the tool used to make the diagnosis. Therefore, all possible means should be made in order to remove any such confounders or variables that could hurt its accuracy. For example, the assumption that all players are "asymptomatic" at baseline, prior to injury, is false. In a review of 260 Canadian collegiate athletes with and without a history of concussion, only 41.2% were found to be asymptomatic at baseline, and actually the overall average number of symptoms was 5![104] This emphasizes the fact that the symptom checklists can be nonspecific. For example, an athlete on any given day may report having headache or forgetfulness, without ever having a concussion. Therefore, the results

of these tools are best interpreted when the athlete's baseline testing is known. Moreover, as an athlete recovers from a concussion, it is improper and misleading for the provider to assume that all players will return to being asymptomatic without knowing their baseline prior to injury.

In a 2014 survey of athletic trainers, 75% performed baseline testing through the use of computer neurocognitive tests (71%), balance assessments (9%), or symptom scales (11%).[105] Not only is baseline testing important for neurocognitive testing, but also in all sideline measures to improve diagnostic accuracy and better monitor recovery. Therefore, all athletes should receive annual baseline testing using the different sideline assessment tools (SCAT, symptom checklist, neurocognitive testing, reaction time, etc.) that is standardized for that specific school university, for concussion diagnosis.[4,24,106]

Similarly, others have suggested the use of retrospective testing, when baseline testing is

ACUTE CONCUSSION EVALUATION (ACE)
PHYSICIAN/CLINICIAN OFFICE VERSION

Gerard Gioia, PhD[1] & Micky Collins, PhD[2]
[1]Children's National Medical Center
[2]University of Pittsburgh Medical Center

Patient Name:_____
DOB:_____ Age:_____
Date:_____ ID/MR#_____

A. Injury Characteristics Date/Time of Injury_____ Reporter: __Patient __Parent __Spouse __Other_____

1. Injury Description _____

_____

1a. Is there evidence of a forcible blow to the head (direct or indirect)? __Yes __No __Unknown
1b. Is there evidence of intracranial injury or skull fracture? __Yes __No __Unknown
1c. Location of Impact: __Frontal __Lft Temporal __Rt Temporal __Lft Parietal __Rt Parietal __Occipital __Neck __Indirect Force
2. Cause: __MVC __Pedestrian-MVC __Fall __Assault __Sports (specify)_____Other_____
3. Amnesia Before (Retrograde) Are there any events just BEFORE the injury that you/ person has no memory of (even brief)? __Yes __No Duration
4. Amnesia After (Anterograde) Are there any events just AFTER the injury that you/ person has no memory of (even brief)? __Yes __No Duration
5. Loss of Consciousness: Did you/ person lose consciousness? __Yes __No Duration
6. EARLY SIGNS: __Appears dazed or stunned __Is confused about events __Answers questions slowly __Repeats Questions __Forgetful (recent info)
7. Seizures: Were seizures observed? No__ Yes___ Detail_____

B. Symptom Check List* Since the injury, has the person experienced <u>any</u> of these symptoms any <u>more than usual</u> today or in the past day?
Indicate presence of each symptom (0=No, 1=Yes). *Lovell & Collins, 1998 JHTR*

PHYSICAL (10)			COGNITIVE (4)			SLEEP (4)			
Headache	0	1	Feeling mentally foggy	0	1	Drowsiness	0	1	
Nausea	0	1	Feeling slowed down	0	1	Sleeping less than usual	0	1	N/A
Vomiting	0	1	Difficulty concentrating	0	1	Sleeping more than usual	0	1	N/A
Balance problems	0	1	Difficulty remembering	0	1	Trouble falling asleep	0	1	N/A
Dizziness	0	1	COGNITIVE Total (0-4) _____			SLEEP Total (0-4) _____			
Visual problems	0	1	EMOTIONAL (4)						
Fatigue	0	1	Irritability	0	1	**Exertion:** Do these symptoms <u>worsen</u> with:			
Sensitivity to light	0	1	Sadness	0	1	Physical Activity __Yes __No __N/A			
Sensitivity to noise	0	1	More emotional	0	1	Cognitive Activity __Yes __No __N/A			
Numbness/Tingling	0	1	Nervousness	0	1	**Overall Rating:** How <u>different</u> is the person acting			
PHYSICAL Total (0-10) _____			EMOTIONAL Total (0-4) _____			compared to his/her usual self? (circle)			
(Add Physical, Cognitive, Emotion, Sleep totals) Total Symptom Score (0-22) _____						Normal 0 1 2 3 4 5 6 Very Different			

C. Risk Factors for Protracted Recovery (check all that apply)

Concussion History? Y ___ N___	√	Headache History? Y ___ N___	√	Developmental History	√	Psychiatric History
Previous # 1 2 3 4 5 6+		Prior treatment for headache		Learning disabilities		Anxiety
Longest symptom duration Days__ Weeks__ Months__ Years__		History of migraine headache __ Personal __ Family_____		Attention-Deficit/ Hyperactivity Disorder		Depression
						Sleep disorder
If multiple concussions, less force caused reinjury? Yes__ No__		_____		Other developmental disorder_____		Other psychiatric disorder _____

List other comorbid medical disorders or medication usage (e.g., hypothyroid, seizures)_____

_____

D. RED FLAGS for acute emergency management: Refer to the emergency department with <u>sudden onset</u> of any of the following:

* Headaches that worsen	* Looks very drowsy/ can't be awakened	* Can't recognize people or places	* Neck pain
* Seizures	* Repeated vomiting	* Increasing confusion or irritability	* Unusual behavioral change
* Focal neurologic signs	* Slurred speech	* Weakness or numbness in arms/legs	* Change in state of consciousness

E. Diagnosis (ICD): __Concussion w/o LOC 850.0 __Concussion w/ LOC 850.1 __Concussion (Unspecified) 850.9 __Other (854) _____
__No diagnosis

F. Follow-Up Action Plan Complete *ACE Care Plan* and provide copy to patient/family.
___ No Follow-Up Needed
___ **Physician/Clinician Office Monitoring**: Date of next follow-up _____
___ **Referral:**
___ Neuropsychological Testing
___ Physician: Neurosurgery____ Neurology____ Sports Medicine____ Physiatrist____ Psychiatrist____ Other_____
___ Emergency Department

ACE Completed by:_____ **MD RN NP PhD ATC** © Copyright G. Gioia & M. Collins, 2006

This form is part of the "Heads Up: Brain Injury in Your Practice" tool kit developed by the Centers for Disease Control and Prevention (CDC).

(a)

Figure 3.10 Acute concussion assessment. *(Continued)*

A concussion (or mild traumatic brain injury (MTBI)) is a complex pathophysiologic process affecting the brain, induced by traumatic biomechanical forces secondary to direct or indirect forces to the head. Disturbance of brain function is related to neurometabolic dysfunction, rather than structural injury, and is typically associated with normal structural neuroimaging findings (i.e., CT scan, MRI). Concussion may or may not involve a loss of consciousness (LOC). Concussion results in a constellation of physical, cognitive, emotional, and sleep-related symptoms. Symptoms may last from several minutes to days, weeks, months or even longer in some cases.

ACE Instructions

The ACE is intended to provide an evidence-based clinical protocol to conduct an initial evaluation and diagnosis of patients (both children and adults) with known or suspected MTBI. The research evidence documenting the importance of these components in the evaluation of an MTBI is provided in the reference list.

A. Injury Characteristics:

1. Obtain **description of the injury** – how injury occurred, type of force, location on the head or body (if force transmitted to head). Different biomechanics of injury may result in differential symptom patterns (e.g., occipital blow may result in visual changes, balance difficulties).

2. Indicate the **cause of injury**. Greater forces associated with the trauma are likely to result in more severe presentation of symptoms.

3/4. **Amnesia:** Amnesia is defined as the failure to form new memories. Determine whether amnesia has occurred and attempt to determine length of time of memory dysfunction – before (retrograde) and after (anterograde) injury. Even seconds to minutes of memory loss can be predictive of outcome. Recent research has indicated that amnesia may be up to 4-10 times more predictive of symptoms and cognitive deficits following concussion than is LOC (less than 1 minute).[1]

5. **Loss of consciousness (LOC)** – If occurs, determine length of LOC.

6. **Early signs.** If present, ask the individuals who know the patient (parent, spouse, friend, etc) about specific signs of the concussion that may have been observed. These signs are typically observed early after the injury.

7. Inquire whether **seizures** were observed or not.

B. Symptom Checklist: [2]

1. Ask patient (and/or parent, if child) to report presence of the four categories of symptoms since injury. It is important to assess all listed symptoms as different parts of the brain control different functions. One or all symptoms may be present depending upon mechanisms of injury.[3] Record "1" for Yes or "0" for No for their presence or absence, respectively.

2. For all symptoms, indicate presence (as experienced within the past 24 hours. Since symptoms can be present premorbidly/at baseline (e.g., inattention, headaches, sleep, sadness), it is important to assess change from their usual presentation.

3. **Scoring:** Sum total number of symptoms present per area, and sum all four areas into Total Symptom Score (score range 0-22). (Note: most sleep symptoms are only applicable after a night has passed since the injury. Drowsiness may be present on the day of injury.) If symptoms are new and present, there is no lower limit symptom score. Any score > 0 indicates positive symptom history.

4. **Exertion:** Inquire whether any symptoms worsen with physical (e.g., running, climbing stairs, bike riding) and/or cognitive (e.g., academic studies, multi-tasking at work, reading or other tasks requiring focused concentration) exertion. Clinicians should be aware that symptoms will typically worsen or re-emerge with exertion, indicating incomplete recovery. Over-exertion may protract recovery.

5. **Overall Rating:** Determine how different the person is acting from their usual self. Circle "0" (Normal) to "6" (Very Different).

C. Risk Factors for Protracted Recovery: Assess the following risk factors as possible complicating factors in the recovery process.

1. **Concussion history:** Assess the number and date(s) of prior concussions, the duration of symptoms for each injury, and whether less biomechanical force resulted in re-injury. Research indicates that cognitive and symptom effects of concussion may be cumulative, especially if there is minimal duration of time between injuries and less biomechanical force results in subsequent concussion (which may indicate incomplete recovery from initial trauma).[4-8]

2. **Headache history:** Assess personal and/or family history of diagnosis/treatment for headaches. Research indicates headache (migraine in particular) can result in protracted recovery from concussion.[8-11]

3. **Developmental history:** Assess history of learning disabilities, Attention-Deficit/Hyperactivity Disorder or other developmental disorders. Research indicates that there is the possibility of a longer period of recovery with these conditions.[12]

4. **Psychiatric history:** Assess for history of depression/mood disorder, anxiety, and/or sleep disorder.[13-16]

D. Red Flags: The patient should be carefully observed over the first 24-48 hours for these serious signs. Red flags are to be assessed as possible signs of deteriorating neurological functioning. Any positive report should prompt strong consideration of referral for emergency medical evaluation (e.g. CT Scan to rule out intracranial bleed or other structural pathology).[17]

E. Diagnosis: The following ICD diagnostic codes may be applicable.

850.0 (Concussion, with no loss of consciousness) – Positive injury description with evidence of forcible direct/ indirect blow to the head (A1a); plus evidence of active symptoms (B) of any type and number related to the trauma (Total Symptom Score >0); no evidence of LOC (A5), skull fracture or intracranial injury (A1b).

850.1 (Concussion, with brief loss of consciousness < 1 hour) – Positive injury description with evidence of forcible direct/ indirect blow to the head (A1a); plus evidence of active symptoms (B) of any type and number related to the trauma (Total Symptom Score >0); positive evidence of LOC (A5), skull fracture or intracranial injury (A1b).

850.9 (Concussion, unspecified) – Positive injury description with evidence of forcible direct/ indirect blow to the head (A1a); plus evidence of active symptoms (B) of any type and number related to the trauma (Total Symptom Score >0); unclear/unknown injury details; unclear evidence of LOC (A5), no skull fracture or intracranial injury.

Other Diagnoses – If the patient presents with a positive injury description and associated symptoms, but additional evidence of intracranial injury (A 1b) such as from neuroimaging, a moderate TBI and the diagnostic category of 854 (Intracranial injury) should be considered.

F. Follow-Up Action Plan: Develop a follow-up plan of action for symptomatic patients. The physician/clinician may decide to (1) monitor the patient in the office or (2) refer them to a specialist. Serial evaluation of the concussion is critical as symptoms may resolve, worsen, or ebb and flow depending upon many factors (e.g., cognitive/physical exertion, comorbidities). Referral to a specialist can be particularly valuable to help manage certain aspects of the patient's condition. (Physician/Clinician should also complete the ACE Care Plan included in this tool kit.)

1. **Physician/Clinician serial monitoring** – Particularly appropriate if number and severity of symptoms are steadily decreasing over time and/or fully resolve within 3-5 days. If steady reduction is not evident, referral to a specialist is warranted.

2. **Referral to a specialist** – Appropriate if symptom reduction is not evident in 3-5 days, or sooner if symptom profile is concerning in type/severity.
   - Neuropsychological Testing can provide valuable information to help assess a patient's brain function and impairment and assist with treatment planning, such as return to play decisions.
   - Physician Evaluation is particularly relevant for medical evaluation and management of concussion. It is also critical for evaluating and managing focal neurologic, sensory, vestibular, and motor concerns. It may be useful for medication management (e.g., headaches, sleep disturbance, depression) if post-concussive problems persist.

(b)

Figure 3.10 (Continued) Acute concussion assessment.

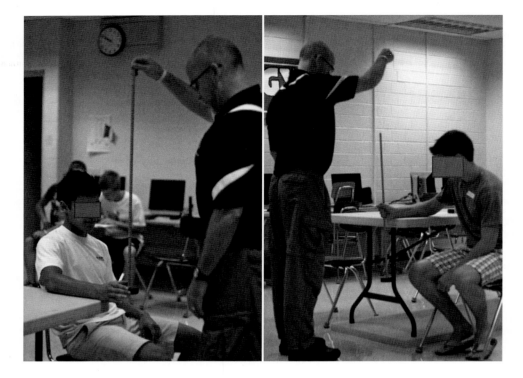

Figure 3.11 **Bedside clinical assessment of reaction time.** (From MacDonald J et al. *Clinical Journal of Sport Medicine.* Jan;25(1):43–8, 2015.)

not available, where the athlete is completing the assessment after the injury, but is requested to reflect upon their symptoms prior to the injury. This retrospective baseline testing is fraught with errors due to bias and therefore must be used cautiously. One such bias, termed "good-old-days bias" is where the athlete inaccurately reflects back to their preinjury symptomatology burden as being less than what it really was.[107]

There are also multiple environmental factors that need to be taken into account in order to improve testing accuracy. It is important that all testing, baseline and post injury, occur in a similar environment and format.[4,108] Obtaining baseline and postinjury assessments with the player away from the field and in the locker room or athletic trainer's office will help to eliminate any external distractions on the athlete. This is especially important following an injury in order to prevent influence on the athlete's symptom reporting by external pressures from coaches, fellow teammates, or parents.[33] Secondly, the tests should always be administered in the same manner. For

example, Meehan et al. performed a study among 73 healthy undergraduate students and noted a change in reported symptoms whether the material was obtained in a checklist or interview format.[63]

Last, as emphasized in the discussion of symptom checklists, it is also important to note that evaluation immediately following exercise can influence testing results.[33,109] Therefore, all assessments should similarly not be obtained immediately following exertion.

Acute management of the concussed player

Once it has been determined that the player has sustained a concussion, what is the next step? The most important initial step for any player who is diagnosed with a concussion based on the multimodal approach described above is, to be removed from play immediately and not allowed to return to activity until a graded "return to play" algorithm has been completed.[4,6,7,14,15,66,89,110–114] This includes all athletic activities (games and/or practices)

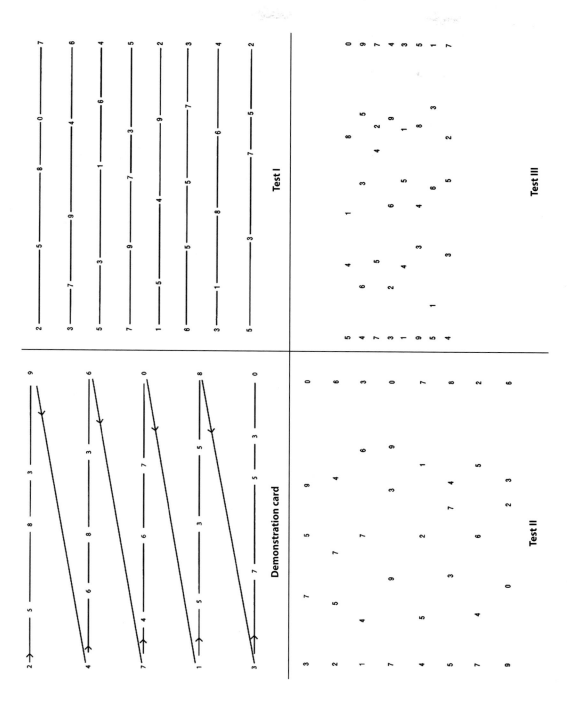

Figure 3.12 King Devick test. (Reproduced from Leong DF et al. *Journal of Optometry* Apr–Jun;8(2):131–9, 2015. CC BY-NC-ND 4.0. http://creativecommons.org/licenses /by-nc-nd/4.0/.)

and has become the standard in all professional athletic leagues, the NCAA, and the National Federation of State High Schools.[24] Further discussed in Chapter 8, the typical adult athlete potentially can return to play as early as 1 week from injury pending clearance from a medical professional, while the child athlete requires a more conservative approach with a minimum return of at least 2 weeks. These current recommendations are a drastic change to the previous guidelines, which allowed players to return to the same competition if their symptoms resolved within 20 min, or if the symptoms were not provoked with exertion.[22,115,116] Now with a greater understanding of the pathophysiology of concussion (Chapter 2),[66,117–124] the known increased concussion risk acutely following injury,[125] the acute harmful effects of repeat concussion on the healing brain (Chapter 8),[126–134] postconcussion syndrome (Chapter 5),[135–137] the growing case reports of second impact syndrome (Chapter 4),[138–143] and the potential long-term risk of Chronic Traumatic Encephalopathy (Chapter 10),[144–167] athletes are to return to play *only* after a graded rehabilitation and medical clearance by a physician (i.e., the return to play protocol).

Second, what determines when the athlete requires transportation to the local hospital for further evaluation? As mentioned, the obvious scenarios, that require an escalation of care is when the player either immediately or after repeat neurological assessments, develops neurological deficits, a change in mental status (obtunded, confused, disoriented, etc.), traumatic seizures, or respiratory/cardiovascular difficulties. This is why continued neurological reassessment is required in all athletes following concussion, as there is always a potential for development of abrupt changes in neurological status in those with intracranial lesions like hematomas. Further, after completion of sideline assessments in athletes that do not develop the previous "red flags," those with severe or worsening symptoms, significant trauma, prolonged loss of consciousness, or prolonged post-traumatic amnesia should also be transported for evaluation in the emergency department of the local hospital.[4,24,111,115,168–170] Also, escalation may be warranted if the care of the athlete exceeds the available equipment on hand and expertise of personnel available.

This may include even the "On-field Secondary Assessment" if there are no medical providers present experienced with administering the SCAT or other sideline assessment tools. The only athletes that potentially could be sent home directly with close monitoring are those subjected to only a mild impact and with near to complete resolution of symptoms. It is imperative that athletes have a reliable caregiver that will be able to monitor them while at home.

Concussion in the emergency department

The emergency department evaluation

In concordance with the most recent Zurich guidelines, the emergency department evaluation should include "a medical assessment, including a comprehensive history and detailed neurological examination with a thorough assessment of mental status, cognitive functioning, gait, and balance" and "a determination of the clinical status of the patient, including whether there has been improvement or deterioration since the time of injury."[5] This assessment is purposefully very similar in appearance to the on-field secondary assessment in order to evaluate the athlete for any clinical changes as they progress in time from the initial injury. For this reason, prior communication between the school and referring hospital system should occur in order to standardize the postconcussive assessment of the athlete. This can easily be done through obtaining the SCAT postinjury and again in the emergency department. Use of an identical tool improves transfer of information regarding the patient's symptoms and neurocognitive status between the different medical provider encounters. Therefore, use of the same standardized on-field, emergency department, and even outpatient multimodal postconcussive assessment provides the provider with a thorough and fluid representation of the athlete's recovery or progressive decline following concussion.

Concussion neuroimaging in the emergency department

Though dated regarding its use of the generic term "structural," the Zurich guidelines emphasizes the role of the emergency department in determining the need for "emergent neuroimaging in order to exclude a more severe brain injury involving a structural abnormality."[5] Though macrostructural pathology is uncommon in concussions, it still can occur and therefore must be ruled out in a subset of patients. These abnormalities include subdural hemorrhage, epidural hemorrhage, traumatic subarachnoid hemorrhage, and diffuse cerebral edema (see Chapter 4). The best imaging choice, taking into account speed of acquisition, to assess intracranial blood products is CT imaging.[23,171] In recent years, there has been a greater effort to reduce radiation exposure, especially in the pediatric population through the use of MR imaging. Available at some institutions is a rapid MRI sequence ("HASTE") that allows image acquisition in less than 5 min and is more sensitive for intraparenchymal lesions.[172–174] This may be considered if the pediatric patient warrants cranial imaging and if this technology is available without any delay in care. As will be discussed in Chapter 9, further advanced neuroimaging techniques have demonstrated their ability to evaluate in vivo microstructural injury, but these types of imaging modalities are highly technical, currently only in the preclinical stage, and therefore not recommended in the acute phase.[175–204]

Retrospective reviews have demonstrated varying prevalence for positive CT head findings in concussed patients more importantly, but only with 0%–1% actually requiring surgical intervention.[205–217] One such study found that abnormal CT head findings were found in 5% versus 30% if the presenting GCS was either 15 or 13, respectively.[208] Therefore, even asymptomatic patients have the potential to possess intracranial blood products, but the likelihood for this changing current management is rather small.[23] For this reason, there have been numerous published guidelines giving recommendations for when to obtain imaging in the concussed patient in efforts to minimize unnecessary scans. Due to the concern for increased risk of future malignancies with repetitive exposure to radiation from various imaging modalities, specifically in the pediatric population, there is an attempt to develop a highly specific and sensitive algorithm through the details of the injury, symptomatology, and clinical findings, that selects the patients most likely to have intracranial

pathology. Consistent criteria throughout these guidelines are that cranial imaging is required in patients with an abnormal neurological exam and should also be considered in those with progressive worsening of symptoms or prolonged loss of consciousness.[210,211] Please refer to Table 3.3 for further discussion of these various guidelines. One may consider not obtaining imaging if the patient is clinically normal (asymptomatic with normal neurological exam), is not elderly or pediatric age, and has no concerning medical history making the patient prone to hemorrhage (antiplatelet or anticoagulation use).[8,23]

Disposition from the emergency department

Following completion of the clinical evaluation, disposition of the athlete is to be determined. Similar to the on-field assessment, all athletes should be monitored for a few hours following concussion to monitor for symptom exacerbation or changes in neurological exam.[24,212] If they have a normal neurological exam, minimal to no symptoms, and a negative head CT (if obtained), consideration for discharge home is conceivable.[23] Interestingly, a study in concussed patients cleared for discharge from the ED were either randomized for overnight admission versus discharge home. Those that received overnight observation were shown to have no difference in long-term outcomes, specifically postconcussive symptoms, in comparison to the group that was discharged home the day of injury.[213]

Currently, there are no detailed guidelines to assist the clinician in determining which athlete requires admission for observation versus those who can be safely discharged home. In a recent article by Caskey et al. regarding the management of the pediatric concussed patient, the recommendation for admission were based on:

1. Positive head CT findings
2. Presence of significant symptoms (headache, nausea, vomiting, etc.) and/or
3. Prolonged loss of consciousness following injury[39]

The vital question to answer is "what is the likelihood that this patient's symptoms or pathology

Table 3.3 Guideline Recommendations for Obtaining CT Imaging in the Adult and Pediatric Patient Following Head Injury

Guideline Source	Recommendation to Obtain Noncontrast Cranial CT
Adult Patient	
4th International Conference on Concussion in Sport	"Prolonged disturbance of conscious state, focal neurological deficit, or worsening symptoms"[5]
American College of Emergency Physicians Neuroimaging Guidelines (ACEP)	Level A recommendations. Patient with loss of consciousness or post traumatic amnesia if one of these are present: headache, vomiting, age >60, intoxication, deficit in short-term memory, evidence of trauma above the clavicle, post-traumatic seizure, GCS score <15, focal neurological deficit, or coagulopathy Level B recommendations: Patient without loss of consciousness or post-traumatic amnesia if with focal neurological deficit, vomiting, severe headache, age >65, physical signs of skull fracture, GCS score <15, coagulopathy, or dangerous mechanism of injury[214]
Canadian head CT rule	GCS <15 at 2 h after injury, suspected open or depressed skull fracture, any sign of basal skull fracture (hemotympanum, "raccoon" eyes, CSF otorrhea/rhinorrhea, battle's sign), vomiting ≥2 episodes, age ≥65 years, pre-impact amnesia >30 min, dangerous mechanism[215,216] Sensitivity: 65% to 100%[207,217–221]
New Orleans rule	In patients with GCS 15, following head trauma, obtain imaging if at least 1 of: headache, vomiting, age >60, alcohol or drug intoxication, persistent anterograde amnesia, visible trauma above the clavicles, or presence of seizures[222] Sensitivity: 88% to 100%[217–221]
Pediatric Patient	
Canadian Assessment of Tomography for Childhood Head Injury (CATCH)	High-risk criteria: GCS does not improve to 15 within 2 h, suspicion of skull fracture on clinical exam, worsening headache, and irritability Medium-risk factors: large scalp hematoma, exam findings of basal skull fracture, dangerous mechanism of injury Sensitivity: 100% (high risk criteria), 98.1% (medium risk criteria)[223]
Pediatric Emergency Care Applied Research Network (PECARN)	Categorized as "high" and "intermediate risk" findings. Recommendation to obtain immediate head CT if had at least 1 high-risk finding. For low risk criteria, recommend either CT scan versus observation first followed by CT if symptoms progress For <2 years old: High-risk findings include altered mental status/abnormal behavior or palpable fracture, while intermediate risk include nonfrontal scalp hematoma, loss of consciousness >5 s, and/or significant mechanism of injury For >2 years old: High-risk findings included altered mental status or signs of skull fracture. With intermediate risk factors including loss of consciousness, vomiting, severe headache, or significant mechanism of injury Preferred due to risk stratification in young patients and also recommendation for conservative approach with observation for more intermediate risk findings[39] Sensitivity: 96.8% to 100%[224–226]
Children's Head Injury Algorithm for the Predication of Important Clinical Events (CHALICE)	History of: loss of consciousness or amnesia >5 min, drowsiness, >3 episodes of emesis, concern for non-accidental trauma, new onset seizure Examination consistent with: GCS <14 or <15 if <1 yo, findings concerning for skull fracture, tense fontanelle, focal neurological deficit, external trauma (ecchymosis, edema, or laceration) >5 cm if <1 year old Mechanism of injury: accident with speed >40 mph, fall >3 m, or high speed injury from projectile[227] Sensitivity: 98%

will progress requiring medical or even surgical intervention?" A prospective study of 203 patients found that 3 (1.5%) had a neurological decline following a concussion/mTBI. These patients were more likely to have a coagulopathy or use anticoagulants, have a lower GCS (13–14), and were older in age.[228] Therefore, history (past medical history, age, mechanism of injury, degree of symptoms, social support), clinical exam (neurological status), and imaging (positive head CT findings, other injuries) should be used to determine the need for overnight observation in an inpatient hospital facility.[229] If admission is warranted, the admitting service (pediatrics, internal medicine, neurology, trauma surgery, or neurosurgery) is determined by the nature of the injury, comorbid conditions, hospital policy, and comfort of accepting physician. Many reviews have discussed the management of even small intracranial hemorrhages, found on CT in the presence of a normal neurological exam, by acute care surgeons without the assistance of neurosurgery.[230,231]

For those admitted for observation with intracranial bleeding found on CT, there is great debate in regards to need for repeat imaging. Many advocate for repeat imaging based on specific features of the cranial pathology; for example, if it is at a high risk to expand, as in the case of a temporal bone fracture near the middle meningeal artery.[23] Through retrospective review, many advocate only repeat imaging if neurological symptoms develop, even if the patient is on antiplatelet or anticoagulation medications, and this also should apply to the outpatient setting.[232–234] For comparison, Almenawer et al. retrospectively reviewed mild TBI patients (GCS 13–15), and stated that a repeat CT scan after 24 h altered the current management in only 0.6% of the patients.

Whether determined safe to be sent home from the playing field, discharged from the emergency department, or inpatient hospital following observation, the instructions are similar: focusing on education (what is a concussion, symptomatology of concussion, etc.), activity restrictions, reasons to seek medical attention, and when to follow-up with a medical provider. What is essential to emphasize is that no player diagnosed with a concussion is to return to sport on the day of injury. The player should maintain adequate hydration, eat a well-balanced diet, be given oral antiemetics as needed, be instructed on the use of acetaminophen for analgesia (refraining from aspirin or nonsteroidal anti-inflammatory medications in the acute period due to the potential increase in hemorrhage risk), and also refrain from neurotoxic agents such as alcohol or illicit drug use.[4,24,31,66,235–239] Within these detailed, written directions, the athlete and parent should also be given instructions specifying "red flags" of when to notify a physician and/or return to a local emergency department.[240] The player should return to the hospital if they develop dramatic worsening of symptoms, new neurological deficit, or change in mental status.

Once arriving home from either the field or hospital, the player is to initiate physical and cognitive rest for at least 48 h followed by a structured "return to learn" process that focuses on activity modification individualized to exacerbation/mitigation of symptoms, detailed in Chapter 8.[4,6,7,14,15,66,89,110–114,241,242] The athlete should then follow up with their primary care physician once asymptomatic or with minimal symptoms, for a graded return to play algorithm. This follow-up visit should not exceed 1–2 weeks from injury in order to evaluate and initiate proper return to activity, but also to identify those with a protracted recovery requiring more aggressive interventions in order to improve recovery.[39,243–245] Some players may also choose to follow-up directly with a specialized sports concussion clinic if available.[236–248] Importantly, all of these recommendations along with potential risks of returning to play early, and also current limitations in evidence must be clearly instructed to the patient and caregiver and documented in the chart, followed by open-ended questions in order to assess their level of understanding.[249]

Conclusion

The acute management of concussion is focused on recognition that the concussion occurred through the use of specific diagnostic tools, removing all players from activity the day of concussion, and then determining the need for an evaluation at a higher level of care. Specific signs and symptoms, like altered mental status and localizing neurological signs, always warrant neuroimaging to rule out a space-occupying lesion within the brain. Once deemed possible for discharge from acute medical observation, the athlete requires home observation and initiation of a rest period. The acute management of concussion is only a small fraction of the further care the athlete will require in regards to outpatient management for postconcussive syndrome management, monitoring their recovery, and return to activity. These topics will be discussed in the following chapters.

References

1. Notebaert AJ, Guskiewicz KM. Current trends in athletic training practice for concussion assessment and management. *Journal of Athletic Training*. 2005; 40(4): 320–325.

2. Guskiewicz KM, Broglio SP. Sport-related concussion: on-field and sideline assessment. *Physical Medicine and Rehabilitation Clinics of North America*. 2011; 22(4): 603–617, vii.

3. Herring SA, Kibler WB, Putukian M. Team Physician Consensus Statement: 2013 update. *Medicine and Science in Sports and Exercise*. 2013; 45(8): 1618–1622.

4. Broglio SP, Cantu RC, Gioia GA et al. National Athletic Trainers' Association position statement: management of sport concussion. *Journal of Athletic Training*. 2014; 49(2): 245–265.

5. McCrory P, Meeuwisse WH, Aubry M et al. Consensus statement on concussion in sport: the 4th International Conference on Concussion in Sport, Zurich, November 2012. *Journal of Athletic Training*. 2013; 48(4): 554–575.

6. McCrory P, Meeuwisse W, Aubry M et al. Consensus statement on Concussion in Sport – The 4th International Conference on Concussion in Sport held in Zurich, November 2012. *Physical Therapy in Sport*. 2013; 14(2): e1–e13.

7. Giza CC, Kutcher JS, Ashwal S et al. Summary of evidence-based guideline update: evaluation and management of concussion in sports: report of the Guideline Development Subcommittee of the American Academy of Neurology. *Neurology*. 2013; 80(24): 2250–2257.

8. Institute of Medicine (IOM) and National Research Council (NRC). In: Graham R, Rivara FP, Ford MA, Spicer CM, eds. *Sports-Related Concussions in Youth: Improving the Science, Changing the Culture*. Washington D.C: The National Academics Press. 2014.

9. Ommaya AK. Head injury mechanisms and the concept of preventive management: a review and critical synthesis. *Journal of Neurotrauma*. 1995; 12(4): 527–546.

10. Stone JL, Patel V, Bailes JE. The history of neurosurgical treatment of sports concussion. *Neurosurgery*. 2014; 75 Suppl 4: S3–s23.

11. Meaney DF, Morrison B, Dale Bass C. The mechanics of traumatic brain injury: a review of what we know and what we need to know for reducing its societal burden. *Journal of Biomechanical Engineering*. 2014; 136(2): 021008.

12. Duhaime AC, Beckwith JG, Maerlender AC et al. Spectrum of acute clinical characteristics of diagnosed concussions in college athletes wearing instrumented helmets: clinical article. *Journal of Neurosurgery*. 2012; 117(6): 1092–1099.

13. Warren WL, Jr., Bailes JE. On the field evaluation of athletic head injuries. *Clinics in Sports Medicine*. 1998; 17(1): 13–26.

14. Harmon KG, Drezner J, Gammons M et al. American Medical Society for Sports Medicine position statement: concussion in sport. *Clinical Journal of Sport Medicine*. 2013; 23(1): 1–18.

15. West TA, Marion DW. Current recommendations for the diagnosis and treatment of concussion in sport: a comparison of three new guidelines. *Journal of Neurotrauma*. 2014; 31(2): 159–168.

16. Pearce AJ, Hoy K, Rogers MA et al. Acute motor, neurocognitive and neurophysiological change following concussion injury in Australian amateur football. A prospective multimodal investigation. *Journal of Science and Medicine in Sport/Sports Medicine Australia*. 2015; 18(5): 500–506.

17. Miles CM. Concussion management: the current landscape. *Journal of the American Academy of Physician Assistants*. 2014; 27(2): 8–9.

18. Putukian M, Kutcher J. Current concepts in the treatment of sports concussions. *Neurosurgery*. 2014; 75 Suppl 4: S64–70.

19. Chameides L, Samson R, Schexnayder S, Hazinski M. Pediatric Advanced Life Support:

Provider Manual. In: *Association TAH, Pediatrics* AAo, eds: First American Heart Association Printing; 2011.

20. Sinz E, Navarro K. Advanced Cardiovascular Life Support: Provider Manual. In: Association TAH, ed: First American Heart Association; 2011.

21. Jung JY. Airway management of patients with traumatic brain injury/C-spine injury. *Korean Journal of Anesthesiology*. 2015; 68(3): 213–219.

22. Concussion (mild traumatic brain injury) and the team physician: a consensus statement. *Medicine and Science in Sports and Exercise*. 2006; 38(2): 395–399.

23. Ropper AH, Gorson KC. Clinical practice. Concussion. *The New England Journal of Medicine*. 2007; 356(2): 166–172.

24. Putukian M. The acute symptoms of sport-related concussion: diagnosis and on-field management. *Clinics in Sports Medicine*. 2011; 30(1): 49–61, viii.

25. *National Athletic Trainer's Association, Appropriate Prehospital Management of the Spine–Injured Athlete, Updated from 1998 document*. nata.org, 2015.

26. Committee on Sports-Related Concussions in Y, Board on Children Y, Families, Institute of M, National Research C. The National Academies Collection: Reports funded by National Institutes of Health. In: Graham R, Rivara FP, Ford MA, Spicer CM, eds. *Sports-Related Concussions in Youth: Improving the Science, Changing the Culture*. Washington D.C.; 2014.

27. Putukian M, Raftery M, Guskiewicz K et al. Onfield assessment of concussion in the adult athlete. *British Journal of Sports Medicine*. 2013; 47(5): 285–288.

28. Guskiewicz KM, Broglio SP. Acute sports-related traumatic brain injury and repetitive concussion. *Handbook of Clinical Neurology*. 2015; 127: 157–172.

29. Echemendia RJ, Giza CC, Kutcher JS. Developing guidelines for return to play: consensus and evidence-based approaches. *Brain Injury*. 2015; 29(2): 185–194.

30. Buckley TA, Burdette G, Kelly K. Concussion-management practice patterns of National Collegiate Athletic Association Division II and III athletic trainers: how the other half lives. *Journal of Athletic Training*. 2015; 50(8): 879–888.

31. Willer B, Leddy JJ. Management of concussion and post-concussion syndrome. *Current Treatment Options in Neurology*. 2006; 8(5): 415–426.

32. Foley C, Gregory A, Solomon G. Young age as a modifying factor in sports concussion management: what is the evidence? *Current Sports Medicine Reports*. 2014; 13(6): 390–394.

33. Dessy A, Rasouli J, Gometz A, Choudhri T. A review of modifying factors affecting usage of diagnostic rating scales in concussion management. *Clinical Neurology and Neurosurgery*. 2014; 122: 59–63.

34. Covassin T, Swanik CB, Sachs ML. Sex differences and the incidence of concussions among collegiate athletes. *Journal of Athletic Training*. 2003; 38(3): 238–244.

35. Covassin T, Elbin RJ. The female athlete: the role of gender in the assessment and management of sport-related concussion. *Clinics in Sports Medicine*. 2011; 30(1): 125–131, x.

36. Reynolds E, Collins MW, Mucha A, Troutman-Ensecki C. Establishing a clinical service for the management of sports-related concussions. *Neurosurgery*. 2014; 75 Suppl 4: S71–81.

37. Reddy CC, Collins MW. Sports concussion: management and predictors of outcome. *Current Sports Medicine Reports*. 2009; 8(1): 10–15.

38. Makdissi M, Davis G, Jordan B, Patricios J, Purcell L, Putukian M. Revisiting the modifiers: how should the evaluation and management of acute concussions differ in specific groups? *British Journal of Sports Medicine*. 2013; 47(5): 314–320.

39. Caskey RC, Nance ML. Management of pediatric mild traumatic brain injury. *Advances in Pediatrics*. 2014; 61(1): 271–286.

40. Gioia GA. Multimodal evaluation and management of children with concussion: using our heads and available evidence. *Brain Injury* 2015; 29(2): 195–206.

41. Junn C, Bell KR, Shenouda C, Hoffman JM. Symptoms of concussion and comorbid disorders. *Current Pain and Headache Reports*. 2015; 19(9): 46.

42. Carney N, Ghajar J, Jagoda A et al. Executive summary of concussion guidelines step 1: systematic review of prevalent indicators. *Neurosurgery*. 2014; 75 Suppl 1: S1–2.

43. McCrory P, Meeuwisse WH, Echemendia RJ, Iverson GL, Dvorak J, Kutcher JS. What is the lowest threshold to make a diagnosis of concussion? *British Journal of Sports Medicine*. 2013; 47(5): 268–271.

44. Barry NC, Tomes JL. Remembering your past: The effects of concussion on autobiographical memory recall. *Journal of Clinical and Experimental Neuropsychology*. 2015; 37(9): 994–1003.

45. Carney N, Ghajar J, Jagoda A et al. Concussion guidelines step 1: systematic review of prevalent indicators. *Neurosurgery*. 2014; 75 Suppl 1: S3–15.

46. Lovell MR, Collins MW, Iverson GL et al. Recovery from mild concussion in high school athletes. *Journal of Neurosurgery*. 2003; 98(2): 296–301.

47. Mrazik M, Naidu D, Lebrun C, Game A, Matthews-White J. Does an individual's fitness level affect baseline concussion symptoms? *Journal of Athletic Training*. 2013; 48(5): 654–658.

48. Makdissi M, Darby D, Maruff P, Ugoni A, Brukner P, McCrory PR. Natural history of concussion in sport: markers of severity and implications for management. *The American Journal of Sports Medicine*. 2010; 38(3): 464–471.

49. Bramley H, Heverley S, Lewis MM, Kong L, Rivera R, Silvis M. Demographics and treatment of adolescent posttraumatic headache in a regional concussion clinic. *Pediatric Neurology*. 2015; 52(5): 493–498.

50. Guskiewicz KM, McCrea M, Marshall SW et al. Cumulative effects associated with recurrent concussion in collegiate football players: the NCAA Concussion Study. *The Journal of the American Medical Association*. 2003; 290(19): 2549–2555.

51. Heyer GL, Young JA, Rose SC, McNally KA, Fischer AN. Post-traumatic headaches correlate with migraine symptoms in youth with concussion. *Cephalalgia*. 2015.

52. Wasserman EB, Kerr ZY, Zuckerman SL, Covassin T. Epidemiology of Sports-related concussions in National Collegiate Athletic Association Athletes from 2009–2010 to 2013–2014: symptom prevalence, symptom resolution time, and return-to-play time. *The American Journal of Sports Medicine*. 2015.

53. Guskiewicz KM, Weaver NL, Padua DA, Garrett WE, Jr. Epidemiology of concussion in collegiate and high school football players. *The American Journal of Sports Medicine*. 2000; 28(5): 643–650.

54. Torres DM, Galetta KM, Phillips HW et al. Sports-related concussion: Anonymous survey of a collegiate cohort. *Neurology Clinical Practice*. 2013; 3(4): 279–287.

55. Pellman EJ, Powell JW, Viano DC et al. Concussion in professional football: epidemiological features of game injuries and review of the literature—part 3. *Neurosurgery*. 2004; 54(1): 81–94.

56. Merritt VC, Rabinowitz AR, Arnett PA. Injury-related predictors of symptom severity following sports-related concussion. *Journal of Clinical and Experimental Neuropsychology*. 2015; 37(3): 265–275.

57. Meehan WP, 3rd, d'Hemecourt P, Comstock RD. High school concussions in the 2008–2009 academic year: mechanism, symptoms, and management. *The American Journal of Sports Medicine*. 2010; 38(12): 2405–2409.

58. Meehan WP, 3rd, Mannix RC, Stracciolini A, Elbin RJ, Collins MW. Symptom severity predicts prolonged recovery after sport-related concussion, but age and amnesia do not. *Journal of Pediatrics*. 2013; 163(3): 721–725.

59. Lau BC, Kontos AP, Collins MW, Mucha A, Lovell MR. Which on-field signs/symptoms predict protracted recovery from sport-related concussion among high school football players? *The American Journal of Sports Medicine*. 2011; 39(11): 2311–2318.

60. Kontos AP, Elbin RJ, Lau B et al. Posttraumatic migraine as a predictor of recovery and cognitive impairment after sport-related concussion. *The American Journal of Sports Medicine*. 2013; 41(7): 1497–1504.

61. Shim J, Smith DH, Van Lunen BL. On-field signs and symptoms associated with recovery duration after concussion in high school and college athletes: a critically appraised topic. *Journal of Sport Rehabilitation*. 2015; 24(1): 72–76.

62. Lau B, Lovell MR, Collins MW, Pardini J. Neurocognitive and symptom predictors of recovery in high school athletes. *Clinical Journal of Sport Medicine*. 2009; 19(3): 216–221.

63. Meehan WP, 3rd, Mannix R, Monuteaux MC, Stein CJ, Bachur RG. Early symptom burden predicts recovery after sport-related concussion. *Neurology*. 2014; 83(24): 2204–2210.

64. Randolph C, Millis S, Barr WB et al. Concussion symptom inventory: an empirically derived scale for monitoring resolution of symptoms following sport–related concussion. *Archives of Clinical Neuropsychology*. 2009; 24(3): 219–229.

65. Sady MD, Vaughan CG, Gioia GA. Psychometric characteristics of the postconcussion symptom inventory in children and adolescents. *Archives of Clinical Neuropsychology*. 2014; 29(4): 348–363.

66. Choe MC, Giza CC. Diagnosis and management of acute concussion. *Seminars in Neurology*. 2015; 35(1): 29–41.

67. McCrea M, Iverson GL, Echemendia RJ, Makdissi M, Raftery M. Day of injury assessment of sport-related concussion. *British Journal of Sports Medicine*. 2013; 47(5): 272–284.

68. Luoto TM, Silverberg ND, Kataja A et al. Sport concussion assessment tool 2 in a civilian trauma sample with mild traumatic brain injury. *Journal of Neurotrauma*. 2014; 31(8): 728–738.

69. Putukian M, Echemendia R, Dettwiler-Danspeckgruber A et al. Prospective clinical assessment using Sideline Concussion Assessment Tool-2 testing in the evaluation of sport-related concussion in college athletes. *Clinical Journal of Sport Medicine*. 2015; 25(1): 36–42.

70. Guskiewicz KM, Register-Mihalik J, McCrory P et al. Evidence-based approach to revising the SCAT2: introducing the SCAT3. *British Journal of Sports Medicine*. 2013; 47(5): 289–293.

71. Schneider KJ, Emery CA, Kang J, Schneider GM, Meeuwisse WH. Examining Sport Concussion Assessment Tool ratings for male and female youth hockey players with and without a history of concussion. *British Journal of Sports Medicine*. 2010; 44(15): 1112–1117.

72. Glaviano NR, Benson S, Goodkin HP, Broshek DK, Saliba S. Baseline SCAT2 assessment of healthy youth student-athletes: preliminary evidence for the use of the child-SCAT3 in children younger than 13 years. *Clinical Journal of Sport Medicine*. 2015; 25(4): 373–379.

73. Snyder AR, Bauer RM. A normative study of the sport concussion assessment tool (SCAT2) in children and adolescents. *The Clinical Neuropsychologist*. 2014; 28(7): 1091–1103.

74. Valovich McLeod TC, Bay RC, Lam KC, Chhabra A. Representative baseline values on the Sport Concussion Assessment Tool 2 (SCAT2) in adolescent athletes vary by gender, grade, and concussion history.

The American Journal of Sports Medicine. 2012; 40(4): 927–933.

75. Zimmer A, Marcinak J, Hibyan S, Webbe F. Normative values of major SCAT2 and SCAT3 components for a college athlete population. *Applied Neuropsychology Adult.* 2015; 22(2): 132–140.

76. Hanninen T, Tuominen M, Parkkari J et al. Sport concussion assessment tool—3rd edition—normative reference values for professional ice hockey players. *Journal of Science and Medicine in Sport/Sports Medicine Australia.* 2015.

77. Maddocks DL, Dicker GD, Saling MM. The assessment of orientation following concussion in athletes. *Clinical Journal of Sport Medicine.* 1995; 5(1): 32–35.

78. McCrea M. Standardized mental status assessment of sports concussion. *Clinical Journal of Sport Medicine.* 2001; 11(3)79: 176–181.

79. Barr WB, McCrea M. Sensitivity and specificity of standardized neurocognitive testing immediately following sports concussion. *Journal of International Neuropsychological Society.* 2001; 7(6): 693–702.

80. McCrea M, Kelly JP, Randolph C et al. Standardized assessment of concussion (SAC): on-site mental status evaluation of the athlete. *The Journal of Head Trauma Rehabilitation.* 1998; 13(2): 27–35.

81. Valovich TC, Perrin DH, Gansneder BM. Repeat administration elicits a practice effect with the balance error scoring system but not with the standardized assessment of concussion in high school athletes. *Journal of Athletic Training.* 2003; 38(1): 51–56.

82. Guskiewicz KM. Balance assessment in the management of sport-related concussion. *Clinics in Sports Medicine.* 2011; 30(1): 89–102, ix.

83. Okonkwo DO, Tempel ZJ, Maroon J. Sideline assessment tools for the evaluation of concussion in athletes: a review. *Neurosurgery.* 2014; 75 Suppl 4: S82–95.

84. Guskiewicz KM, Riemann BL, Perrin DH, Nashner LM. Alternative approaches to the assessment of mild head injury in athletes. *Medicine and Science in Sports and Exercise.* 1997; 29(7 Suppl): S213–221.

85. Harmon KG, Drezner JA, Gammons M et al. American Medical Society for Sports Medicine position statement: concussion in sport. *British Journal of Sports Medicine.* 2013; 47(1): 15–26.

86. Schneiders AG, Sullivan SJ, Gray AR, Hammond-Tooke GD, McCrory PR. Normative values for three clinical measures of motor performance used in the neurological assessment of sports concussion. *Journal of Science and Medicine in Sport/Sports Medicine Australia.* 2010; 13(2): 196–201.

87. Gioia GA, Collins M, Isquith PK. Improving identification and diagnosis of mild traumatic brain injury with evidence: psychometric support for the acute concussion evaluation. *The Journal of Head Trauma Rehabilitation.* 2008; 23(4): 230–242.

88. Zuckerbraun NS, Atabaki S, Collins MW, Thomas D, Gioia GA. Use of modified acute concussion evaluation tools in the emergency department. *Pediatrics.* 2014; 133(4): 635–642.

89. Terrell TR, Cox CB, Bielak K, Casmus R, Laskowitz D, Nichols G. Sports Concussion Management: part II. *Southern Medical Journal.* 2014; 107(2): 126–135.

90. Eckner JT, Kutcher JS, Broglio SP, Richardson JK. Effect of sport-related concussion on clinically measured simple reaction time. *British Journal of Sports Medicine.* 2014; 48(2): 112–118.

91. Reddy S, Eckner JT, Kutcher JS. Effect of acute exercise on clinically measured reaction time in collegiate athletes. *Medicine and Science in Sports and Exercise.* 2014; 46(3): 429–434.

92. Eckner JT, Whitacre RD, Kirsch NL, Richardson JK. Evaluating a clinical measure of reaction

time: an observational study. *Perceptual and Motor Skills*. 2009; 108(3): 717–720.

93. Parker TM, Osternig LR, van Donkelaar P, Chou LS. Recovery of cognitive and dynamic motor function following concussion. *British Journal of Sports Medicine*. 2007; 41(12): 868–873.

94. Eckner JT, Kutcher JS, Richardson JK. Effect of concussion on clinically measured reaction time in 9 NCAA division I collegiate athletes: a preliminary study. *PM & R*. 2011; 3(3): 212–218.

95. Maugans TA, Farley C, Altaye M, Leach J, Cecil KM. Pediatric sports-related concussion produces cerebral blood flow alterations. *Pediatrics*. 2012; 129(1): 28–37.

96. MacDonald J, Wilson J, Young J et al. Evaluation of a simple test of reaction time for baseline concussion testing in a population of high school athletes. *Clinical Journal of Sport Medicine*. 2015; 25(1): 43–48.

97. Galetta KM, Morganroth J, Moehringer N et al. Adding vision to concussion testing: a prospective study of sideline testing in youth and collegiate athletes. *Journal of Neuro-Ophthalmology*. 2015; 35(3): 235–241.

98. Vernau BT, Grady MF, Goodman A et al. Oculomotor and neurocognitive assessment of youth ice hockey players: baseline associations and observations after concussion. *Developmental Neuropsychology*. 2015; 40(1): 7–11.

99. Leong DF, Balcer LJ, Galetta SL, Evans G, Gimre M, Watt D. The King-Devick test for sideline concussion screening in collegiate football. *Journal of Optometry*. 2015; 8(2): 131–139.

100. King D, Hume P, Gissane C, Clark T. Use of the King-Devick test for sideline concussion screening in junior rugby league. *Journal of the Neurological Sciences*. 2015; 357(1–2): 75–79.

101. Seidman DH, Burlingame J, Yousif LR et al. Evaluation of the King-Devick test as a concussion screening tool in high school

football players. *Journal of the Neurological Sciences*. 2015; 356(1–2): 97–101.

102. Tjarks BJ, Dorman JC, Valentine VD et al. Comparison and utility of King-Devick and ImPACT(R) composite scores in adolescent concussion patients. *Journal of the Neurological Sciences*. 2013; 334(1–2): 148–153.

103. King D, Gissane C, Hume PA, Flaws M. The King-Devick test was useful in management of concussion in amateur rugby union and rugby league in New Zealand. *Journal of the Neurological Sciences*. 2015; 351(1–2): 58–64.

104. Shehata N, Wiley JP, Richea S, Benson BW, Duits L, Meeuwisse WH. Sport concussion assessment tool: baseline values for varsity collision sport athletes. *British Journal of Sports Medicine*. 2009; 43(10): 730–734.

105. Williams RM, Welch CE, Weber ML, Parsons JT, Valovich McLeod TC. Athletic trainers' management practices and referral patterns for adolescent athletes after sport-related concussion. *Sports Health*. 2014; 6(5): 434–439.

106. Merritt VC, Rabinowitz AR, Arnett PA. Personality factors and symptom reporting at baseline in collegiate athletes. *Developmental Neuropsychology*. 2015; 40(1): 45–50.

107. Yang CC, Yuen KM, Huang SJ, Hsiao SH, Tsai YH, Lin WC. "Good-old-days" bias: a prospective follow-up study to examine the preinjury supernormal status in patients with mild traumatic brain injury. *Journal of Clinical and Experimental Neuropsychology*. 2014; 36(4): 399–409.

108. Meier TB, Brummel BJ, Singh R, Nerio CJ, Polanski DW, Bellgowan PS. The underreporting of self-reported symptoms following sports-related concussion. *Journal of Science and Medicine in Sport/Sports Medicine Australia*. 2015; 18(5): 507–511.

109. Balasundaram AP, Sullivan JS, Schneiders AG, Athens J. Symptom response following acute bouts of exercise in concussed and non-concussed individuals—a systematic narrative review. *Physical Therapy in Sport*. 2013; 14(4): 253–258.

110. Rivera RG, Roberson SP, Whelan M, Rohan A. Concussion evaluation and management in pediatrics. *MCN The American Journal of Maternal Child Nursing.* 2015; 40(2): 76–86; quiz E75–76.

111. Rose SC, Weber KD, Collen JB, Heyer GL. The diagnosis and management of concussion in children and adolescents. *Pediatric Neurology.* 2015; 53(2): 108–118.

112. Terrell TR, Nobles T, Rader B et al. Sports concussion management: part I. *Southern Medical Journal.* 2014; 107(2): 115–125.

113. Levin HS, Diaz-Arrastia RR. Diagnosis, prognosis, and clinical management of mild traumatic brain injury. *The Lancet Neurology* 2015; 14(5): 506–517.

114. Herring SA, Cantu RC, Guskiewicz KM et al. Concussion (mild traumatic brain injury) and the team physician: a consensus statement—2011 update. *Medicine and Science in Sports and Exercise.* 2011; 43(12): 2412–2422.

115. Guskiewicz KM, Bruce SL, Cantu RC et al. National Athletic Trainers' Association Position Statement: Management of Sport-Related Concussion. *Journal of Athletic Training.* 2004; 39(3): 280–297.

116. Gomez JE, Hergenroeder AC. New guidelines for management of concussion in sport: special concern for youth. *The Journal of Adolescent Health.* 2013; 53(3): 311–313.

117. Smith DH, Meaney DF, Shull WH. Diffuse axonal injury in head trauma. *The Journal of Head Trauma Rehabilitation.* 2003; 18(4): 307–316.

118. Siedler DG, Chuah MI, Kirkcaldie MT, Vickers JC, King AE. Diffuse axonal injury in brain trauma: insights from alterations in neurofilaments. *Frontiers in Cellular Neuroscience.* 2014; 8: 429.

119. Povlishock JT, Pettus EH. Traumatically induced axonal damage: evidence for enduring changes in axolemmal permeability with associated cytoskeletal change.

Acta Neurochirurgica Supplement. 1996; 66: 81–86.

120. Pettus EH, Povlishock JT. Characterization of a distinct set of intra-axonal ultrastructural changes associated with traumatically induced alteration in axolemmal permeability. *Brain Research* 1996; 722(1–2): 1–11.

121. McKee AC, Daneshvar DH. The neuropathology of traumatic brain injury. *Handbook of Clinical Neurology* 2015; 127: 45–66.

122. Maxwell WL, McCreath BJ, Graham DI, Gennarelli TA. Cytochemical evidence for redistribution of membrane pump calcium-ATPase and ecto-Ca-ATPase activity, and calcium influx in myelinated nerve fibres of the optic nerve after stretch injury. *Journal of Neurocytology.* 1995; 24(12): 925–942.

123. Maxwell WL, Graham DI. Loss of axonal microtubules and neurofilaments after stretch-injury to guinea pig optic nerve fibers. *Journal of Neurotrauma.* 1997; 14(9): 603–614.

124. Farkas O, Lifshitz J, Povlishock JT. Mechanoporation induced by diffuse traumatic brain injury: an irreversible or reversible response to injury? *Journal of Neuroscience* 2006; 26(12): 3130–3140.

125. McCrea M, Guskiewicz K, Randolph C et al. Effects of a symptom-free waiting period on clinical outcome and risk of reinjury after sport-related concussion. *Neurosurgery.* 2009; 65(5): 876–882.

126. Laurer HL, Bareyre FM, Lee VM et al. Mild head injury increasing the brain's vulnerability to a second concussive impact. *Journal of Neurosurgery.* 2001; 95(5): 859–870.

127. Bolton AN, Saatman KE. Regional neurodegeneration and gliosis are amplified by mild traumatic brain injury repeated at 24–hour intervals. *Journal of Neuropathology and Experimental Neurology.* 2014; 73(10): 933–947.

128. Huang L, Coats JS, Mohd-Yusof A et al. Tissue vulnerability is increased following repetitive mild traumatic brain injury in the rat. *Brain Research.* 2013; 1499: 109–120.

129. Friess SH, Ichord RN, Ralston J et al. Repeated traumatic brain injury affects composite cognitive function in piglets. *Journal of Neurotrauma.* 2009; 26(7): 1111–1121.

130. Weber JT. Experimental models of repetitive brain injuries. *Progress in Brain Research.* 2007; 161: 253–261.

131. Longhi L, Saatman KE, Fujimoto S et al. Temporal window of vulnerability to repetitive experimental concussive brain injury. *Neurosurgery.* 2005; 56(2): 364–374.

132. Goddeyne C, Nichols J, Wu C, Anderson T. Repetitive mild traumatic brain injury induces ventriculomegaly and cortical thinning in juvenile rats. *Journal of Neurophysiology.* 2015; 113(9): 3268–3280.

133. Raghupathi R, Mehr MF, Helfaer MA, Margulies SS. Traumatic axonal injury is exacerbated following repetitive closed head injury in the neonatal pig. *Journal of Neurotrauma.* 2004; 21(3): 307–316.

134. Donovan V, Kim C, Anugerah AK et al. Repeated mild traumatic brain injury results in long-term white-matter disruption. *Journal of Cerebral Blood Flow and Metabolism.* 2014; 34(4): 715–723.

135. Boake C, McCauley SR, Levin HS et al. Diagnostic criteria for postconcussional syndrome after mild to moderate traumatic brain injury. *The Journal of Neuropsychiatry and Clinical Neurosciences.* 2005; 17(3): 350–356.

136. World Heatlh Organization: ICD 10 Classification of Mental and Behavioral Disorders: Diagnostic Criteria for Research. *Geneva: World Health Organization.*

137. Tator CH, Davis HS, Dufort PA et al. Postconcussion syndrome: demographics and predictors in 221 patients. *Journal of Neurosurgery.* 2016: 1–11.

138. Cantu RC. Second-impact syndrome. *Clinics in Sports Medicine.* 1998; 17(1): 37–44.

139. Cantu RC, Gean AD. Second-impact syndrome and a small subdural hematoma: an uncommon catastrophic result of repetitive head injury with a characteristic imaging appearance. *Journal of Neurotrauma.* 2010; 27(9): 1557–1564.

140. McQuillen JB, McQuillen EN, Morrow P. Trauma, sport, and malignant cerebral edema. *The American Journal of Forensic Medicine and Pathology.* 1988; 9(1): 12–15.

141. McCrory PR, Berkovic SF. Second impact syndrome. *Neurology.* 1998; 50(3): 677–683.

142. Kelly JP, Nichols JS, Filley CM, Lillehei KO, Rubinstein D, Kleinschmidt-DeMasters BK. Concussion in sports. Guidelines for the prevention of catastrophic outcome. *The Journal of the American Medical Association.* 1991; 266(20): 2867–2869.

143. Hebert O, Schlueter K, Hornsby M, Van Gorder S, Snodgrass S, Cook C. The diagnostic credibility of second impact syndrome: A systematic literature review. *Journal of Science and Medicine in Sport/Sports Medicine Australia.* 2016.

144. McKee AC, Daneshvar DH. The neuropathology of traumatic brain injury. *Handbook of Clinical Neurology.* 2015; 127: 45–66.

145. Omalu BI, DeKosky ST, Minster RL, Kamboh MI, Hamilton RL, Wecht CH. Chronic traumatic encephalopathy in a National Football League player. *Neurosurgery.* 2005; 57(1): 128–134.

146. Omalu BI, DeKosky ST, Hamilton RL et al. Chronic traumatic encephalopathy in a national football league player: part II. *Neurosurgery.* 2006; 59(5): 1086–1092.

147. Montenigro PH, Corp DT, Stein TD, Cantu RC, Stern RA. Chronic traumatic encephalopathy: historical origins and current perspective. *Annual Review of Clinical Psychology.* 2015; 11: 309–330.

148. Omalu BI, Hamilton RL, Kamboh MI, DeKosky ST, Bailes J. Chronic traumatic encephalopathy (CTE) in a National Football League Player: Case report and emerging medicolegal practice questions. *Journal of Forensic Nursing.* 2010; 6(1): 40–46.

149. Maroon JC, Winkelman R, Bost J, Amos A, Mathyssek C, Miele V. Chronic traumatic encephalopathy in contact sports: a systematic review of all reported pathological cases. *PLoS One*. 2015; 10(2): e0117338.

150. Geddes JF, Vowles GH, Nicoll JA, Revesz T. Neuronal cytoskeletal changes are an early consequence of repetitive head injury. *Acta Neuropathologica*. 1999; 98(2): 171–178.

151. Lepreux S, Auriacombe S, Vital C, Dubois B, Vital A. Dementia pugilistica: a severe tribute to a career. *Clinical Neuropathology*. 2015; 34(4): 193–198.

152. Omalu B, Hammers JL, Bailes J et al. Chronic traumatic encephalopathy in an Iraqi war veteran with posttraumatic stress disorder who committed suicide. *Neurosurgical Focus*. 2011; 31(5): E3.

153. Omalu BI, Bailes J, Hammers JL, Fitzsimmons RP. Chronic traumatic encephalopathy, suicides and parasuicides in professional American athletes: the role of the forensic pathologist. *The American Journal of Forensic Medicine and Pathology*. 2010; 31(2): 130–132.

154. Omalu BI, Fitzsimmons RP, Hammers J, Bailes J. Chronic traumatic encephalopathy in a professional American wrestler. *Journal of Forensic Nursing*. 2010; 6(3): 130–136.

155. Aotsuka A, Kojima S, Furumoto H, Hattori T, Hirayama K. [Punch drunk syndrome due to repeated karate kicks and punches]. *Rinsho Shinkeigaku = Clinical Neurology*. 1990; 30(11): 1243–1246.

156. Baugh CM, Stamm JM, Riley DO et al. Chronic traumatic encephalopathy: neurodegeneration following repetitive concussive and subconcussive brain trauma. *Brain Imaging and Behavior*. 2012; 6(2): 244–254.

157. Stein TD, Alvarez VE, McKee AC. Chronic traumatic encephalopathy: a spectrum of neuropathological changes following repetitive brain trauma in athletes and military personnel. *Alzheimer's Research and Therapy*. 2014; 6(1): 4.

158. Roberts GW, Allsop D, Bruton C. The occult aftermath of boxing. *Journal of Neurology, Neurosurgery, and Psychiatry*. 1990; 53(5): 373–378.

159. Roberts GW, Whitwell HL, Acland PR, Bruton CJ. Dementia in a punch-drunk wife. *Lancet (London, England)*. 1990; 335(8694): 918–919.

160. Baugh CM, Robbins CA, Stern RA, McKee AC. Current understanding of chronic traumatic encephalopathy. *Current Treatment Options in Neurology*. 2014; 16(9): 306.

161. Mez J, Stern RA, McKee AC. Chronic traumatic encephalopathy: where are we and where are we going? *Current Neurology and Neuroscience Reports*. 2013; 13(12): 407.

162. Clinton J, Ambler MW, Roberts GW. Posttraumatic Alzheimer's disease: preponderance of a single plaque type. *Neuropathology and Applied Neurobiology*. 1991; 17(1): 69–74.

163. McKee AC, Stein TD, Kiernan PT, Alvarez VE. The neuropathology of chronic traumatic encephalopathy. *Brain Pathology (Zurich, Switzerland)*. 2015; 25(3): 350–364.

164. McKee AC, Cantu RC, Nowinski CJ et al. Chronic traumatic encephalopathy in athletes: progressive tauopathy after repetitive head injury. *Journal of Neuropathology and Experimental Neurology*. 2009; 68(7): 709–735.

165. McKee AC, Stern RA, Nowinski CJ et al. The spectrum of disease in chronic traumatic encephalopathy. *Brain*. 2013; 136(Pt 1): 43–64.

166. Omalu B, Bailes J, Hamilton RL et al. Emerging histomorphologic phenotypes of chronic traumatic encephalopathy in American athletes. *Neurosurgery*. 2011; 69(1): 173–183.

167. Tartaglia MC, Hazrati LN, Davis KD et al. Chronic traumatic encephalopathy and other neurodegenerative proteinopathies. *Frontiers in Human Neuroscience*. 2014; 8: 30.

168. Guskiewicz KM, Bruce SL, Cantu RC et al. Research based recommendations on management of sport related concussion: summary of the National Athletic Trainers' Association position statement. *British Journal of Sports Medicine*. 2006; 40(1): 6–10.

169. Guskiewicz KM, Bruce SL, Cantu RC et al. Recommendations on management of sport-related concussion: summary of the National Athletic Trainers' Association position statement. *Neurosurgery*. 2004; 55(4): 891–895.

170. Casa DJ, Guskiewicz KM, Anderson SA et al. National athletic trainers' association position statement: preventing sudden death in sports. *Journal of Athletic Training*. 2012; 47(1): 96–118.

171. Koo AH, LaRoque RL. Evaluation of head trauma by computed tomography. *Radiology*. 1977; 123(2): 345–350.

172. Buttram SD, Garcia-Filion P, Miller J et al. Computed tomography vs magnetic resonance imaging for identifying acute lesions in pediatric traumatic brain injury. *Hospital Pediatrics*. 2015; 5(2): 79–84.

173. Mehta H, Acharya J, Mohan AL, Tobias ME, LeCompte L, Jeevan D. Minimizing radiation exposure in evaluation of pediatric head trauma: use of rapid MR imaging. *AJNR American Journal of Neuroradiology*. 2016; 37(1): 11–18.

174. Roguski M, Morel B, Sweeney M et al. Magnetic resonance imaging as an alternative to computed tomography in select patients with traumatic brain injury: a retrospective comparison. *Journal of Neurosurgery Pediatrics*. 2015; 15(5): 529–534.

175. Carman AJ, Ferguson R, Cantu R et al. Expert consensus document: Mind the gaps-advancing research into short-term and long-term neuropsychological outcomes of youth sports-related concussions. *Nature Reviews Neurology*. 2015; 11(4): 230–244.

176. Chamard E, Lefebvre G, Lassonde M, Theoret H. Long-term abnormalities in the corpus callosum of female concussed athletes. *Journal of Neurotrauma*. 2016; 33(13): 1220–1226.

177. Dean PJ, Sato JR, Vieira G, McNamara A, Sterr A. Long-term structural changes after mTBI and their relation to post-concussion symptoms. *Brain Injury*. 2015: 1–8.

178. Orr CA, Albaugh MD, Watts R et al. Neuroimaging biomarkers of a history of concussion observed in asymptomatic young athletes. *Journal of Neurotrauma*. 2015.

179. Waljas M, Lange RT, Hakulinen U et al. Biopsychosocial outcome after uncomplicated mild traumatic brain injury. *Journal of Neurotrauma*. 2014; 31(1): 108–124.

180. Henry LC, Tremblay J, Tremblay S et al. Acute and chronic changes in diffusivity measures after sports concussion. *Journal of Neurotrauma*. 2011; 28(10): 2049–2059.

181. Helmer KG, Pasternak O, Fredman E et al. Hockey Concussion Education Project, Part 1. Susceptibility-weighted imaging study in male and female ice hockey players over a single season. *Journal of Neurosurgery*. 2014; 120(4): 864–872.

182. Mayer AR, Ling J, Mannell MV et al. A prospective diffusion tensor imaging study in mild traumatic brain injury. *Neurology*. 2010; 74(8): 643–650.

183. Miles L, Grossman RI, Johnson G, Babb JS, Diller L, Inglese M. Short-term DTI predictors of cognitive dysfunction in mild traumatic brain injury. *Brain Injury*. 2008; 22(2): 115–122.

184. Messe A, Caplain S, Paradot G et al. Diffusion tensor imaging and white matter lesions at the subacute stage in mild traumatic brain injury with persistent neurobehavioral impairment. *Human Brain Mapping*. 2011; 32(6): 999–1011.

185. Murugavel M, Cubon V, Putukian M et al. A longitudinal diffusion tensor imaging study assessing white matter fiber tracts after sports-related concussion. *Journal of Neurotrauma*. 2014; 31(22): 1860–1871.

186. Rutgers DR, Toulgoat F, Cazejust J, Fillard P, Lasjaunias P, Ducreux D. White matter abnormalities in mild traumatic brain injury: a diffusion tensor imaging study. *AJNR American Journal of Neuroradiology*. 2008; 29(3): 514–519.

187. Rutgers DR, Fillard P, Paradot G, Tadie M, Lasjaunias P, Ducreux D. Diffusion tensor imaging characteristics of the corpus callosum in mild, moderate, and severe traumatic brain injury. *AJNR American Journal of Neuroradiology*. 2008; 29(9): 1730–1735.

188. Pasternak O, Koerte IK, Bouix S et al. Hockey Concussion Education Project, Part 2. Microstructural white matter alterations in acutely concussed ice hockey players: a longitudinal free-water MRI study. *Journal of Neurosurgery*. 2014; 120(4): 873–881.

189. Sasaki T, Pasternak O, Mayinger M et al. Hockey Concussion Education Project, Part 3. White matter microstructure in ice hockey players with a history of concussion: a diffusion tensor imaging study. *Journal of Neurosurgery*. 2014; 120(4): 882–890.

190. Chong CD, Schwedt TJ. White matter damage and brain network alterations in concussed patients: a review of recent diffusion tensor imaging and resting-state functional connectivity data. *Current Pain and Headache Reports*. 2015; 19(5): 485.

191. Shin SS, Pathak S, Presson N et al. Detection of white matter injury in concussion using high-definition fiber tractography. *Progress in Neurological Surgery*. 2014; 28: 86–93.

192. Wozniak JR, Krach L, Ward E et al. Neurocognitive and neuroimaging correlates of pediatric traumatic brain injury: a diffusion tensor imaging (DTI) study. *Archives of Clinical Neuropsychology*. 2007; 22(5): 555–568.

193. Wilde EA, McCauley SR, Hunter JV et al. Diffusion tensor imaging of acute mild traumatic brain injury in adolescents. *Neurology*. 2008; 70(12): 948–955.

194. Toth A, Kovacs N, Perlaki G et al. Multimodal magnetic resonance imaging in the acute and sub-acute phase of mild traumatic brain injury: can we see the difference? *Journal of Neurotrauma*. 2013; 30(1): 2–10.

195. Virji-Babul N, Borich MR, Makan N et al. Diffusion tensor imaging of sports-related concussion in adolescents. *Pediatric Neurology*. 2013; 48(1): 24–29.

196. Metting Z, Cerliani L, Rodiger LA, van der Naalt J. Pathophysiological concepts in mild traumatic brain injury: diffusion tensor imaging related to acute perfusion CT imaging. *PLoS One*. 2013; 8(5): e64461.

197. Goswami R, Dufort P, Tartaglia MC et al. Frontotemporal correlates of impulsivity and machine learning in retired professional athletes with a history of multiple concussions. *Brain Structure and Function*. 2015.

198. Bazarian JJ, Zhu T, Zhong J et al. Persistent, long-term cerebral white matter changes after sports-related repetitive head impacts. *PLoS One*. 2014; 9(4): e94734.

199. Bazarian JJ, Zhu T, Blyth B, Borrino A, Zhong J. Subject-specific changes in brain white matter on diffusion tensor imaging after sports-related concussion. *Magnetic Resonance Imaging*. 2012; 30(2): 171–180.

200. McAllister TW, Ford JC, Flashman LA et al. Effect of head impacts on diffusivity measures in a cohort of collegiate contact sport athletes. *Neurology*. 2014; 82(1): 63–69.

201. Davenport EM, Whitlow CT, Urban JE et al. Abnormal white matter integrity related to head impact exposure in a season of high school varsity football. *Journal of Neurotrauma*. 2014; 31(19): 1617–1624.

202. Koerte IK, Ertl-Wagner B, Reiser M, Zafonte R, Shenton ME. White matter integrity in the brains of professional soccer players without a symptomatic concussion. *The Journal of the American Medical Association*. 2012; 308(18): 1859–1861.

203. Myer GD, Yuan W, Barber Foss KD et al. The effects of external jugular compression applied during head impact exposure on longitudinal changes in brain

neuroanatomical and neurophysiological biomarkers: a preliminary investigation. *Frontiers in Neurology.* 2016; 7: 74.

204. Myer GD, Yuan W, Barber Foss KD et al. Analysis of head impact exposure and brain microstructure response in a season-long application of a jugular vein compression collar: a prospective, neuroimaging investigation in American football. *British Journal of Sports Medicine.* 2016.

205. Stein SC, Ross SE. Mild head injury: a plea for routine early CT scanning. *The Journal of Trauma.* 1992; 33(1): 11–13.

206. Zyluk A, Mazur A, Piotuch B, Safranow K. Analysis of the reliability of clinical examination in predicting traumatic cerebral lesions and skull fractures in patients with mild and moderate head trauma. *Polski Przeglad Chirurgiczny.* 2013; 85(12): 699–705.

207. Albers CE, von Allmen M, Evangelopoulos DS, Zisakis AK, Zimmermann H, Exadaktylos AK. What is the incidence of intracranial bleeding in patients with mild traumatic brain injury? A retrospective study in 3088 Canadian CT head rule patients. *BioMed Research International.* 2013; 2013: 453978.

208. Borg J, Holm L, Cassidy JD et al. Diagnostic procedures in mild traumatic brain injury: results of the WHO Collaborating Centre Task Force on Mild Traumatic Brain Injury. *Journal of Rehabilitation Medicine.* 2004(43 Suppl): 61–75.

209. Bramley H, McFarland C, Lewis MM et al. Short-term outcomes of sport- and recreation-related concussion in patients admitted to a pediatric trauma service. *Clinical Pediatrics.* 2014; 53(8): 784–790.

210. Ellis MJ, Leiter J, Hall T et al. Neuroimaging findings in pediatric sports–related concussion. *Journal of Neurosurgery Pediatrics.* 2015; 16(3): 241–247.

211. McCrea HJ, Perrine K, Niogi S, Hartl R. Concussion in sports. *Sports Health.* 2013; 5(2): 160–164.

212. Atabaki SM. Updates in the general approach to pediatric head trauma and concussion.

Pediatric Clinics of North America. 2013; 60(5): 1107–1122.

213. Borg J, Holm L, Peloso PM et al. Non-surgical intervention and cost for mild traumatic brain injury: results of the WHO Collaborating Centre Task Force on Mild Traumatic Brain Injury. *Journal of Rehabilitation Medicine.* 2004(43 Suppl): 76–83.

214. Jagoda AS, Bazarian JJ, Bruns JJ, Jr. et al. Clinical policy: neuroimaging and decision-making in adult mild traumatic brain injury in the acute setting. *Annals of Emergency Medicine.* 2008; 52(6): 714–748.

215. Stiell IG, Wells GA, Vandemheen K et al. The Canadian CT Head Rule for patients with minor head injury. *Lancet (London, England).* 2001; 357(9266): 1391–1396.

216. Stiell IG, Lesiuk H, Wells GA et al. The Canadian CT Head Rule Study for patients with minor head injury: rationale, objectives, and methodology for phase I (derivation). *Annals of Emergency Medicine.* 2001; 38(2): 160–169.

217. Kavalci C, Aksel G, Salt O et al. Comparison of the Canadian CT head rule and the new orleans criteria in patients with minor head injury. *World Journal of Emergency Surgery.* 2014; 9: 31.

218. Stiell IG, Clement CM, Rowe BH et al. Comparison of the Canadian CT Head Rule and the New Orleans Criteria in patients with minor head injury. *The Journal of the American Medical Association.* 2005; 294(12): 1511–1518.

219. Smits M, Dippel DW, de Haan GG et al. External validation of the Canadian CT Head Rule and the New Orleans Criteria for CT scanning in patients with minor head injury. *The Journal of the American Medical Association.* 2005; 294(12): 1519–1525.

220. Schachar JL, Zampolin RL, Miller TS, Farinhas JM, Freeman K, Taragin BH. External validation of the New Orleans Criteria (NOC), the Canadian CT Head Rule (CCHR) and

the National Emergency X-Radiography Utilization Study II (NEXUS II) for CT scanning in pediatric patients with minor head injury in a non-trauma center. *Pediatric Radiology*. 2011; 41(8): 971–979.

221. Korley FK, Morton MJ, Hill PM et al. Agreement between routine emergency department care and clinical decision support recommended care in patients evaluated for mild traumatic brain injury. *Academic Emergency Medicine*. 2013; 20(5): 463–469.

222. Haydel MJ, Preston CA, Mills TJ, Luber S, Blaudeau E, DeBlieux PM. Indications for computed tomography in patients with minor head injury. *The New England Journal of Medicine*. 2000; 343(2): 100–106.

223. Osmond MH, Klassen TP, Wells GA et al. CATCH: a clinical decision rule for the use of computed tomography in children with minor head injury. *Canadian Medical Association Journal*. 2010; 182(4): 341–348.

224. Kuppermann N, Holmes JF, Dayan PS et al. Identification of children at very low risk of clinically-important brain injuries after head trauma: a prospective cohort study. *Lancet (London, England)*. 2009; 374(9696): 1160–1170.

225. Mihindu E, Bhullar I, Tepas J, Kerwin A. Computed tomography of the head in children with mild traumatic brain injury. *The American Surgeon*. 2014; 80(9): 841–843.

226. Faris G, Byczkowski T, Ho M, Babcock L. Prediction of persistent post-concussion symptoms in youth using a neuroimaging decision rule. *Academic Pediatrics*. 2015.

227. Dunning J, Daly JP, Lomas JP, Lecky F, Batchelor J, Mackway-Jones K. Derivation of the children's head injury algorithm for the prediction of important clinical events decision rule for head injury in children. *Archives of Disease in Childhood*. 2006; 91(11): 885–891.

228. Seddighi AS, Motiei-Langroudi R, Sadeghian H et al. Factors predicting early deterioration

in mild brain trauma: a prospective study. *Brain Injury*. 2013; 27(13–14): 1666–1670.

229. Ratcliff JJ, Adeoye O, Lindsell CJ et al. ED disposition of the Glasgow Coma Scale 13 to 15 traumatic brain injury patient: analysis of the Transforming Research and Clinical Knowledge in TBI study. *The American Journal of Emergency Medicine*. 2014; 32(8): 844–850.

230. Joseph B, Aziz H, Sadoun M et al. The acute care surgery model: managing traumatic brain injury without an inpatient neurosurgical consultation. *The Journal of Trauma and Acute Care Surgery*. 2013; 75(1): 102–105.

231. Overton TL, Shafi S, Cravens GF, Gandhi RR. Can trauma surgeons manage mild traumatic brain injuries? *American Journal of Surgery*. 2014; 208(5): 806–810.

232. McCammack KC, Sadler C, Guo Y, Ramaswamy RS, Farid N. Routine repeat head CT may not be indicated in patients on anticoagulant/antiplatelet therapy following mild traumatic brain injury. *The Western Journal of Emergency Medicine*. 2015; 16(1): 43–49.

233. Almenawer SA, Bogza I, Yarascavitch B et al. The value of scheduled repeat cranial computed tomography after mild head injury: single-center series and meta-analysis. *Neurosurgery*. 2013; 72(1): 56–62.

234. Rubino S, Zaman RA, Sturge CR et al. Outpatient follow-up of nonoperative cerebral contusion and traumatic subarachnoid hemorrhage: does repeat head CT alter clinical decision-making? *Journal of Neurosurgery*. 2014; 121(4): 944–949.

235. Simma B, Lutschg J, Callahan JM. Mild head injury in pediatrics: algorithms for management in the ED and in young athletes. *The American Journal of Emergency Medicine*. 2013; 31(7): 1133–1138.

236. Petraglia AL, Maroon JC, Bailes JE. From the field of play to the field of combat: a review of the pharmacological management

of concussion. *Neurosurgery.* 2012; 70(6): 1520–1533.

237. Mychasiuk R, Hehar H, van Waes L, Esser MJ. Diet, age, and prior injury status differentially alter behavioral outcomes following concussion in rats. *Neurobiology of Disease.* 2015; 73: 1–11.

238. Mychasiuk R, Hehar H, Ma I, Esser MJ. Dietary intake alters behavioral recovery and gene expression profiles in the brain of juvenile rats that have experienced a concussion. *Frontiers in Behavioral Neuroscience.* 2015; 9: 17.

239. Appelberg KS, Hovda DA, Prins ML. The effects of a ketogenic diet on behavioral outcome after controlled cortical impact injury in the juvenile and adult rat. *Journal of Neurotrauma.* 2009; 26(4): 497–506.

240. Tavender EJ, Bosch M, Gruen RL et al. Understanding practice: the factors that influence management of mild traumatic brain injury in the emergency department—a qualitative study using the Theoretical Domains Framework. *Implementation Science.* 2014; 9: 8.

241. Upchurch C, Morgan CD, Umfress A, Yang G, Riederer MF. Discharge instructions for youth sports-related concussions in the emergency department, 2004 to 2012. *Clinical Journal of Sport Medicine.* 2015; 25(3): 297–299.

242. Hwang V, Trickey AW, Lormel C et al. Are pediatric concussion patients compliant with discharge instructions? *The Journal of Trauma and Acute Care Surgery.* 2014; 77(1): 117–122.

243. Hartwell JL, Spalding MC, Fletcher B, O'Mara M S, Karas C. You cannot go home: routine concussion evaluation is not enough. *The American Surgeon.* 2015; 81(4): 395–403.

244. Bock S, Grim R, Barron TF et al. Factors associated with delayed recovery in athletes with concussion treated at a pediatric neurology concussion clinic. *Child's Nervous System.* 2015; 31(11): 2111–2116.

245. Benedict PA, Baner NV, Harrold GK et al. Gender and age predict outcomes of cognitive, balance and vision testing in a multidisciplinary concussion center. *Journal of the Neurological Sciences.* 2015; 353(1–2): 111–115.

246. Kinnaman KA, Mannix RC, Comstock RD, Meehan WP, 3rd. Management of pediatric patients with concussion by emergency medicine physicians. *Pediatric Emergency Care.* 2014; 30(7): 458–461.

247. Resch JE, Kutcher JS. The acute management of sport concussion in pediatric athletes. *Journal of Child Neurology.* 2015; 30(12): 1686–1694.

248. Makdissi M, Cantu RC, Johnston KM, McCrory P, Meeuwisse WH. The difficult concussion patient: what is the best approach to investigation and management of persistent (>10 days) postconcussive symptoms? *British Journal of Sports Medicine.* 2013; 47(5): 308–313.

249. Malhotra RK. Legal issues of return to play after a concussion. *Continuum (Minneapolis, Minn).* 2014; 20(6 Sports Neurology): 1688–1691.

CHAPTER 4

Severe head injuries

Introduction

A review of the National Center for Catastrophic Sports Injuries from 1990 to 2010 estimated that there are 1,205,000 high school and collegiate players participating in competitive football yearly.[1] Within that 20-year span, there were a total of 243 football fatalities, of those, 100 (41.2%) and 62 (25.5%) were of injuries involving the cerebrum. Therefore, within a 1-year period, there is a 0.0003% risk of death from a cranial injury while playing football. Though this may appear to be a small number, the ultimate goal is to reduce the annual fatality rate in football due to cerebral causes to zero.

Although this text's focus is on concussion, it is important to briefly discuss the continuum of head injuries involving those of a severe and even catastrophic nature. In general, TBI can be divided into diffuse (i.e., diffuse axonal injury) and focal injuries (i.e., intra and extraparenchymal hemorrhage). Though uncommon, because it is a diffuse injury, concussion can also include the presence of focal lesions. Within this chapter, we will introduce the various focal lesions and other post-traumatic sequela, such as seizures and arterial dissections, which can potentially occur following a concussion and further contribute to significant morbidity and mortality of the athlete. Lastly, we will discuss the entity of Second Impact Syndrome and describe its presentation, pathophysiology, and management.

Skull fractures

Skull fractures occur due to direct blunt trauma to the skull. The incidence of this type of injury in athletics has seen a dramatic reduction due to the implementation and improvement in protective equipment, specifically helmets. For example, in American football, the yearly fatality rate dropped from 9.5 (from 1945 to 1975) to 5–6 during the 1980s, likely due to the improvement in football helmets and the precipitous reduction in skull fractures.[1] Skull fractures can be characterized as depressed or comminuted if bony fragments extend into the cranial vault. Depressed skull fractures can further be subdivided into simple or complex, depending on whether the overlying scalp is closed or open. Skull fractures are rare in sports, but when they occur, they are usually as a result of player-to-ground collision or player-to-player collisions in nonhelmeted sports.

Athletes with a diagnosis of a skull fracture rarely present asymptomatically, and will more often display focal tenderness, edema (swelling), bruising (ecchymosis), or a deformity overlying the fracture site. Specific clinical exam findings also may help point to the location of fracture. Patients may develop "raccoon eyes" (bilateral periorbital ecchymosis) or "battle's sign" (ecchymosis behind the ear overlying the mastoid process) in the setting of basal skull fractures[2] (Figure 4.1). Ultimate diagnosis of a skull fracture is determined through a skull x-ray or head CT (Figure 4.2).

All skull fractures should involve consultation and evaluation by a neurosurgeon. Most commonly, athletes will present with a simple nondepressed skull fracture that can be managed conservatively with pain analgesia until the fracture heals. Surgical intervention for depressed skull fractures should be considered if the following criteria are present[3]:

◆ The skull is depressed greater than the calvarial thickness.
◆ Presence of cosmetic deformity.

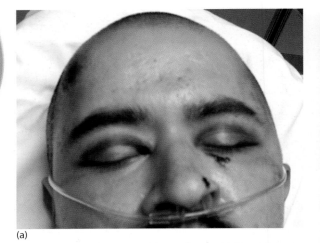

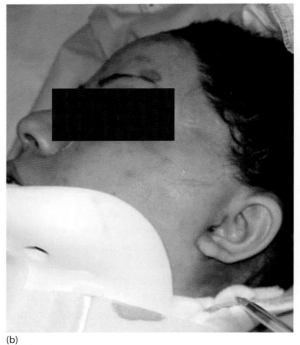

(a)

(b)

Figure 4.1 Typical "Raccoon's Eyes" and "Battle's sign" seen with skull base fractures. (a) "Raccoon's eyes." (From McPheeters RA et al. *West J Emerg Med.* Feb;11(1):97, 2010.) (b) "Battle sign." (From Sanaei-Zedeh H et al. *NZJM* May;122:1295, 2009. With permission New Zealand Medical Association.)

◆ Complex depressed fracture requiring debridement.

◆ A decline in neurological status that can be attributable to the presence of hematoma or skull fragments.

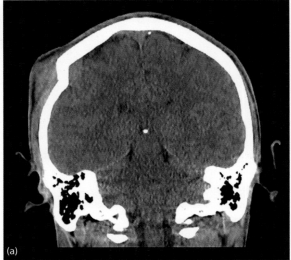

(a)

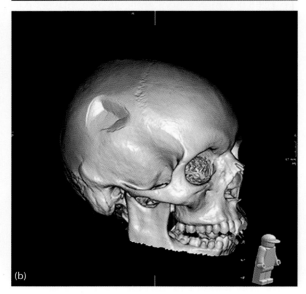

(b)

Figure 4.2 Depressed parietal skull fracture seen on noncontrast CT appreciated on (a) coronal plane and (b) 3-D reconstruct. (From Rincon S et al. *Handb Clin Neurol.* 135:447–77, 2016.)

◆ Concern for sinus injury or dural laceration involvement (CSF leak or presence of pneumocephalus).

Hemorrhagic contusion/traumatic intracerebral hemorrhage

A hemorrhagic contusion/traumatic intracerebral hemorrhage (TICH) occurs from a sudden acceleration/deceleration event causing the cerebrum to move or slosh, striking against the bony edges of the skull leading to hemorrhage. This may occur in a coup, directly adjacent to where the head was struck, or contrecoup, at the opposite side of the cerebrum (Figure 4.3). Over the course of 24–72 h, the contusion can evolve, becoming enlarged or hemorrhagic, and involve a larger portion of the cerebrum. Also, in up to 10% of patients with GCS<8, delayed intracerebral bleeding may occur as a result of a new hemorrhage extending into a previous injury site.[4] Depending on the location and size of the hemorrhage, the patient's condition may vary from being asymptomatic to being in a comatose state.

Definitive diagnosis of intracerebral hemorrhage requires visualization of a hyperdense (bright) lesion within the parenchyma on CT (Figure 4.4). Management of hemorrhagic contusions typically involve nonoperative measures unless there is progressive neurological deterioration, mass effect, medically refractory elevations in intracranial pressure (ICP) secondary to the TICH, or the TICH volume is greater than 50 cm, prompting surgical decompression and/or evacuation.[5]

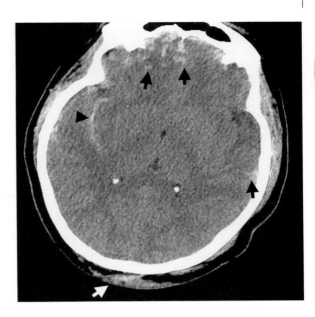

Figure 4.4 Bifrontal hemorrhagic contusions seen on a noncontrast axial CT following a blow to the occiput, as indicated by soft tissue swelling (white arrow), characteristic contrecoup hemorrhagic contusions are seen in the inferior frontal and temporal lobes (black arrows). Also note the subarachnoid hemorrhage SAH (arrowhead) in the right Sylvian fissure, which is a poor prognostic indicator. (From Kim JJ et al. *Neurotherapeutics.* Jan;8(1):39–53, 2011.)

Traumatic subarachnoid hemorrhage

Traumatic subarachnoid hemorrhage (tSAH) is hemorrhage resulting from tearing of blood vessels that are present within the space between the pia and dura mater (Figure 4.5). Though trauma is the most common cause of subarachnoid hemorrhage, it may also occur due to arterial aneurysmal rupture. However, the location of hemorrhage due to arterial aneurismal rupture is classically located in the basilar cisterns and Sylvian fissure, which usually differs from tSAH location (high cortical convexity). tSAH is typically associated with more severe head injury, however a study by Deepika et al. showed that in a cohort of 1149 mTBI patients, isolated tSAH had no influence on overall outcomes at 1 year.[6]

Patients may be asymptomatic on presentation with tSAH or complain of headache, nausea, vomiting, or have a spectrum of neurological

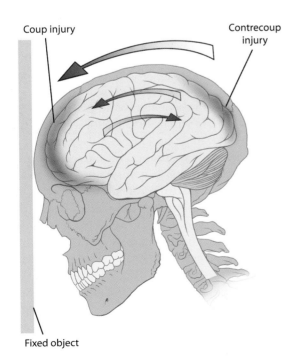

Coup injury

Contrecoup injury

Fixed object

Figure 4.3 Depiction of coup (adjacent) and contrecoup (opposite) injury.

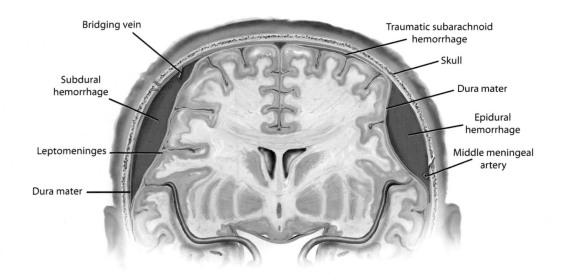

Figure 4.5 Cartoon depiction of location and cause of traumatic subarachnoid hemorrhage, subdural hematoma, and epidural hematoma.

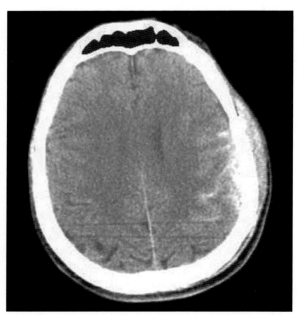

Figure 4.6 Left cortical traumatic subarachnoid hemorrhage seen on a noncontrast axial CT. (From Rincon S et al. *Handb Clin Neurol.* 135:447–77, 2016.)

deficits depending on the extent of injury or location. CT imaging of the head will display a thin hyperdense lesion in the supratentorial cortical area, unlike aneurysmal SAH that exists within the deep cisterns or Sylvian fissure (Figure 4.6). Though tSAH may expand, usually in the presence of anticoagulants, they are rarely symptomatic and management is conservative in nature.[7]

Epidural hematoma

An epidural hematoma, EDH, usually occurs due to a fracture in the squamous portion of the temporal bone causing laceration to the underlying middle meningeal artery, or less commonly a dural sinus. Blood then accumulates within the space between the dura mater and calvarium (Figure 4.5).

The classic presentation of an EDH involves a lucid interval after injury that follows with a dramatic decline in consciousness. Depending on the size, rate of expansion, and intracranial anatomy, patients may have a varying clinical exam. Therefore the spectrum of presentation of an EDH may vary from either the patient being fully awake and alert to even being obtunded or in a comatose state. For example, as an EDH expands, the uncus can get pushed against the oculomotor nerve (causing ipsilateral pupillary dilation), the ipsilateral cerebral peduncle (causing contralateral hemiparesis), and the brainstem (leading to coma, respiratory apnea, and subsequent death) (Figure 4.7). As a variant, the brainstem may be pushed far enough that the contralateral cerebral peduncle squeezes against the tentorium causing ipsilateral hemiparesis, termed "Kernahan's notch."

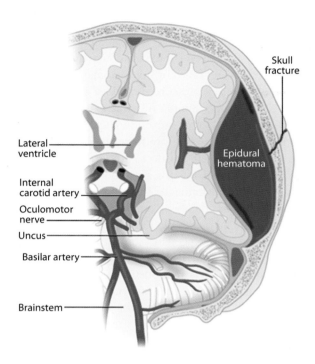

Figure 4.7 Uncal herniation with compression of the ipsilateral oculomotor nerve and cerebral peduncle of the brainstem due to mass effect from a left-sided epidural hematoma. (From Wright DW, Merck LH. Head trauma in adults and children. Chapter 254. In: Tintinalli JE, Stapczynski J, Ma O, Cline DM, Cydulka RK, Meckler GD, T. eds. *Tintinalli's Emergency Medicine: A Comprehensive Study Guide*, 7e. New York, NY: McGraw-Hill, 2011.)

Imaging of an EDH is significant for a hyperdense convex/lentiform shaped lesion adjacent to the skull that usually does not extend beyond skull sutures (Figure 4.8). With immediate recognition and surgical intervention, the mortality for EDH is 12%.[8] Any patient with neurological symptoms should have surgical evacuation of the EDH via craniotomy. If the patient is neurologically intact an EDH should still be considered to be surgically managed if[9]:

◆ EDH > 15 mm in thickness
◆ Midline shift > 5 mm
◆ Volume > 30 cm³

Subdural hematoma

A subdural hematoma, SDH, is caused by an acceleration/deceleration moment of the brain that leads

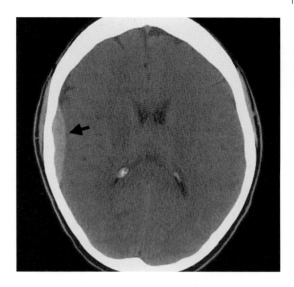

Figure 4.8 Axial noncontrast CT in brain windows shows a lentiform, high attenuation collection (arrow) adjacent to the right temporal lobe, consistent with an epidural hematoma caused by injury to a branch of the middle meningeal artery. (From Kim JJ et al. *Neurotherapeutics.* Jan;8(1):39–53, 2011.)

to tearing of bridging veins or formation of parenchymal lesions and accumulation of blood underneath the dura mater (Figure 4.5). Likely as a result of improvement in cranial protection and reduction in skull fractures, a SDH is now three times more likely than an epidural hematoma.[10] Unlike EDHs, SDHs typically do not have a lucid interval and in general present with poorer neurological exams due to the underlying parenchymal injury. For this reason, SDH also typically have worse outcomes than EDH. With prompt surgical evacuation (<4 h from injury), the mortality from a SDH is <30% but if the evacuation is delayed >4 h, the mortality dramatically rises to 90%.[11] For this reason, prompt evaluation and determination for need for surgical intervention is paramount to mortality reduction.

A SDH is distinct from an EDH because there is no structural limitation to the blood spreading along the hemisphere; this is what gives it a hyperdense concave/crescent shape adjacent to the brain parenchyma on clinical imaging (Figure 4.9). Neurosurgical consultation should be obtained to determine the surgical intervention is needed for SDH if[12]:

◆ Poor neurological status or decline in GCS by two points related to SDH

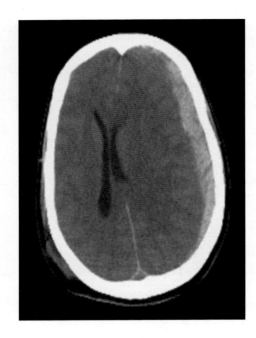

Figure 4.9 Typical concave shaped left-sided acute subdural hematoma seen on noncontrast axial CT. (From Rincon S et al. *Handb Clin Neurol.* 135:447–77, 2016.)

- SDH > 10 mm in thickness
- Midline shift > 5 mm
- Pupillary changes (dilated and fixed)
- ICP elevation that is refractory to medical management

Management of focal mass lesions

All of the above mass lesions require similar prehospital and hospital management guided by the 2007 recommendations in the American Association of Neurological Surgeons and Congress of Neurological Surgeons, and more recently released guidelines by the American College of Surgeons in 2015.[13,14] It is recommended for the reader to refer to these publications for a more thorough discussion of management of severe brain injury.

The management approach to a patient with severe brain injury is to determine the extent of injury, need for surgical intervention (as detailed above for each lesion), and to prevent further injury through medical and surgical means. The focus of initial management should be to avoid hypoxia (goal: maintain O_2 saturation greater than 95%), hypotension (goal: systolic blood pressure >100 mmHg),

hypoglycemia (goal: glucose 80–180 mg/dL), and hypocarbia (goal: PCO_2 35–45).[14] Maintaining these parameters has been shown to reduce negative outcomes in severe TBI. Further, management of elevated intracranial pressure should be executed in a graded approach. Simple measures such as raising the head of the bed or preventing neck constriction, facilitating venous outflow from the brain, should be initial steps. If unsuccessful, the therapeutic escalation should involve sedation and/or analgesia, ventricular drainage, mannitol or hypertonic saline, muscular paralysis, and barbiturate coma.[13,14] Prophylactic hyperventilation has been shown to reduce cerebral oxygenation and therefore should only be used as a temporary emergent measure in a patient who is demonstrating active cerebral herniation syndrome. Patients with structural injury on head CT and a GCS score of 3–8 often require ICP monitoring. Also, level 3 guidelines recommend that those with severe TBI, but with a normal CT scan, should still receive ICP monitoring if the patient presents[13] with: (see Figure 4.10)

- Age greater than 40 years
- Posturing on neurological examination
- Episode of systolic blood pressure below 90 mmHg

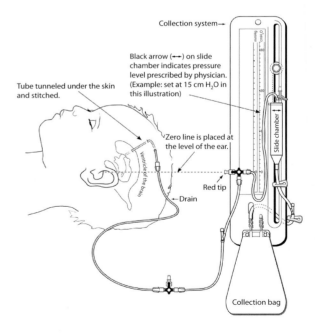

Figure 4.10 External ventricular drain for cerebrospinal fluid drainage.

If the increase in intracranial pressure is not successfully managed medically, then consideration is given for surgical decompression. An Australian randomized controlled study, "DECRA," was published in 2011 and showed that patients with increased ICP that were managed with surgical intervention did have a reduction in ICP, however, did not show improvements in 6-month mortality compared to those without surgical intervention.[15] Therefore, this study questioned the usefulness of decompression in those patients with elevated ICP.[15] This study has received great criticism due to dissimilar neurological examinations between the two cohorts, a high crossover rate to surgical intervention, and divergent management in comparison to clinical practice.[16] A more recent randomized controlled study, Randomized Evaluation of Surgery with Craniectomy for Uncontrollable Elevation of Intracranial Pressure or "RESCUEicp," has finalized recruitment and results are currently pending.[17]

Arterial dissection

In athletics, an arterial dissection can occur due to rapid hyperextension/rotation of the neck or even from direct blunt trauma (Figure 4.11). Usually involving a high cervical carotid or vertebral artery, a layer within the wall of a blood vessel, tunica intima, tears away from the more inner layer, tunica media. People with increased risk of developing an arterial dissection are those with a hereditary condition (like Ehlers-Danlos, Marfan, Autosomal Dominant Polycystic Kidney disease, osteogenesis imperfecta), hypertension, diabetes, hyperlipidemia, or recent migraine.[18] The most concerning aspect of arterial dissection is that it causes narrowing of the blood vessel, which in turn reduces distal blood flow and can also cause plaque formation with subsequent distal embolization causing a stroke (Figure 4.12).

Suwanwela et al. published that 18.6% of moderate to severe TBI patients had the presence of an internal carotid dissection.[19] Presumably, the incidence in sports is dramatically lower, but there is currently no published data other than case reports. Numerous case studies have been published for both internal carotid and vertebral

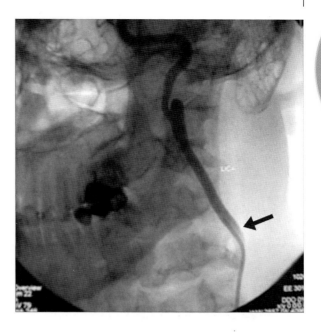

Figure 4.11 Carotid artery dissection seen on a lateral projeciton.

artery dissections causing strokes among athletes participating in rugby,[20,21] scuba diving,[22,23] wake boarding,[24] jogging,[25] taekwondo,[26] swimming/diving,[18,27] soccer,[28,29] kick boxing,[30] baseball/softball,[18,31] and weightlifting,[18] leading to significant morbidity and even mortality.

Typical presentation is dependent on the location of the dissection. Vertebral artery dissections tend to present immediately while carotid dissections develop symptoms roughly 1 to 24 h following the intimal tear.[2,18] Injury to the carotid artery can be asymptomatic, with pain only, or be manifested by more pronounced neurological symptoms like aphasia, hemiparesis/plegia, sensory difficulties, or Horner's syndrome (anhydrosis, miosis, and ptosis resulting from injury of the sympathetic plexus that surrounds the carotid artery; see Figure 4.13). Similarly, vertebral artery injury can present asymptomatically, with headache (classically at the base of the skull), or with ataxia, poor coordination, nystagmus, swallowing difficulties, hemiparesis/plegia, nystagmus, or Horner's syndrome due to involvement of the brainstem, cranial nerve nuclei, and cerebellum. Presentation with any one of these symptoms warrants arterial imaging with either MRI or CT

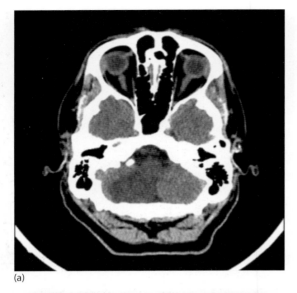

(a)

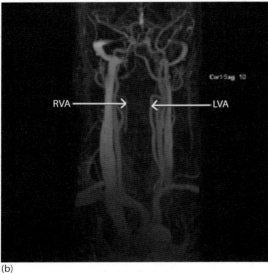

(b)

Figure 4.12 **Vertebral artery dissection causing distal embolic stroke.** (a) Computed tomography scan of the brain showing right posterior inferior cerebellar artery infarct. (b) Magnetic resonance angiography showing vertebral artery dissection (anterior perspective). LVA, left vertebral artery; RVA, right vertebral artery. (Slowey M et al. Case report on vertebral artery dissection in mixed martial arts. *Emerg Med Australas.* 2012 Apr;24. (2):203–6. Copyright Wiley-VCH Verlag GmbH & Co. KGaA. Reproduced with permission.)

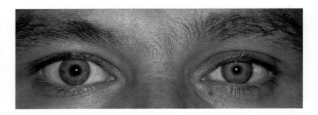

Figure 4.13 **Left sided Horner's syndrome.** Characterized by ptosis (drooping eyelid), miosis (small pupil), and anhydrosis (absence of sweating) to one side of the face. (From Mazzucco S, Rizzuto N. *Neurology.* Mar 14;66(5):E19, 2006.)

angiography. Diagnosis of an arterial dissection requires the patient to receive either medical therapy (antiplatelet or anticoagulation), or in some cases endovascular stenting depending on the nature of the dissection.

Seizures

The presence of seizures following a brain injury have been shown to be prevalent, especially in cases of severe TBI. Arndt et al. studied a cohort of mild to severe pediatric TBI ICU patients and found that 43% had ictal events on electroencephalogram (EEG) while inpatient.[32] Through staggering high in severe TBI, limited data exists with regards to the incidence of seizures in mTBI, and more specifically, in sports-related concussions immediately following injury and also at long term follow. In a review of 102 video-recorded concussions in an Australian football league, there were a total of 25 athletes with tonic posturing and 6 with clonic posturing immediately after impact.[33] Gilad et al. reported that in 2005 patients who suffered from a "whiplash injury/mTBI" from either a fall or motor vehicle accident, 0.18% of them were found to develop seizures at 1-year follow-up.[34] These two examples only give a small glimpse into the prevalence of post traumatic seizures and epilepsy in sports related concussion. It has been postulated through preclinical models that post-traumatic seizures and epilepsy occur due to neuronal excitability from metabolic derangements, cellular edema, and cerebral scar formation along with alterations in inhibitory interneurons and sprouting of hyperexcitable neurons.[35–39]

When determining the management of seizures, it is important to differentiate ictal events with relation to the time from injury. Ictal events that occur upon impact, or during the early post-traumatic period are handled differently than late post-traumatic seizures. Impact seizures, also termed "convulsive motor phenomena or tonic posturing," occur directly following a concussive blow to the head that results in loss of consciousness with the seizure episode lasting less than a minute. This benign single event does not have any correlation to the severity of concussive injury or development of epilepsy, and therefore has not been recommended to warrant the initiation of anticonvulsants medications. But, if the seizure reoccurs or happens days following injury, then antiepileptic medications should be instituted.[37,40,41] Interestingly, the occurrence of an impact seizure has been demonstrated to increase the risk of postconcussive syndrome (PCS).[42,43] Heidari et al. determined in a group of 176 mTBI patients that the presence of impact seizures following an injury increased the risk of PCS sixfold at 1 month.[43]

For moderate to severe TBI, patients may develop immediate seizures (occurring within 24 h from injury), early post-traumatic seizures (within 1 week from injury), and late post-traumatic seizures (greater than 1 week from injury). Current consensus guidelines recommend the prophylactic use of phenytoin/fosphenytoin for 1 week following severe TBI in all patients in efforts to reduce the risk of immediate and early post-traumatic seizures.[13,44] Phenytoin is only given for 1 week because clinical studies have observed a limited effect of phenytoin on late post-traumatic seizures and also has been associated with long-term detrimental cognitive effects.[45,46] Other preclinical (animal) and clinical TBI research has shown similar efficacy in seizure prevention with Levetiracetam, being advantageous as this antiepileptic medication has a better side-effect profile than phenytoin.[47,48] Any patient that develops clinical seizures, or is found to have ictal events on EEG, will require standard medical therapy for seizure management, as well as an evaluation by a neurologist. It is important to note that the risk of epilepsy following a concussive injury is rather low and therefore, any patient

with poorly controlled epilepsy following concussion should be evaluated for pseudoseizures.[49] Pseudoseizures, also known as nonepileptic or psychogenic seizures, are characterized as clinically appearing like a seizure, however they do not have the abnormal electrical activity seen on EEG.

Second impact syndrome

Introduction

There is substantial preclinical evidence that following a concussive injury, neurons are thrown into a metabolically disturbed state where further injury is detrimental to their recovery.[50–62] Case reports describe players sustaining even very mild head trauma shortly after an initial concussive injury loading to a hyperemic state of vascular dysregulation, substantial vasodilation, and cerebral edema, ultimately causing cerebral herniation and death, often within minutes.[63–68] This has been termed as Second Impact Syndrome (SIS), also known as malignant cerebral edema. A review by Cantu et al. from 1980 to 1993 documented a total of 35 probable cases of SIS.[63]

Presentation

Case reports have noted that second impact syndrome occurs when a player sustains an initial concussive injury and subsequently returns to contact sport prior to resolution of symptoms or complete recovery from the initial concussion. The athlete may be subjected to either a high impact force or even a very minor tackle or blow to the head causing initiation of this lethal cascade of events. The player may stand up after the incident and even walk to the side lines complaining of headache and/or vomiting, but within minutes, collapses to the ground. Upon initial evaluation, the athlete is found to have symptoms of cerebral herniation: comatose state, blown/nonreactive pupils, and respiratory failure.[68,69] Of all the reviewed cases, SIS tends to be observed in adolescent to young adult males occurring roughly within 4 weeks from initial injury, and has been seen in the sports of football, boxing, rugby, and karate.[64,68,70,71]

Pathophysiology

To understand the theory behind SIS, it is important to review the basics of vascular autoregulation of the brain. As systemic blood pressure decreases, cerebral oxygenation is reduced, and arterial CO_2 increases. The cerebral vasculature has an important physiological response to this change in efforts to provide continuous oxygenation with minimal fluctuations. In more detail, as the partial pressure of CO_2 increases, the cerebral vessels dilate resulting in increased blood flow to the brain, ensuring stable oxygen delivery (Figure 4.14). The brain protects itself from fluctuations in systemic blood pressure through this intrinsic property of cerebral vasculature.[72,73]

Following mTBI, this autoregulatory vascular response is impaired and believed to be a contributor to the symptoms following concussion, like headaches.[72–92] Both clinical studies in mTBI and sports concussion have demonstrated loss of this autoregulation from 31 h to 2 months after injury with recovery by 1 year, assessed by both ultrasonic and fMRI techniques.[74,75,88,89,93] Interestingly, Junger et al. studied mTBI patients 48 h after injury to demonstrate this alteration was present in up to 28% of individuals. It is believed that this abnormal vascular autoregulatory physiology, following an initial concussion, then causes an altered response with a second blow to the head that perpetuates massive vascular engorgement and substantial cerebral edema (Figure 4.14).[2,64,65,69,94] Ultimately, this state of dysautoregulation and hyperperfusion leads to cerebral herniation, respiratory arrest, and death.

"First impact" syndrome

It is important to note that SIS is an incredibly rare phenomenon that is poorly understood due to the lack of sound clinical evidence. In a team composed of 50 players, it would take 4100 seasons for one case of SIS to be seen.[68] Even in Australian

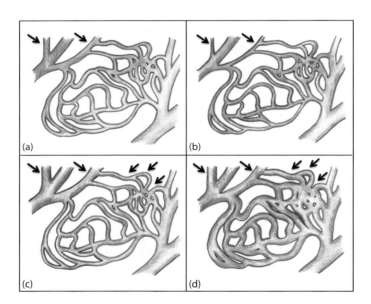

Figure 4.14 **Autoregulation of brain arterioles and pathophysiology.** Baseline (a): When blood pressure is normal, brain arteriole blood vessels are neither constricted nor dilated. Increased blood pressure. (b): The brain seeks to maintain constant blood flow. The brain arteriole blood vessels constrict. Decreased blood pressure (c): As pressure falls, brain arteriole dilation occurs. Blood flow to the brain remains unchanged. Dysautoregulation or second impact syndrome (d): A serious disruption occurs. The brain acts as if blood pressure is low when it is not low; it is normal or may be elevated. Brain arteriole blood vessels dilate and blood rushes in the brain and results in a massive rise in intracranial pressure. Within minutes, the brain can herniate, resulting in coma. (Montenigro PH, Bernick C, Cantu RC. Clinical features of repetitive traumatic brain injury and chronic traumatic encephalopathy. *Brain Pathol.* 2015 May;25(3). 304–17. Copyright Wiley-VCH Verlag GmbH & Co. KGaA. Reproduced with permission.)

football, where the concussion risk is higher than American football, there is a paucity of literature of SIS.[66,95] There is also a lack of European literature on SIS in boxing, in which the athlete receives countless blows to the head.[66,69,95] Though not outright refuted, authors have emphasized caution in assigning the diagnosis of SIS and the importance of thorough documentation of athletes' initial concussion in order to better understand the link

between the two.[68] This thorough documentation is important because it will allow us to better understand whether this catastrophic brain injury is truly a result of a 'second impact' to the brain, or, if it is an isolated entity which can occur upon first impact.

Upon review of nationwide cases and recent news reports, we noted that not all of these catastrophic brain injuries were preceded by a

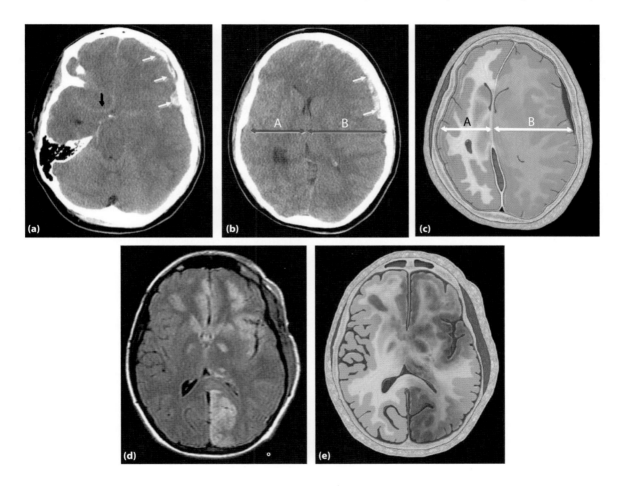

Figure 4.15 Typical imaging findings of dysautoregulation/second-impact syndrome (DSIS). (a and b) Admission noncontrast axial CT images, and (c) artist's rendition demonstrate a small heterogeneous left frontal subdural hematoma (SDH; white arrows), that causes complete effacement of the basal cisterns and brainstem distortion. Note the subtle linear increased density in the region of the circle of Willis (black arrow), consistent with "pseudo-subarachnoid hemorrhage," resulting from the marked elevation in intracranial pressure. Although there is preservation of the gray–white matter differentiation, there is asymmetric enlargement of the left hemisphere, consistent with hyperemic cerebral swelling (dysautoregulation). Note how side A is smaller than side B, even though the left hemisphere is mildly compressed by the overlying SDH. The extent of mass effect and midline shift is disproportional to the volume of the SDH (compare with Figures 4.3 and 4.4). This 3-day-postoperative FLAIR MR image (d), and the artist's rendition (e), demonstrate bilateral multifocal ischemic lesions involving several vascular territories, including the left posterior cerebral artery, thalamus, insular cortex, basal ganglia, and orbitofrontal cortex. Diffusion-weighted MR images were positive for acute ischemic injury, and the gradient-echo sequence excluded hemorrhage in these areas (not shown).

documented concussion. This could either be due to poor documentation of the initial concussion, or, as mentioned above, bring light to another entity of its own. Further, malignant brain edema following TBI in children, without need for a previous injury, is a known phenomenon.[94] Therefore, it may be appropriate to consider this pathophysiological entity to occur following one initial injury due to either age related physiology or genetics, not requiring a "priming" initial concussion, and therefore properly termed "First Impact Syndrome."[96]

A single initial impact can cause a transient increase in ICP and reduction in cerebral blood flow.[97,98] This signals the vasculature to compensate through increasing blood flow with vasodilation; but due to the impaired vascular response, a massive hyperemic state occurs leading to profound brain edema and herniation.[71,99–101] Therefore, without proper documentation of a patient's exposure to a first concussion, it may be more plausible and appropriate to use the term "First Impact Syndrome" in those athletes with a similar clinical picture but without a previous history of concussion.

Imaging

Neuroimaging is significant for immense cerebral edema (sulcal effacement, obliteration of cisterns, and cerebral herniation) and usually small subdural or traumatic subarachnoid hemorrhages, possibly an epiphenomenon, out of proportion to the extensive cerebral shift that is present (Figure 4.15).[64,70,71,102] Weinstein et al. published a case report where a player received imaging following the first concussion and then subsequently after the second injury that instigated SIS. It is important to note that the initial head CT was negative for any mass lesion to account for or precipitate the later SIS.[102]

Clinical management

Management of SIS entails placement of an advanced airway in the setting of impending central respiratory failure and an ICP monitoring device if GCS is less than 8.[69] Similar to the tiered approach to managing ICP of a space-occupying lesion, SIS will likely require a similar but more aggressive escalation of care. Measures to alleviate ICP include patient positioning (with head elevated and ensuring nothing is constricting the neck), aggressive hyperosmolar therapy (hypertonic saline and/or mannitol), sedation, acute hyperventilation (if signs of herniation), and possible surgical decompression.[13] A case report by Potts et al. demonstrated how aggressive ICP lowering techniques resulted in a nonfatal outcome of SIS.[103] Nevertheless, even with aggressive measures, SIS has been shown to have up to 50% mortality and 100% morbidity.[104]

Prevention

In a review of the National Center for Catastrophic Sports Injuries from 1989 to 2002, there were a total of 8 deaths per year from 94 severe head injuries in football.[105] Of these deaths, 59% of the deceased players had a previous history of head injury, and of those, 71% of these occurred within the same season. It was also found that 39% of these players were playing with residual concussive symptoms at the time of death.[105] An even more recent review of catastrophic sports injuries from 1990 to 2010 found that 16.1% of deceased players had a history of a concussion within 1 month of their death.[1] As these figures indicate, there appears to be a correlation between early return to play and catastrophic events, but with such a low occurrence, it has been difficult to make any definitive conclusions. Due to the rapid and highly fatal nature of this process, focus has been directed on determining proper return to play guidelines in order to help prevent the occurrence of SIS.[68] The difficulty with our current evidence is that there exist many gaps in our knowledge concerning measures for recovery and proper determination for return to activity.

Conclusion

Though a rarity, catastrophic head injuries do occur in competitive sports. For this reason, it is important for those managing concussion to be aware of the different entities that can occur following a blunt head impact. Only through appropriate use of sport-specific equipment, appropriate preparedness by onfield medical personnel, responding EMS, and emergency medical physicians, the establishment of appropriate return to activity recommendations, and proper

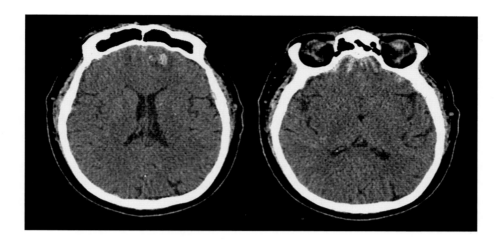

Figure 4.16 Axial CT scans of a 17-year-old boy with bifrontal cerebral contusions after single impact.

education to student athletes and parents, can the prevalence of catastrophic injuries in sports be reduced.

Case studies

Case 1

A 17-year-old high school football player sustained a single head impact after tackling an opponent.

He had progressive headache and subsequently collapsed, but remained awake. On presentation to the emergency department, his CT head was significant for bifrontal cerebral contusions prompting inpatient admission (Figure 4.16). During hospitalization, the patient remained neurologically intact and did not require any aggressive medical or surgical interventions. Within 3 days, all of the player's symptoms resolved. But, due to the hemorrhagic

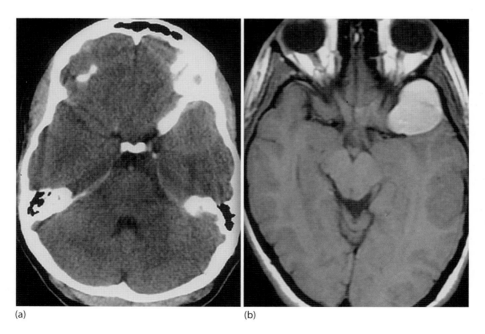

(a)　　　　　　　　　(b)

Figure 4.17 (a) CT scan showing the left middle cranial fossa with a mildly hyperdense lesion representing hemorrhage within a temporal arachnoid cyst. (b) T1-weighted magnetic resonance imaging scan delineating the hemorrhagic cyst. (From Prabhu VC, Bailes JE. *Neurosurgery.* Jan;50(1):195–7, 2002.)

injury, he was prohibited from return to football or other contact activities.

Case 2

A high school female soccer athlete headed the ball during a routine play in a competition, causing her to be "stunned" but not lose consciousness. After evaluation, she was removed from play and received an uncomplicated, prompt graded return to activity. Unfortunately, 6 weeks after the incident, the player developed an acute onset seizure with right-sided numbness. CT brain imaging demonstrated a large subdural hematoma resulting from a ruptured arachnoid cyst (Figure 4.17). An arachnoid cyst is filled with cerebrospinal fluid encased within a layer of arachnoid. This usually asymptomatic, benign lesion is commonly found incidentally but may cause subdural hematomas due to bridging veins being draped over the cyst wall. Due to the patient's neurological deficits, a craniotomy was performed to remove the hematoma and fenestrate the cyst wall. Despite her full recovery, she did not return to soccer.

Case 3

A 17-year-old high school football player was hit when returning a kick-off during a game. He walked off the field and shortly thereafter,

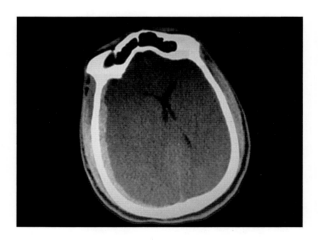

Figure 4.18 Legend: Axial CT scan of a 17-year-old boy with a large right subdural hematoma with midline shift due to a major blunt force head impact in football. (From Bailes J et al. *J Neurosurg Pediatr.* Jan;19(1):116–121, 2017.)

vomited and collapsed. Intubation and successful cardiopulmonary resuscitation was performed enroute when patient noted to be pulseless. Initial neurological assessment demonstrated fixed and dilated pupils and minimal movement to stimulation. Medical measures to reduce intracranial pressure were instituted. The patient's CT head was significant for a right-sided subdural hematoma with diffuse cerebral edema (Figure 4.18). Shortly thereafter, the patient was found to have pulseless electrical activity. Following repeated rounds of unsuccessful CPR, the patient was declared dead of important note, the player's family denied any known recent history of concussive injuries, therefore suggestive of "First Impact Syndrome."

References

1. Boden BP, Breit I, Beachler JA, Williams A, Mueller FO. Fatalities in high school and college football players. *The American Journal of Sports Medicine*. 2013; 41(5): 1108–1116.

2. Morris SA, Jones WH, Proctor MR, Day AL. Emergent treatment of athletes with brain injury. *Neurosurgery*. 2014; 75 Suppl 4: S96–s105.

3. Bullock MR, Chesnut R, Ghajar J et al. Surgical management of depressed cranial fractures. *Neurosurgery*. 2006; 58(3 Suppl): S56–60; discussion Si–iv.

4. Gudeman SK, Kishore PR, Miller JD, Girevendulis AK, Lipper MH, Becker DP. The genesis and significance of delayed traumatic intracerebral hematoma. *Neurosurgery*. 1979; 5(3): 309–313.

5. Bullock MR, Chesnut R, Ghajar J et al. Surgical management of traumatic parenchymal lesions. *Neurosurgery*. 2006; 58(3 Suppl): S25–46; discussion Si–iv.

6. Deepika A, Munivenkatappa A, Devi BI, Shukla D. Does isolated traumatic subarachnoid hemorrhage affect outcome in patients with mild traumatic brain injury? *The Journal of Head Trauma Rehabilitation*. 2013; 28(6): 442–445.

7. Albers CE, von Allmen M, Evangelopoulos DS, Zisakis AK, Zimmermann H, Exadaktylos AK. What is the incidence of intracranial bleeding in patients with mild traumatic brain injury? A retrospective study in 3088 Canadian CT head rule patients. *BioMed Research International*. 2013; 2013: 453978.

8. Rivas JJ, Lobato RD, Sarabia R, Cordobes F, Cabrera A, Gomez P. Extradural hematoma: analysis of factors influencing the courses of 161 patients. *Neurosurgery*. 1988; 23(1): 44–51.

9. Bullock MR, Chesnut R, Ghajar J et al. Surgical management of acute epidural hematomas. *Neurosurgery*. 2006; 58(3 Suppl): S7–15; discussion Si–iv.

10. Warren WL, Jr., Bailes JE. On the field evaluation of athletic head injuries. *Clinics in Sports Medicine*. 1998; 17(1): 13–26.

11. Seelig JM, Becker DP, Miller JD, Greenberg RP, Ward JD, Choi SC. Traumatic acute subdural hematoma: major mortality reduction in comatose patients treated within four hours. *The New England Journal of Medicine*. 1981; 304(25): 1511–1518.

12. Bullock MR, Chesnut R, Ghajar J et al. Surgical management of acute subdural hematomas. *Neurosurgery*. 2006; 58(3 Suppl): S16–24; discussion Si–iv.

13. Guidelines for the management of severe traumatic brain injury. *Journal of Neurotrauma*. 2007; 24 Suppl 1: S1–106.

14. Surgeons ACo. Best Practices in the management of Traumatic Brain Injury. *TQIP*. 2015: 30.

15. Cooper DJ, Rosenfeld JV, Murray L et al. Decompressive craniectomy in diffuse traumatic brain injury. *The New England Journal of Medicine*. 2011; 364(16): 1493–1502.

16. Honeybul S, Ho KM, Lind CR. What can be learned from the DECRA study. *World Neurosurgery*. 2013; 79(1): 159–161.

17. Hutchinson PJ, Corteen E, Czosnyka M et al. Decompressive craniectomy in traumatic brain injury: the randomized multicenter RESCUEicp study (http: //www.rescueicp .com/). *Acta Neurochirurgica Supplement*. 2006; 96: 17–20.

18. Dharmasaroja P, Dharmasaroja P. Sports-related internal carotid artery dissection: pathogenesis and therapeutic point of view. *The Neurologist*. 2008; 14(5): 307–311.

19. Suwanwela C, Suwanwela N. Intracranial arterial narrowing and spasm in acute head injury. *Journal of Neurosurgery*. 1972; 36(3): 314–323.

20. Miyata M, Yamasaki S, Hirayama A, Tamaki N. Traumatic middle cerebral artery occlusion. *No Shinkei Geka Neurological Surgery*. 1994; 22(3): 253–257.

21. Cuellar TA, Lottenberg L, Moore FA. Blunt cerebrovascular injury in rugby and other contact sports: case report and review of the literature. *World Journal of Emergency Surgery: WJES*. 2014; 9: 36.

22. Skurnik YD, Sthoeger Z. Carotid artery dissection after scuba diving. *The Israel Medical Association Journal: IMAJ*. 2005; 7(6): 406–407.

23. Hafner F, Gary T, Harald F, Pilger E, Groell R, Brodmann M. Dissection of the internal carotid artery after SCUBA-diving: a case report and review of the literature. *The Neurologist*. 2011; 17(2): 79–82.

24. Fridley J, Mackey J, Hampton C, Duckworth E, Bershad E. Internal carotid artery dissection and stroke associated with wakeboarding. *Journal of Clinical Neuroscience*. 2011; 18(9): 1258–1260.

25. Macdonald DJ, McKillop EC. Carotid artery dissection after treadmill running. *British Journal of Sports Medicine*. 2006; 40(4): e10.

26. Pary LF, Rodnitzky RL. Traumatic internal carotid artery dissection associated with taekwondo. *Neurology*. 2003; 60(8): 1392–1393.

27. Furtner M, Werner P, Felber S, Schmidauer C. Bilateral carotid artery dissection caused by springboard diving. *Clinical Journal of Sport Medicine*. 2006; 16(1): 76–78.

28. Motohashi O, Kameyama M, Kon H, Fujimura M, Onuma T. A case of vertebral artery occlusion following heading play in soccer. *No Shinkei Geka Neurological Surgery*. 2003; 31(4): 431–434.

29. Reess J, Pfandl S, Pfeifer T, Kornhuber HH. Traumatic occlusion of the internal carotid artery as an injury sequela of socce. *Sportverletzung Sportschaden: Organ der Gesellschaft fur Orthopadisch-Traumatologische Sportmedizin*. 1993; 7(2): 88–89.

30. Echaniz-Laguna A, Fleury MC, Petrow P, Arnould G, Beaujeux R, Warter JM. Internal carotid artery dissection caused by a kick during French boxing. *Presse Medicale*. 2001; 30(14): 683.

31. Schievink WI, Atkinson JL, Bartleson JD, Whisnant JP. Traumatic internal carotid artery dissections caused by blunt softball injuries. *The American Journal of Emergency Medicine*. 1998; 16(2): 179–182.

32. Arndt DH, Lerner JT, Matsumoto JH et al. Subclinical early posttraumatic seizures detected by continuous EEG monitoring in a consecutive pediatric cohort. *Epilepsia*. 2013; 54(10): 1780–1788.

33. McCrory PR, Berkovic SF. Video analysis of acute motor and convulsive manifestations in sport-related concussion. *Neurology*. 2000; 54(7): 1488–1491.

34. Gilad R, Boaz M, Sadeh M, Eilam A, Dabby R, Lampl Y. Seizures after very mild head or spine trauma. *Journal of Neurotrauma*. 2013; 30(6): 469–472.

35. Pitkanen A, Immonen RJ, Grohn OH, Kharatishvili I. From traumatic brain injury to posttraumatic epilepsy: what animal models tell us about the process and treatment options. *Epilepsia*. 2009; 50 Suppl 2: 21–29.

36. Prince DA, Parada I, Scalise K, Graber K, Jin X, Shen F. Epilepsy following cortical injury: cellular and molecular mechanisms as targets for potential prophylaxis. *Epilepsia*. 2009; 50 Suppl 2: 30–40.

37. Schwartzkroin PA, Baraban SC, Hochman DW. Osmolarity, ionic flux, and changes in brain excitability. *Epilepsy Research*. 1998; 32(1–2): 275–285.

38. Hunt RF, Scheff SW, Smith BN. Posttraumatic epilepsy after controlled cortical impact injury in mice. *Experimental Neurology*. 2009; 215(2): 243–252.

39. Lu DC, Zador Z, Yao J, Fazlollahi F, Manley GTMDPD. Aquaporin-4 reduces posttraumatic seizure susceptibility by promoting astrocytic glial scar formation in mice. *Journal of Neurotrauma*. 2011.

40. Ropper AH, Gorson KC. Clinical practice. Concussion. *The New England Journal of Medicine*. 2007; 356(2): 166–172.

41. Concussion (mild traumatic brain injury) and the team physician: a consensus statement. *Medicine and Science in Sports and Exercise*. 2006; 38(2): 395–399.

42. Ganti L, Khalid H, Patel PS, Daneshvar Y, Bodhit AN, Peters KR. Who gets post-concussion syndrome? An emergency department-based prospective analysis. *International Journal of Emergency Medicine*. 2014; 7: 31.

43. Heidari K, Asadollahi S, Jamshidian M, Abrishamchi SN, Nouroozi M. Prediction of neuropsychological outcome after mild traumatic brain injury using clinical parameters, serum S100B protein and findings on computed tomography. *Brain Injury*. 2015; 29(1): 33–40.

44. Haltiner AM, Newell DW, Temkin NR, Dikmen SS, Winn HR. Side effects and mortality associated with use of phenytoin for early posttraumatic seizure prophylaxis. *Journal of Neurosurgery*. 1999; 91(4): 588–592.

45. Young B, Rapp RP, Norton JA, Haack D, Tibbs PA, Bean JR. Failure of prophylactically administered phenytoin to prevent late posttraumatic seizures. *Journal of Neurosurgery*. 1983; 58(2): 236–241.

46. Dikmen SS, Temkin NR, Miller B, Machamer J, Winn HR. Neurobehavioral effects of

phenytoin prophylaxis of posttraumatic seizures. *The Journal of the American Medical Association*. 1991; 265(10): 1271–1277.

47. Caballero GC, Hughes DW, Maxwell PR, Green K, Gamboa CD, Barthol CA. Retrospective analysis of levetiracetam compared to phenytoin for seizure prophylaxis in adults with traumatic brain injury. *Hospital Pharmacy*. 2013; 48(9): 757–761.

48. Chen YH, Huang EY, Kuo TT et al. Levetiracetam prophylaxis ameliorates seizure epileptogenesis after fluid percussion injury. *Brain Research*. 2016.

49. Salinsky M, Storzbach D, Goy E, Evrard C. Traumatic brain injury and psychogenic seizures in veterans. *The Journal of Head Trauma Rehabilitation*. 2015; 30(1): E65–70.

50. Creed JA, DiLeonardi AM, Fox DP, Tessler AR, Raghupathi R. Concussive brain trauma in the mouse results in acute cognitive deficits and sustained impairment of axonal function. *Journal of Neurotrauma*. 2011; 28(4): 547–563.

51. Choe MC, Giza CC. Diagnosis and management of acute concussion. *Seminars in Neurology*. 2015; 35(1): 29–41.

52. Giza CC, Kutcher JS, Ashwal S et al. Summary of evidence-based guideline update: evaluation and management of concussion in sports: report of the Guideline Development Subcommittee of the American Academy of Neurology. *Neurology*. 2013; 80(24): 2250–2257.

53. Reynolds E, Collins MW, Mucha A, Troutman-Ensecki C. Establishing a clinical service for the management of sports-related concussions. *Neurosurgery*. 2014; 75 Suppl 4: S71–81.

54. Laurer HL, Bareyre FM, Lee VM et al. Mild head injury increasing the brain's vulnerability to a second concussive impact. *Journal of Neurosurgery*. 2001; 95(5): 859–870.

55. Bolton AN, Saatman KE. Regional neurodegeneration and gliosis are amplified by mild traumatic brain injury repeated at 24-hour intervals. *Journal of Neuropathology and Experimental Neurology*. 2014; 73(10): 933–947.

56. Huang L, Coats JS, Mohd-Yusof A et al. Tissue vulnerability is increased following repetitive mild traumatic brain injury in the rat. *Brain Research*. 2013; 1499: 109–120.

57. Friess SH, Ichord RN, Ralston J et al. Repeated traumatic brain injury affects composite cognitive function in piglets. *Journal of Neurotrauma*. 2009; 26(7): 1111–1121.

58. Weber JT. Experimental models of repetitive brain injuries. *Progress in Brain Research*. 2007; 161: 253–261.

59. Longhi L, Saatman KE, Fujimoto S et al. Temporal window of vulnerability to repetitive experimental concussive brain injury. *Neurosurgery*. 2005; 56(2): 364–374.

60. Goddeyne C, Nichols J, Wu C, Anderson T. Repetitive mild traumatic brain injury induces ventriculomegaly and cortical thinning in juvenile rats. *Journal of Neurophysiology*. 2015; 113(9): 3268–3280.

61. Raghupathi R, Mehr MF, Helfaer MA, Margulies SS. Traumatic axonal injury is exacerbated following repetitive closed head injury in the neonatal pig. *Journal of Neurotrauma*. 2004; 21(3): 307–316.

62. Donovan V, Kim C, Anugerah AK et al. Repeated mild traumatic brain injury results in long-term white-matter disruption. *Journal of Cerebral Blood Flow and Metabolism*. 2014; 34(4): 715–723.

63. Cantu RC. Second-impact syndrome. *Clinics in Sports Medicine*. 1998; 17(1): 37–44.

64. Cantu RC, Gean AD. Second-impact syndrome and a small subdural hematoma: an uncommon catastrophic result of repetitive head injury with a characteristic imaging appearance. *Journal of Neurotrauma*. 2010; 27(9): 1557–1564.

65. McQuillen JB, McQuillen EN, Morrow P. Trauma, sport, and malignant cerebral edema. *The American Journal of Forensic Medicine and Pathology*. 1988; 9(1): 12–15.

66. McCrory PR, Berkovic SF. Second impact syndrome. *Neurology*. 1998; 50(3): 677–683.

67. Kelly JP, Nichols JS, Filley CM, Lillehei KO, Rubinstein D, Kleinschmidt-DeMasters BK. Concussion in sports. Guidelines for the prevention of catastrophic outcome. *The Journal of the American Medical Association*. 1991; 266(20): 2867–2869.

68. Hebert O, Schlueter K, Hornsby M, Van Gorder S, Snodgrass S, Cook C. The diagnostic credibility of second impact syndrome: A systematic literature review. *Journal of Science and Medicine in Sport*. 2016.

69. Bey T, Ostick B. Second impact syndrome. *The Western Journal of Emergency Medicine*. 2009; 10(1): 6–10.

70. Mori T, Katayama Y, Kawamata T. Acute hemispheric swelling associated with thin subdural hematomas: pathophysiology of repetitive head injury in sports. *Acta Neurochirurgica Supplement*. 2006; 96: 40–43.

71. McLendon LA, Kralik SF, Grayson PA, Golomb MR. The controversial second impact syndrome: a review of the literature. *Pediatric Neurology*. 2016; 62: 9–17.

72. Gardner AJ, Tan CO, Ainslie PN et al. Cerebrovascular reactivity assessed by transcranial Doppler ultrasound in sport-related concussion: a systematic review. *British Journal of Sports Medicine*. 2015; 49(16): 1050–1055.

73. Tan CO, Meehan WP, 3rd, Iverson GL, Taylor JA. Cerebrovascular regulation, exercise, and mild traumatic brain injury. *Neurology*. 2014; 83(18): 1665–1672.

74. Chan ST, Evans KC, Rosen BR, Song TY, Kwong KK. A case study of magnetic resonance imaging of cerebrovascular reactivity: a powerful imaging marker for mild traumatic brain injury. *Brain Injury*. 2015; 29(3): 403–407.

75. Mutch WA, Ellis MJ, Graham MR et al. Brain MRI CO_2 stress testing: a pilot study in patients with concussion. *PLoS One*. 2014; 9(7): e102181.

76. Wang Y, Nelson LD, LaRoche AA et al. Cerebral blood flow alterations in acute sport-related concussion. *Journal of Neurotrauma*. 2016; 33(13): 1227–1236.

77. MacFarlane MP, Glenn TC. Neurochemical cascade of concussion. *Brain Injury*. 2015; 29(2): 139–153.

78. Villapol S, Byrnes KR, Symes AJ. Temporal dynamics of cerebral blood flow, cortical damage, apoptosis, astrocyte-vasculature interaction and astrogliosis in the pericontusional region after traumatic brain injury. *Frontiers in Neurology*. 2014; 5: 82.

79. Yu GX, Mueller M, Hawkins BE et al. Traumatic brain injury in vivo and in vitro contributes to cerebral vascular dysfunction through impaired gap junction communication between vascular smooth muscle cells. *Journal of Neurotrauma*. 2014; 31(8): 739–748.

80. Sword J, Masuda T, Croom D, Kirov SA. Evolution of neuronal and astroglial disruption in the peri-contusional cortex of mice revealed by in vivo two-photon imaging. *Brain*. 2013; 136(Pt 5): 1446–1461.

81. Len TK, Neary JP. Cerebrovascular pathophysiology following mild traumatic brain injury. *Clinical Physiology and Functional Imaging*. 2011; 31(2): 85–93.

82. Auerbach PS, Baine JG, Schott ML, Greenhaw A, Acharya MG, Smith WS. Detection of concussion using cranial accelerometry. *Clinical Journal of Sport Medicine*. 2015; 25(2): 126–132.

83. Caskey RC, Nance ML. Management of pediatric mild traumatic brain injury. *Advances in Pediatrics*. 2014; 61(1): 271–286.

84. Militana AR, Donahue MJ, Sills AK et al. Alterations in default-mode network connectivity may be influenced by cerebrovascular changes within 1 week of sports related concussion in college varsity athletes: a pilot study. *Brain Imaging and Behavior*. 2015.

85. Wang Y, Nelson LD, LaRoche AA et al. Cerebral blood flow alterations in acute sport-related concussion. *Journal of Neurotrauma*. 2015; 33(13): 1227–1236.

86. Maugans TA, Farley C, Altaye M, Leach J, Cecil KM. Pediatric sports-related concussion produces cerebral blood flow alterations. *Pediatrics*. 2012; 129(1): 28–37.

87. Len TK, Neary JP, Asmundson GJ et al. Serial monitoring of CO_2 reactivity following sport concussion using hypocapnia and hypercapnia. *Brain Injury*. 2013; 27(3): 346–353.

88. Junger EC, Newell DW, Grant GA et al. Cerebral autoregulation following minor head injury. *Journal of Neurosurgery*. 1997; 86(3): 425–432.

89. Strebel S, Lam AM, Matta BF, Newell DW. Impaired cerebral autoregulation after mild brain injury. *Surgical Neurology*. 1997; 47(2): 128–131.

90. Bartnik-Olson BL, Holshouser B, Wang H et al. Impaired neurovascular unit function contributes to persistent symptoms after concussion: a pilot study. *Journal of Neurotrauma*. 2014; 31(17): 1497–1506.

91. Meier TB, Bellgowan PS, Singh R, Kuplicki R, Polanski DW, Mayer AR. Recovery of cerebral blood flow following sports-related concussion. *The Journal of the American Medical Association Neurology*. 2015; 72(5): 530–538.

92. Wang Y, West JD, Bailey JN et al. Decreased cerebral blood flow in chronic pediatric mild TBI: an MRI perfusion study. *Developmental Neuropsychology*. 2015; 40(1): 40–44.

93. Doshi H, Wiseman N, Liu J et al. Cerebral hemodynamic changes of mild traumatic brain injury at the acute stage. *PLoS One*. 2015; 10(2): e0118061.

94. Bruce DA, Alavi A, Bilaniuk L, Dolinskas C, Obrist W, Uzzell B. Diffuse cerebral swelling following head injuries in children: the syndrome of "malignant brain edema."

Journal of Neurosurgery. 1981; 54(2): 170–178.

95. McCrory P, Davis G, Makdissi M. Second impact syndrome or cerebral swelling after sporting head injury. *Current Sports Medicine Reports*. 2012; 11(1): 21–23.

96. Bailes J, Patel V, Farhat H, Sindelar B, Stone J. Football fatalities: the first impact syndrome. *Journal of Neurosurgery Pediatrics*. 2016; 19(1): 116–121.

97. Langfitt TW, Tannanbaum HM, Kassell NF. The etiology of acute brain swelling following experimental head injury. *Journal of Neurosurgery*. 1966; 24(1): 47–56.

98. Saunders RL, Harbaugh RE. The second impact in catastrophic contact-sports head trauma. *The Journal of the American Medical Association*. 1984; 252(4): 538–539.

99. Obrist WD, Langfitt TW, Jaggi JL, Cruz J, Gennarelli TA. Cerebral blood flow and metabolism in comatose patients with acute head injury. Relationship to intracranial hypertension. *Journal of Neurosurgery*. 1984; 61(2): 241–253.

100. Overgaard J, Tweed WA. Cerebral circulation after head injury. Part 2: The effects of traumatic brain edema. *Journal of Neurosurgery*. 1976; 45(3): 292–300.

101. Overgaard J, Tweed WA. Cerebral circulation after head injury. 1. Cerebral blood flow and its regulation after closed head injury with emphasis on clinical correlations. *Journal of Neurosurgery*. 1974; 41(5): 531–541.

102. Weinstein E, Turner M, Kuzma BB, Feuer H. Second impact syndrome in football: new imaging and insights into a rare and devastating condition. *Journal of Neurosurgery Pediatrics*. 2013; 11(3): 331–334.

103. Potts MA, Stewart EW, Griesser MJ, Harris JD, Gelfius CD, Klamar K. Exceptional neurologic recovery in a teenage football player after second impact syndrome with a thin subdural hematoma. *PM & R*. 2012; 4(7): 530–532.

104. Casa DJ, Guskiewicz KM, Anderson SA et al. National athletic trainers' association position statement: preventing sudden death in sports. *Journal of Athletic Training*. 2012; 47(1): 96–118.

105. Boden BP, Tacchetti RL, Cantu RC, Knowles SB, Mueller FO. Catastrophic head injuries in high school and college football players. *The American Journal of Sports Medicine*. 2007; 35(7): 1075–1081.

CHAPTER 5

Postconcussive syndrome

Introduction

The majority of athletes have complete symptom resolution from 7 to 10 days following a concussion.[1-4] In a small minority of individuals, the somatic, cognitive, and affective postconcussive symptoms become protracted and persist beyond the acute phase. This has been termed as postconcussive or postconcussion syndrome (PCS). In this chapter, we will review the debated definition and epidemiology, the proposed pathophysiological mechanism, specific factors that increase an athlete's risk of developing PCS, and also the clinical management of common postconcussive symptoms that are persistent in PCS.

Definition

In general terms, PCS is a prolonged recovery from concussion characterized by persistence in clinical symptomatology. It is important to note the difference in nomenclature between postconcussive *symptoms* and postconcussive *syndrome*. Postconcussive symptoms are the many single, subjective clinical signs occurring after concussion, while a syndrome is a specific group of symptoms commanding a diagnostic entity.[5]

Over the past two decades, the definition of PCS has varied widely with different subtleties for diagnosis. Criteria PCS has been defined by the International Statistical Classification of Diseases and Related Health Problems (ICD-10),[6,7] the Diagnostic and Statistical Manual of Mental Disorders (DSM),[8] and also in published academic literature.[9] ICD-10 required that the diagnosis of PCS involve a "history of head trauma with loss of consciousness, preceding the onset of symptoms by a period of up to four weeks." The patient must then have three or more symptoms of headache, dizziness, fatigue, malaise, insomnia, emotional changes, concentration and memory difficulties, and reduced tolerance to alcohol that effects daily activities.

More recently, the DSM revised their classification of PCS, in the DSM-V, to include a more thorough description of concussion and also to create subgroupings among the symptoms. Per the DSM-V, PCS requires "evidence of traumatic brain injury, that is, an impact to the head or other mechanisms of rapid movement or displacement of the brain within the skull with one of the following: loss of consciousness, post-traumatic amnesia, disorientation and confusion, and neurological signs." This injury must then be accompanied by either symptoms of: physical disturbance (headache, fatigue, sleep disorders, vertigo/dizziness, tinnitus or hyperacusis, photosensitivity, anosmia, reduced tolerance to psychotropic medications), emotional symptoms (irritability, easy frustration, tension and anxiety, affective lability), personality changes (disinhibition, apathy, suspiciousness, aggression), and/or neurological symptoms.

Research groups have varied between strict use of either the above mentioned DSM or ICD criteria of PCS, created their own definition, or did not specify which criteria they used. Tator et al. proposed their own classification scheme of PCS requiring three or more specific symptoms persisting beyond 1 month from injury but appropriately excluded any individuals that had an intracranial lesion present on imaging.[9] This was in an attempt to obtain a more homogenous and typical concussion population.

As outlined and emphasized in Table 5.1, these classification schemes have many similarities, but

Table 5.1 Classification of PCS

	ICD-10	DSM-IV	DSM-V	Tator et al.[9]
Details	Postconcussional syndrome: history of head trauma with loss of consciousness, preceding the onset of symptoms by a period of up to 4 weeks	Postconcussional disorder: requires concussion history along with neurocognitive deficit	Major or mild neurocognitive disorder due to TBI: Evidence of TBI, that is, an impact to the head or other mechanisms of rapid movement or displacement of the brain within the skull with one of the following: • Loss of consciousness • Post traumatic amnesia • Disorientation and confusion • Neurological signs	Post-concussion syndrome: concussion not associated with mod-severe TBI or intracranial lesion
No. of Symptoms	≥3	≥3	Does not specify	≥3
Duration	Does not specify	>3 mo	Does not specify	>1 mo
Symptoms	• Headache • Dizziness • Fatigue/malaise/insomnia • Emotional changes • Concentration and memory difficulties • Reduced tolerance to alcohol • Preoccupation with above symptoms	• Headache • Dizziness/Vertigo • Fatigue/sleep disorder • Emotional changes/depression/anxiety • Personality changes	• **Physical disturbance** (headache, fatigue, sleep disorders; vertigo/dizziness, tinnitus or hyperacusis, photosensitivity, anosmia, reduced tolerance to psychotropic medications) • **Emotional** (irritability, easy frustration, tension and anxiety, affective lability) • **Personality changes** (disinhibition, apathy, suspiciousness, aggression) • **Neurological symptoms**	• Memory deficits • Concentration difficulties • Fatigue • Sleep problems • Mental fogginess • Confusion • Feeling slowed down • Learning difficulties • Increased thinking time • Problem solving difficulties • Slowed response speed • Irritability • Depression • Anxiety • Emotionality • Personality changes • Aggression • Headaches • Imbalance • Dizziness • Nausea/Vomiting • Sensitivity to light/noise • Vision changes • Neck pain • Tinnitus • Pressure in head • Lightheadedness • Vertigo • Numbness • Loss of appetite • Increased sensitivity to alcohol • Speech problems • Seizures • Stomach ache • Panic attacks • Frustration • Restlessness • Apathy

also great differences. The ICD-10, DSM-IV and V, and Tator et al. recognize the need for PCS to occur in relation to a traumatic/concussive event. But what is the "concussive event?" The ICD-10 necessitates "head trauma with loss of consciousness" which is an outdated statement because research has indicated that loss of consciousness only occurs in roughly 10% of concussions and is not needed for diagnosis.[3,10] Appropriately, the DSM-V included a definition of concussion to accurately describe both direct and indirect head trauma that can cause a concussive injury. Also in reference to the initial injury, only the ICD-10 defined the need for the symptoms required for the diagnosis of PCS to occur within a specific period of time (4 weeks from head trauma). In a review of 350 patients following mTBI, all patients had development of symptoms within 72 h of injury.[11] Though having a defined period is a favorable attribute, a 4-week time frame does appear excessive and this extended window period potentially can lead to athletes improperly labeled with PCS. Lastly, all four of the diagnostic criteria for PCS individually include a specific diverse set of symptoms.[12] Among the specific symptoms, there is a lack of agreement in total number and duration needed for diagnosis of PCS.

These inconsistent diagnostic criteria for PCS create confusion among clinicians to make a proper diagnosis and also makes it impossible to compare results from clinical studies.[13] It has been demonstrated that the ICD-10 compared with the DSM-IV criteria has a five- to sixfold higher incidence in PCS diagnosis within the same cohort of 178 adults with mild-moderate TBI.[6,14] Therefore, it is important to establish a standardized and succinct definition of PCS that includes an appropriate definition for concussive injury, duration of chronicity of concussive symptoms, similar to Tator et al.'s criteria, and also a scientifically validated set of symptoms. In the future, advancements in technology and research may generate serum and/or neuroimaging biomarkers for a more definitive objective diagnosis of PCS.

Epidemiology

It has been quoted that the occurrence of PCS following a sports-related concussion is between 10% and 21%.[5,15–17] Therefore, of the 3.8 million reported

concussions per year, between 380,000 and 570,000 athletes suffer from PCS annually.[5,15,18] Due to the great underreporting of concussions (up to 50%[19]), this value is likely a gross underestimation. For comparison, in studies assessing patients who presented to an emergency department with mTBI due to motor vehicle accidents and falls, between 40% and 62% had PCS beyond 3 months from injury; strikingly, 82% had at least one postconcussive symptom still persistent at 1 year.[20–23] Specifically within the pediatric mTBI population, the incidence of PCS at 3 months has been estimated to be between 11% and 29%.[24–27] But importantly, these studies all reviewed those who suffered an mTBI and not specifically a sports-related concussion; therefore, this likely includes those with intracranial lesions seen on head CT, which is not consistent with sports-related concussion.

There are many issues that make providing an accurate incidence of PCS very difficult. As previously mentioned, there is not a standardized diagnostic criterion for PCS; and those that exist, have inconsistent, nonvalidated symptoms. Secondly, the symptoms used in such classification schemes are not specific to concussion and can be seen in noncranial injuries, those with premorbid psychiatric conditions, and uninjured healthy individuals.[6,28,29] Diagnosis of PCS in healthy controls has been published to be between 20% and 60% and is most likely to occur in those with a preexisting psychiatric or migraine history.[30–34] The gross underreporting of concussions, limitations to the various diagnostic criterion, and high false positive rate in diagnosis, inter- and even intrastudy subject variability, makes analysis, interpretation, and applicability challenging. Therefore, a true incidence of PCS can only be speculated.

Predictors of prolonged symptoms/PCS

Numerous retrospective and prospective clinical studies have evaluated athletes following concussive injury to determine which factors would most likely result in a prolonged recovery and diagnosis of PCS.[5,35] We will review the modifiable and nonmodifiable risk factors of PCS including demographics, injury characteristics, post-injury factors, and premorbid medical conditions that have been shown to have an association with the development of PCS. It is important for anyone caring for a concussed athlete to recognize these factors in order to provide early and more aggressive management of their symptoms in efforts to impede a potentially prolonged course towards recovery.[36]

Demographics

The various demographic features that have been found to contribute to the development of PCS are age, gender, previous concussion history, and family history. Age appears to negatively affect concussion outcomes in a bimodal distribution.[37] Studies that subdivided younger children, adolescents, and college aged athletes showed that younger athletes are at an increased susceptibility to concussion, have worse outcomes with more prolonged symptoms and deficits in neuropsychological and balance testing following injury, more likely to, develop PCS in comparison to collegiate athletes, and have a longer return to play,[26,38–55]; however, this has not been demonstrated in all studies.[56] It has been postulated that children's worse outcomes in TBI could possibly be attributed to the incomplete myelination within their developing brains, increased water content causing higher strain forces, larger head to body ratio, reduced neck musculature, different skill level, and access to the latest equipment.[11,57–62] When evaluating a broader range of ages, studies have also demonstrated that those roughly older than middle age are more likely to have worse postconcussive symptoms with an increased chance of diagnosis of PCS at 3 months.[63–69]

A second consistent nonmodifiable predictor of poor outcome following concussive injury is female sex.[9,29,37,38,40,41,48,50,63–65,67,69–84] Though there is a higher rate of concussions among males due to the sheer volume of male athletes, females at both high school and collegiate levels have been demonstrated to have a higher incidence of concussive injury in comparison to male counterparts.[38,40,50,70,71] Besides the increased susceptibility, women athletes have also been consistently found to be more likely to report greater and more prolonged symptoms following concussive injury, worse performance on neurocognitive testing after injury, prolonged return to play (in one study, 35 days compared to 22 days in male counterpart,

p <0.001),[85] and are more likely to develop chronic PCS.[9,29,37,41,48,63–65,67,71–83,85–88] In a retrospective review of 266 adolescents, woman athletes were three times more likely to require academic accommodations, four times more likely to receive pharmacological therapies for symptom management, and eight times more likely to require some form of vestibular therapy.[78] But, not all studies have universally seen a difference in recovery related to the sex of the athlete, and this has commonly been attributed to a higher baseline of postconcussive symptoms seen in female athletes prior to injury.[89–91]

There are multiple theories as to why female athletes have been found to have worse outcomes following a concussive injury. First, female athletes in general have demonstrated, even at baseline, to have a greater number and severity of symptoms than male athletes, stressing the importance of documented baseline testing.[71] Besides the suggested social influences potentiating reporting bias between the sexes,[39,69] there is evidence that even physiological alterations make the woman athlete more susceptible to injury and also secondary injury. It has been proposed that a woman's neck muscles are smaller and less able to modulate head movement following a blunt force and also that the presence of estrogen and progesterone affects the secondary injury following a concussive injury.[39,69,90]

Another greatly studied risk modifier in concussion recovery is the number of previous concussions the athlete has experienced. It has been well studied that an athlete with a history of multiple concussions is more likely to experience another concussion, have a higher symptom burden upon further concussive injury, have prolonged recovery of symptoms and return to play, and is more likely to develop PCS.[17,37–39,43,91–100] In a prospective review of 280 student athletes aged 11–22 years old, those with a history of previous concussion compared with athletes without a history of concussion, took an average of almost 1 month to recover versus 2 weeks (p = 0.02).[17] Furthermore, Tator et al. retrospectively found within a cohort of athletes with PCS that 80% had at least one previous concussion.[96]

The vast literature on this subject points to the acceptance that previous history does effect the recovery of the athlete upon further concussive injuries. But what is the precise number of total concussions that places the athlete at risk for a prolonged recovery and development of PCS? A review of 596 high school and collegiate concussed athletes sub grouped based on the number of previous concussions found that only those with a history of more than three concussions were found to have a prolonged recovery on ImPACT testing after a recent concussion.[95] But, Tator et al. found that up to 23.1% of athletes suffering from PCS had a history of only one concussion.[9,96] Though all of these studies have inherent biases (selection bias, retrospective nature, recall bias, etc.), it alludes to the fact that exposure to repetitive concussions effects recovery. The inability to find consistent, absolute cutoff values may be due to the individualized differences between all athletes. Therefore, it is important to assess each athlete on a case-by-case nature to determine how they are recovering from their concussion and whether more aggressive management or even a discussion concerning retirement from sport should be made.

Psychiatric conditions

Roughly, 11%–25% of athletes are found to have a psychiatric illness diagnosed following injury with an increased incidence in the female sex, those with greater initial symptom score, preinjury psychiatric history, and family history.[9,101] This highly prevalent comorbid condition has been consistently shown as a strong predictor of PCS development, established by both retrospective and prospective reviews of concussed athletes.[41,65,75,96,97,102] Even regarding patients with a family history of psychiatric illnesses, an analysis of 40 concussed student athletes revealed that those with a family history of mood disorder had a threefold higher chance of developing PCS following a concussion.[97]

In further detail, preinjury depression has consistently been shown as a risk factor of PCS, and in one study, increasing the risk by 18 fold.[25,39,67,73,74,97,103–109] Unlike the accepted chemical imbalance associated with typical psychiatric disorders without concussive injuries, recent work in advanced neuroimaging techniques demonstrated a structural alteration that distinguished athletes with depression from those without, following a concussion. Through both susceptibility weighted imaging (used to analyze presence of micro hemorrhage), diffusion tensor imaging (assesses white

mater structural injury), and functional MRI, the athletes that developed PCS were more likely to have greater number and volume of microhemorrhages,[110] reduced parenchymal volume,[111] white matter changes specifically in the prefrontal cortex, corpus callosum, and nucleus accumbens,[111] and reduced neuronal activation in the prefrontal cortex and striatum.[112]

Also, the presence of premorbid anxiety disorder, anxious personality, attention deficit hyperactivity disorder (ADHD), post-traumatic stress disorder (PTSD), learning disability and migraine history prior to injury increases the risk of poor outcome following concussion and the likelihood of PCS.[25,39,67,73,74,87,96,103,108,113–121] For example, Bonfield et al. compared 48 patients with mTBI and ADHD in comparison to 45 patients with mTBI without ADHD to demonstrate that those with premorbid ADHD were 10-fold more likely to be moderately disabled following injury.[116]

Injury characteristics

Specific day of injury details like loss of consciousness (LOC)/altered consciousness, extent of injury, severity and existence of specific symptoms, and presence of seizures have all been found to be predictive of development of PCS. Multiple studies have shown that an alteration of consciousness or amnesia is predictive of the development of PCS,[9,21,122–126] but this has not been universally accepted.[41,87,127] Therefore, asking about LOC, though not required for concussion diagnosis, is an important detail to obtain. Nevertheless, the true long-term clinical significance is not completely understood.

Intuitively, different features that would denote a more severe injury would likely lead to increased prevalence of PCS, but this has not been seen uniformly. Though not common in concussive injury, one study found that the presence of subarachnoid hemorrhage on a CT scan in cohort of 176 mTBI patients was predictive of PCS at 1 month from injury.[128] However, another study using MRI and DTI imaging, a more sensitive test for structural brain abnormalities, did not correlate the presence of abnormal findings with the development of PCS at 1 month or 1 year from injury.[31] Similarly, S-100 (refer to Chapter 10, a calcium binding protein studied as a potential biomarker for TBI) has been found to be of strong predictive value as a screening test for the presence of intracranial hematomas, contusions, and subarachnoid hemorrhage.[129–134] Therefore, in concert with the previous findings, Heidari et al. found that an elevation of S-100 6 h following mTBI was a significant predictor of PCS at 1 month from injury which correlated with an increased likelihood of intracranial hemorrhage (odds ratio = 2.2).[128] Currently, the use of serum biomarkers has not become standard clinical practice, but in the near future this may assist early recognition in those athletes that are at higher risk of prolonged recovery following concussion. Lastly, co-existence of extracranial injuries has also been shown to be predictive of developing PCS which is intuitive because this infers exposure to a greater blunt force.[9,31,87]

Upon initial assessment of any concussed athlete, a main focus to the history is determining the mechanism of injury and presence, extent, and character of symptoms they are experiencing following the injury. This guides clinical treatment and is a marker of recovery, as the total number and severity of symptoms acutely after injury has shown predictive value of developing PCS.[38,87,126,127] Grubenhoff et al. performed a prospective longitudinal study of patients, 8–18 years old, presenting to the emergency department following a concussive injury.[135] It was noted that those with a concussion symptom inventory score greater than 10 were three times more likely to have PCS at 1 month from injury. Therefore, athletes with acute high symptom burden should warrant earlier therapeutic interventions to address their symptoms in efforts to prevent long-term sequelae. Along with recognition of symptom burden, the presence of specific symptoms has also been found to be predictive of prolonged recovery. Specifically, immediate headache, early proprioceptive deficits, cognitive symptoms, and dizziness following injury was found to be predictive of increased symptom burden, extended recovery, and development of PCS.[26,127,128,136–138]

Therefore, all athletes should be questioned about the day of injury characteristics like LOC, symptoms burden, and presence of extracranial injuries.

Postinjury factors

When caring for any athlete after a concussion, it should be emphasized that although they have had a brain injury, they will likely have a full recovery. It is important to stress the recovery process because a negative outlook can lead to worse outcomes. Termed as the "nocebo effect," it is when a person becomes intensely vigilant and focuses on their symptoms actually causing an increased symptom burden.[139] Multiple studies have demonstrated this direct relationship between negative injury perception, increased postconcussive symptom burden, and likelihood of PCS development at 3 and 6 months.[140–146] Therefore, during the care of a concussed athlete, it is imperative that attention is focused on the psychological factors that could influence their recovery, such as their outlook on recovery, social support, and coping techniques.[147]

Lastly, the presence of litigation has been linked to not only poor neuropsychological testing (NPT) results but also an increase in the risk of PCS diagnosis.[9,148,149] A meta-analysis of 39 studies, totaling 1463 cases of mTBI by Belanger et al. revealed that those patients involved in litigation were more likely to have persistent cognitive deficits on NPT beyond 3 months from injury.[148] Attentiveness should be directed on an athlete's effort and attempts to intentionally underperform or "sand-bag" neuropsychological tests if they are involved in litigation.

This discussion clearly emphasizes that there are many preinjury, injury, and postinjury risk factors in developing PCS. Therefore, being cognizant of these various aspects when managing an athlete may prompt more early and aggressive interventions following a concussive injury to prevent a prolonged recovery.

Pathophysiology

Detailed in Chapter 2, the biomechanics and pathology of concussion involves a force that is applied to the head; resulting in motion of the brain leading to axonal strain and possibly cavitation with commencement of a chain of events associated by: neuronal mechanoporation, electrolyte influx/effluxes, excessive neurotransmitter release, axonal injury, energy mismatch due to inefficient mitochondrial functioning, alterations in cerebral blood flow, neuroinflammation, and blood–brain barrier breakdown. It was deduced that the immediate postconcussive symptoms are a result of this acute neurometabolic response, but there was great uncertainty to the underlying cause of chronic symptoms associated with PCS. This is because we are still not fully knowledgeable of the complete window of recovery at a cellular level. It was only presumed that the structural, functional, vascular, and inflammatory alterations would not persist at chronic time points (months to years). Therefore, as repeated studies continued to demonstrate the recurring conclusion that PCS was directly related and strongly influenced by premorbid mental health disorders and postinjury perceptions, PCS as a unique diagnostic entity, aside from a psychological response, began to become questioned.[11,106–109,150–153] Now with chronic time points being assessed in TBI animal models, we have begun to recognize the occurrence and persistence of the neurometabolic response following injury. Further, advancements in neuroimaging have allowed researchers to commence clinical investigations comparing concussed athletes who recovered within a typical acute time course (7–10 days) versus those that developed PCS. Interestingly, the same structural, functional, vascular, and inflammatory acute alterations that occur in response to a concussive injury have also been shown to be persistent and more prominent in those suffering from PCS.

Those who develop PCS following injury have been demonstrated to have both a greater neuronal structural and functional change in comparison to those with only transient symptoms.[154–158] Structurally, Smits et al. compared 20 concussed athletes with 12 matched controls to find that those with more extensive and persistent postconcussive symptoms at 1 month correlated with the degree of structural white matter injury seen on diffusion tensor imaging (DTI).[159] Further work with functional MRI (fMRI), DTI, and magnetic resonance spectroscopy has led to a proposed hypothesis of how structural and functional alterations lead to the development of postconcussive symptoms and PCS. Researchers studied individuals following a concussive injury at 1–3 weeks, 6 months, and 1 year and demonstrated that structural alterations, mostly in the corona radiata and corpus callosum, were more prevalent and severe in those who developed PCS.[156–158] With the addition of fMRI imaging, it was further noted that these athletes also demonstrated increased activation in attention related areas. This led to the hypothesis that the increased activation in brain areas in response to task-related or cognitive activities is a reactionary compensation for the damaged areas in order to maintain baseline cognitive capacity. Unfortunately, this regionalized, heightened neuronal activity in turn leads to increased cognitive exertion, further stressing the injured brain, and this postulated to be the cause of the somatic and fatigue symptoms of PCS. Similarly, but not specifically studying PCS, Rogers et al. observed event related potentials (ERPs, measure of electrical activity following a stimulus on electroencephalogram) in 10 mild TBI patients on average 15 months from injury in comparison to 10 control patients.[154] On repetitive testing, the control group showed "learning" in which certain, nonessential task related areas of the brain had a reduction of activity following successive trials while the concussed group displayed a lesser extent of attenuation. Again, this failure of attenuation requires the athlete to maintain higher mental effort in comparison to an uninjured athlete, and therefore amounting to the cognitive symptomatology.

Therefore, if athletes who develop more structural/functional injury are more prone to develop PCS, would it mean that those athletes who are exposed to greater axonal strain forces are at an increased risk for PCS? From a biomechanical perspective, Oeur et al. performed finite element modeling to reconstruct the injurious mechanism in nine patients (three per group) who either had a concussion with expected recovery, concussion with development of PCS, and head trauma resulting in a subdural hematoma.[160] Those with transient symptoms, PCS, or presence of subdural hemorrhage had an increasing calculated rotational and linear acceleration, respectively. Likely due to the underpowered nature of the study, statistical significance was only found between those with transient symptoms versus those that developed a subdural hemorrhage. Similar findings were obtained by Post et al. who compared injury reconstructions of a cohort of patients who presented to an ED with PCS to those of published literature of neuronal strain in concussive injury.[161] Though finite element modeling has many limitations, the theory that higher linear and rotational acceleration forces correlate with PCS offers the potential to predict PCS with the use of helmet sensors. However, this requires further work and technological advances.

Along with the neurometabolic reaction after injury, a robust neuroinflammatory response occurs following a concussive injury. The immune system's reparative attempt can become unchecked and place the body into a state of constant destruction, postulated as the underlying cause of chronic traumatic encephalopathy. Similarly, the neuronal and vascular responses to inflammation could potentiate postconcussive symptoms, and if unremitting, cause PCS.[162–165] A fascinating recent animal study demonstrated that following head injury, an inflammatory response characterized by increased mast cells in the skull leading to a hypersensitivity to pain could contribute to postconcussive headaches.[165] Further preclinical and clinical research is needed in order to determine the association between chronic inflammation and the development of PCS.

Lastly, a concussive injury also causes the cerebral vasculature to have impaired responses to carbon dioxide.[166,167] Normally the cerebral vessels dilate when exposed to increasing carbon dioxide in order to increase blood flow and oxygen delivery to the brain. Loss of proper cerebral perfusion autoregulation has been demonstrated not only acutely following concussion, as discussed in Chapter 2, but has also been demonstrated in clinical studies of patients with persistent symptoms following TBI.[168–171] Therefore, postconcussive symptoms, like headaches and fatigue, in response to cognitive activity may occur due to an inappropriate reactively of the cerebral vasculature.[167,172] A fascinating clinical study by Agrawal et al. obtained single-photon emission computed tomography (SPECT) 72 h following a concussive injury. Those that were found to have hypoperfusion, specifically of the mesial temporal lobe, were more likely to develop PCS at 3 months ($p = 0.0003$).[170] This study by Agrawal et al. not only supports the theory of impaired vascular response and perfusion in PCS, it also exhibits a potential predictive PCS biomarker.

The structural, functional, inflammatory, and vascular alterations following concussion have been shown to persist and potentially contribute to the development of symptoms leading to PCS. But, the strong relationship between those with premorbid mental health illnesses and PCS cannot be ignored. Though preclinical and clinical work has better defined the neuronal pathophysiological causes that potentially result in PCS, we still

do not fully appreciate what the duration of these structural changes are and how they are affected or influenced by premorbid or postinjury psychological disorders. Therefore, the question that arises is to what extent PCS is due to neurogenic versus psychogenic triggers; and, is there a specific susceptibility threshold (premorbid conditions, genetics, environmental influences, and concussion exposure) between this heterogeneous interplay.

Since the diagnosis of postconcussive *syndrome* is purely clinical, determined by nonspecific symptoms that have great overlap with psychiatric and psychological disorders, it is futile to debate the exact neurogenic and psychogenic interaction that exists within PCS until we develop a more objective way to diagnose it.[153,173,174] Until then, it is essential for the clinician to understand that those with premorbid psychiatric disorders and various postinjury psychological characteristics are at a higher risk of prolonged recovery following concussive injury and therefore necessitate screening and aggressive intervention if discovered.

Focused management of PCS clinical symptoms

As detailed in Chapter 3, there are a multitude of postconcussive symptoms that may occur following a concussive injury. These symptoms have been traditionally grouped into either somatic, cognitive, psychiatric/affective, and sleep-related/fatigue symptoms.[11,36,175] Depending on the criteria, the persistence of these for greater than 1 or 3 months confirms diagnosis of PCS. The components of therapy for those unfortunate athletes who suffer with chronic symptoms should entail *1)* early intervention, *2)* a multifaceted team approach at a specialized center, *3)* the combination of conservative, supportive, and pharmacological interventions to improve daily functioning, and *4)* the identification of risk factors (medical history, mental health issues, severity of injury, etc.) of PCS requiring more aggressive and early intervention.[5,11,176,177]

With no single FDA approved therapy to treat PCS as a whole, the mainstay of treatment is focused on specific symptom management.[117,175] The mean number of total symptoms experienced by an athlete suffering from PCS is 8.1.[9] With this high volume of clinical symptoms, it is clearly challenging to address each separately; but fortunately, there is considerable interplay between symptoms and therefore, treatment of one usually results in improvement of others.[178] Therefore, it is important to discuss which symptoms are most debilitating for the athlete and select specific clinical interventions that target two or three of the athlete's main complaints. Also, any initiation of pharmacological interventions should involve the use of the lowest possible dose with increasing titration based on symptom severity.[175] The prescribing physician should choose agents with an understanding of their side effect profile in order to optimize their therapy with the use of the fewest drugs possible, and also to not worsen other symptoms, such as fatigue or slowed cognition.

Lastly, any athlete that is suffering from a protracted recovery or those that have preexisting factors that would increase their susceptibility to an elongated recovery, as detailed above, should receive neuropsychological testing along with repeated symptom checklists.[5,179] Use of a symptom checklist should focus specifically on the improvement of a specific symptom and not the total symptom checklist score.[11] This allows the person caring for an athlete with PCS to objectively quantify their recovery, gauge treatment efficacy, and importantly, use the score to provide a source of quantifiable encouragement for the athlete. This encouragement is essential for recovery.

Somatic symptoms

Somatic symptoms following concussion can include headache, nausea/vomiting, vertigo, and visual difficulties (please refer to Chapter 6 for discussion in management of vestibular and visual deficits). The most common somatic symptom is the development of a headache, occurring in 89% of athletes after concussion, which is more prevalent in female athletes.[15,180] Headaches tend to also be the first symptom experienced, and the most prolonged in nature, and can be clustered with photophobia, phonophobia, nausea, vomiting, dizziness, and neck pain.[181,182]

To properly manage a headache, it is important to note that there are many different pain generators and types of headaches. Pain generators of headaches can also be numerous in nature, such as: central in origin, extracranial (sinuses, eyes, temporomandibular joint), cervical (facet/

zygapophyseal joints, disc herniation), neurogenic (peripheral nerve irritation/injury such as supraorbital, trochlear, greater, and lesser occipital nerve), and myofascial (cervical muscular strain).[163] The term "sports concussion headache" is a broad, all-encompassing term that includes sub classes of headaches that occur following a concussion such as tension, cluster, migrainous, cervicogenic, medication overuse headache, and other types.[163] This is also assuming that one has already ruled out anxiety, sleep difficulties, physical exertion, or even dehydration as the culprit to the headache.[181] Generally, headaches can be managed similarly with pharmacological agents, but specific pain generators require directly tailored interventions to provide relief. Most headaches can be managed by a general practitioner, but patients that do not respond to first-line therapy should be referred to a concussion specialty clinic with a neurologist versed in both noninvasive and invasive headache treatments.

The management of headaches should involve a stepwise progression in pharmacological agents along with simple behavioral conservative measures. Following a concussion, the initial management of a headache should include rest and acetaminophen over aspirin or NSAIDs as not to increase the theoretical hemorrhage risk.[175,181,183,184] Subsequently, in the acute phase (3 days to 2 weeks after injury), acetaminophen or nonsteroidal anti-inflammatory medications (ibuprofen, naproxen, diclofenac) may be used, rather than opiate medications.[117,181,183–185] If the patient is still with persistent headaches beyond 2 weeks, an escalation in agents is likely required, furthermore, a referral to a specialized clinic or neurologist should be placed. Abortive pharmacotherapy such as triptans (i.e. sumatriptan, zolmitriptan, rizatriptan) or ergots (i.e. dihydroergotamine) along with prophylactic medications such as tricyclic antidepressants (i.e. amitriptyline, nortriptyline), anticonvulsants (i.e. topiramate, valproic acid, gabapentin), vitamin B12, magnesium, and beta blockers (i.e. propranolol, metoprolol) or calcium channel blockers can be considered (refer to Table 5.2).[117,163,175,181,183–190] A recent review by Bramley et al. found that amitriptyline was the most commonly prescribed medication in the pediatric concussed patient, with a reported 82% improvement.[180] Headaches, specifically migrainous in nature, may illicit nausea/vomiting, and therefore

Table 5.2   Pharmacotherapy for Headaches

Symptom	Class	Medication	Brand Names	Dosing	Side Effects
Headache	Analgesics	Acetaminophen	Tylenol	500 to 1000 mg 3–4 times daily (maximum daily dose, 4000 mg)	Usually rare; at high doses/ overdoses, vomiting, liver and kidney failure
		Aspirin	Bayer, Bufferin, Ecotrin	81 or 325 mg daily	GI upset, ulcers, bleeding, nausea, headache
	NSAIDs	Ibuprofen	Advil, Motrin	600–800 mg 3 times daily	GI upset, GI ulcers, GI bleeding, dizziness, nausea, vomiting, loss of appetite, arrhythmia, confusion; prolonged use in concussion patients can lead to rebound headaches
		Naproxen	Aleve, Naprosyn	550–850 mg twice daily	
		Diclofenac	Voltaren, Cataflam	50–100 mg daily (divided doses)	
	Antidepressants	Amitriptyline	Elavil, Endep, Vanatrip	10–25 mg QHS; titrate up for effect (usually doses of # 150 mg)	Nausea, GI upset, weakness, blurred vision, changes in appetite, drowsiness, dizziness, arrhythmia, motor tics, seizures, hallucination, unusual bleeding
		Nortriptyline	Aventyl, Pamelor	10–25 mg QHS; titrate as above	
	Anticonvulsants	Valproic acid	Depakene, Depakote	250 mg twice daily; can titrate up in increments of 250 mg for effect; (maximum daily dose, 1500 mg)	Drowsiness, dizziness, headache, diarrhea, constipation, heartburn, appetite changes, weight changes, back pain, agitation, mood swings
		Topiramate	Topamax, Topiragen	15–25 mg QHS and slowly raised to as high as 100 mg twice daily	Lack of coordination, impaired memory/ concentration, irritability, headache, weakness, motor tic, GI upset, hair loss, appetite changes
		Gabapentin	Neurontin, Gabarone, Vanatrex, Horizant	300 mg 3 times daily and may be slowly raised as high as 1200 mg 3 times daily	Dizziness, headache, blurred vision, anxiety, memory problems, motor tics, increased appetite
	b-Adrenergic antagonists	Propranolol	Inderal, Innopran	40–320 mg daily (divided doses)	Abdominal cramps, fatigue, insomnia, nausea, depression, impotence, lightheadedness, slow heart rate, low blood pressure, cold extremities, shortness of breath or wheezing; not to be used in patients with asthma

(Continued)

Table 5.2 (Continued)   Pharmacotherapy for Headaches

Symptom	Class	Medication	Brand Names	Dosing	Side Effects
		Metoprolol	Lopressor, Toprol	25 mg twice daily; can increase dose up to 100 mg twice daily if needed	
	Ergot preparations (abortive)	Dihydroergotamine	DHE45, Migranal	Intranasal vs IM/SQ vs IV (0.5–1 mg, maximum, 2 mg/d)	Abnormal skin sensations, anxiety, diarrhea, dizziness, flushing, sweating, nausea, vomiting
	Triptans (abortive)	Sumatriptan	Imitrex, Alsuma	Oral: 25–100 mg prn; intranasal: 10–20 mg BID prn; SQ: 6 mg	Unusual taste (nasal formulation), paresthesias, hyperesthesia, dizziness, chest tightness, dizziness, vertigo, tingling, hypertension, injection site reactions, flushing, chest pressure, heaviness, jaw or neck pain
		Zolmitriptan Rizatriptan	Zomig Maxalt	Oral: 5–10 mg; intranasal: 5 mg 5–10 mg; can repeat dose 2 h from first dose (maximum, 30 mg/d)	

Note: GI, gastrointestinal; NSAIDs, nonsteroidal antiinflammatory drugs; prn, as needed; QHS, at bedtime; SQ, subcutaneous.
Source: Petraglia AL, Maroon JC, Bailes JE. From the field of play to the field of combat: a review of the pharmacological management of concussion. *Neurosurgery.* 2012 Jun;70(6):1520–33.

anti-emetic/nausea pharmacological agents may be considered like ondansetron or promethazine.

Aside from the pharmacological agents, simple behavioral approaches for headaches may should always be implemented like a symptom diary, improving sleep quality, reducing caffeine intake, proper hydration and nutrition, and stress/anxiety management.[163,184,186,191] Other conservative, non-pharmacological approaches may include cognitive therapy, biofeedback measures, and physical therapy.[163,184,186,191]

Lastly, though most headaches can be managed as described above, it is always necessary to rule out medication overuse headache, cervicogenic headache, and occipital neuralgia because the treatment modalities are different. In a review by Petraglia et al. of 104 adolescent, concussed patients with persistent headaches, 69% had resolution of their headaches following complete cessation of analgesic medications.[175] Therefore, any athlete with persistent, difficult to manage symptoms who are found to be taking frequent doses should attempt a trial of cessation from analgesia to rule out medication overuse headaches.[163]

Cervicogenic headaches are headache symptoms secondary to pain triggers coming from the neck such as peripheral nerves, cervical spine, or musculature. Therefore, it is imperative to perform a neck exam on all patients with persistent headaches and determine if the pain is elicited with neck movement.[163,192,193] Further workup may require advanced neuroimaging if there are concerns seen on a detailed examination like neurological deficits in the extremities, radicular pain, etc. Clinical management of cervicogenic headaches of musculoskeletal nature includes therapies such as warm compresses, muscle relaxants, physical therapy, massage therapy, acupuncture, biofeedback, manipulation, or trigger point injections.[163,175,181,189,194,195]

A specific type of cervicogenic headache due to peripheral nerve irritation is occipital neuralgia. This is due to either direct neck trauma or a whiplash injury that causes injury to the greater or lesser occipital nerves.[163] Pain is severe and shooting along the craniocervical junction may be reproduced with movement of the head or palpation of the greater occipital nerve (2 cm lateral and 2 cm inferior to the external occipital protuberance) and can also be associated with eye pain and tinnitus.[163,196] Initial conservative measures include massage therapy, nonsteroidal muscle relaxers, gabapentin, or tricyclic antidepressants.[163] Athletes with refractory symptoms should be referred to a neurologist or pain management specialist for pharmacological management, consideration for local injections, and possible surgical intervention if more noninvasive measures are unsuccessful.[163,181,186,197]

Fatigue/sleep-related symptoms

Preclinical and clinical research has investigated the effects of concussion on sleep and mentation and their high incidence in those suffering with PCS.[198] Discussed within this chapter and further detailed in Chapter 2, the neurometabolic cascade causes neuronal, electrical, inflammatory, and vascular changes affecting the functioning of the neuron. These persistent microscopic disturbances generate neuronal inefficiency and the brain attempts to compensate by recruiting or increasing activity in other areas of the brain. This compensation taxes the brain on a global scale increasing symptom burden and potentially arousing clinical signs of acute and chronic cognitive slowing.[199]

Besides the direct effect of a concussion on cognitive functioning, the injury and clinical symptomatology also affects proper sleep performance of the athlete. Studies have demonstrated that acutely, animals have an increase in sleep following injury and this is also correlated with changes in brain wave activity measured by electrocorticography.[200,201] Further retrospective and prospective clinical studies have found that children, adolescents, and adults following concussion have an acute increased sleep duration, but eventually transition from hypersomnia to insomnia with poor sleep efficiency due to increased sleep latency and frequent awakenings.[11,202–207] This amounts to a vicious cycle of poor sleep quality worsening the already present cognitive fatigue and effective symptoms, leading to subjective daytime tiredness and even objective worsening in reaction time, neuropsychological testing, and symptom checklist scoring.[208–210] It is difficult to determine the full extent of the effects that fatigue and sleep-related symptoms have on neurocognitive testing because even healthy athletes show statistically significant differences on baseline testing when they receive too little or too much sleep prior to testing.[211,212]

Risk factors for developing chronic insomnia following a head injury correlated strongly with high symptom burden, dizziness, headaches, anxiety, depression, and even recurrent TBIs.[213] Though studied in a military cohort, Bryan et al. found that those with increasing exposure to TBIs were more likely to develop insomnia, documenting that the rate of insomnia in soldiers without TBI was 5.6%, 20.4% following one TBI, and 50% with a history of two TBIs.[214]

Treatment of cognitive issues, fatigue, and sleep disorders involve similar conservative measures, but different pharmacological agents depending on the specific complaint the athlete has. Simple behavioral modifications include sleep hygiene education such as consistent sleep and awake times, limiting screen use or stimulating activities prior to sleep (television, cell phone use, texting, exercising, etc.), and reduction in caffeine, alcohol, and nicotine.[11,184,186,215] Assessment and referral to a clinical therapist should be considered for issues such as anxiety, depression, and social withdrawal.[11] Lastly, cognitive behavioral therapy and light therapy have both been shown efficacy in those suffering with cognitive and sleep difficulties following concussion.[11,184,186,189,216]

Conservative measures can be instituted acutely and continued with chronically symptomatic athletes, but persistent symptoms warrant escalation to pharmacological agents. Due to the limited research on pharmaceutical interventions specifically for concussive injury, these are only recommendations based on the limited data from concussion and moderate to severe TBI literature. Medications that have been suggested for use in cognition and arousal following a concussion/TBI are neurostimulants (i.e. amantadine, dextroamphetamine, modafinal, methylphenidate, atomoxetine), selective serotonin reuptake inhibitors (i.e sertraline, fluoxetine), and acetylcholinesterase inhibitors (i.e donepezil, rivastigmine, galantamine)[175,184,186,215,217–227] (refer to Table 5.3).[175] In patients whose complaints appear to be more sleep-related, the use of both nonbenzodiazepine sedatives and herbal remedies are advocated (Table 5.4).[175] Benzodiazepines, such as lorazepam, clonazepam, and diazepam, are highly addictive and alter the normal sleep architecture

Table 5.3   Pharmacotherapy for Cognitive Symptoms

Class	Medication	Brand Names	Dosing	Side Effects
Neurostimulants	Methylphenidate	Ritalin, Concerta, Metadate	5 mg twice daily; can titrate up total daily dose by 5 mg every 2 wk to a maximum of 20 mg twice daily	Insomnia, decreased appetite, GI upset, headaches, dizziness, motor tics, irritability, anxiousness, tearfulness
	Dextroamphetamine	Adderall, Dexadrine ProCentra	5 mg daily; can titrate up for effect (maximum daily dose, 40 mg)	Anxiety, GI upset, insomnia, irritability, euphoria, starting episodes
	Modafanil	Provigil	100 mg every morning; can increase by 100 mg using divided doses (maximum daily dose, 400 mg)	Headache, dizziness, feeling nervous or agitated, nausea, diarrhea, insomnia, dry mouth, hallucinations, depression
	Amantadine	Symadine, Symmetrel	100–400 mg daily	Dizziness, blurred vision, anxiety, insomnia
	Atomoxetine	Strattera	40 mg daily (single or divided doses); can titrate up for effect (maximum daily dose 100 mg)	Dry mouth, irritability, nausea, decreased appetite, constipation, dizziness, sweating, dysuria, sexual problems, weight changes, palpitations, tachycardia
Selective serotonin reuptake inhibitors	Sertraline	Zoloft	25 mg daily; can increase weekly in 25-mg increments (maximum daily dose, 200 mg)	Aggressiveness, strange changes in behavior, extreme changes in mood, insomnia, nausea, dry mouth, decreased libido, dizziness, diarrhea
	Fluoxetine	Prozac	20 mg daily; can increase maintenance dose up to 80 mg daily	Anxiety, nausea, motor tics, decreased appetite, weakness
Acetylcholinesterase inhibitors	Donepezil	Aricept	5–10 mg daily	Severe diarrhea, severe nausea or vomiting, weight loss, stomach pain, fainting spells, bradycardia, difficulty passing urine, worsening of asthma, stomach ulcers
	Rivastigmine	Exelon	1.5 mg twice daily; can be titrated for effect (maximum daily dose, 200 mg)	Diarrhea, dizziness, drowsiness, headache, loss of appetite, nausea, stomach upset, vomiting
	Galantamine	Razadyne	4 mg twice daily initially, then increased to goal 8 to 12 mg twice daily (also available in extended-release form)	Diarrhea, dizziness, headache, loss of appetite, nausea, stomach upset, drowsiness, weight loss
Others	Cytidine diphosphate choline	Citicoline	250–500 mg daily	Increased body temperature, sweating, nausea loss of appetite

Note: GI: gastrointestinal.

Source: Petraglia AL, Maroon JC, Bailes JE. From the field of play to the field of combat: a review of the pharmacological management of concussion. *Neurosurgery.* 2012 Jun;70(6):1520–33.

and therefore are not recommended for routine use.[184,186,228] Nonbenzodiazepine derivatives, such as zolpidem, are good short-term, first line agents to aid those with sleep difficulties because they decrease sleep latency and nocturnal awakenings.[11,175,184,228] Caution should be exercised when used in the elderly due to potential side effects of confusion and altered mental status.[228]

Melatonin, an herbal remedy, has been frequently used as a sleep aid due to its lack of

Table 5.4 Pharmacotherapy for Sleep Disturbances

Class	Medication	Brand Names	Dosing	Side-Effects
Sedative-hypnotics	Zolpidem	Ambien, Edluar, Zolpimist	5 mg QHS; can increase to 10 mg QHS if poor results	Drowsiness, headache, dizziness, lightheadedness, unsteady walking, difficulty with coordination, constipation, diarrhea, heartburn, stomach pain, changes in appetite, paresthesias, unusual dreams
Serotonin modulators	Trazodone	Desyrel, Oleptro	25–50 mg QHS	Headache or heaviness in head, nausea, vomiting, bad taste in mouth, stomach pain, diarrhea, constipation, changes in appetite or weight, weakness, nervousness, decreased, concentration, confusion, nightmares, tinnitus
Benzodiazepines	Lorazepam	Ativan	0.5 mg twice daily	Sedation, dizziness, weakness, unsteadiness, depression, loss of orientation, headache, respiratory depression; caution should be used because these medications can cause physical dependence
	Clonazepam	Ceberclon, Klonopin, Valpax	0.25–0.5 mg twice daily	
	Diazepam	Valium, Valrelease	2–10 mg daily	
Supplement	elatonin	Health Aid Melatonin, VesPro Melatonin SGard	0.3–5 mg QHS	Daytime sleepiness, sleepwalking, confusion, headache, dizziness, abdominal discomfort

Note: QHS, at bedtime.
Source: Petraglia AL, Maroon JC, Bailes JE. From the field of play to the field of combat: a review of the pharmacological management of concussion. *Neurosurgery.* 2012 Jun;70(6):1520–33.

rebound effects, unlike the other medications mentioned.[11,175,184,186,215,228] Interestingly, melatonin has been found to have a neuroprotective effect in TBI, stroke, and spinal cord injury in animal models due to its antioxidative and anti-inflammatory properties.[229–231] For these reasons, the use of melatonin has been advocated for in concussion, but there exists limited evidence to prove its clinical effectiveness in humans.[11,184,186,215,228] Currently, there is active enrollment for a randomized controlled clinical study for the use of melatonin in athletes with PCS.[232]

Psychiatric/affective symptoms

As discussed previously, there is a direct correlation between those with preexisting conditions, like depression, anxiety disorder, or ADHD, that places the athlete more prone to a protracted recovery following concussion.[25,39,67,73,74,87,97,105–111,115–119] It has also been shown that concussion alone increases the risk of developing postinjury depression, anxiety disorder, and ADHD.[115,117,233–238] Max

et al. studied a cohort of children following a mTBI and found that roughly 28%–36% developed a *new* psychiatric disorder at 6 months, which interestingly directly correlated with frontal white matter injury seen on MRI and reduced neurocognitive performance.[239,240] Regarding specific psychiatric conditions, Iverson et al. reviewed 6529 school-aged children to show that those with a history of ADHD were more likely to have had a history of a concussion ($p < 0.00001$).[233] These results begin to pose the interesting question of the directionality of cause and effect between concussions and psychiatric conditions.[115] Does a single or repetitive concussion increase the risk of mental health disorders in someone that otherwise would not have developed the condition? Or, does the development of depression or anxiety disorder following a concussion only occur in those with preexisting conditions or those with increased susceptibility, such as genetic or environmental influences? At this time, evidences is limited and further research is required.

Whether it was the "chicken or the egg," the management of a psychiatric/effective disorder is similar whether it was existing prior to or developed following the concussion. Specifically, due to the strong psychological effect in worsening somatic, cognitive, and sleep symptoms, all athletes should be screened for depression and anxiety, and these should be promptly addressed if present.[3,174,241] Comanagement should be considered with a clinical psychologist and psychiatrist in order to offer both conservative measures in concert with pharmaceutical agents.[11,174] Conservative measures for anxiety and depressive symptoms include relaxation training, anxiety reduction techniques, biofeedback, education, implementation of coping mechanisms, and cognitive behavioral therapy.[106,242–245]

Cognitive behavioral therapy (CBT) has been shown to aid in treating depression but has limited evidence following a concussive injury.[106,188,246] Silverberg et al. randomized 28 patients, considered high-risk for development of PCS, to be enrolled in CBT within 6 weeks of injury and observed almost a 50% reduction in patients developing PCS at 3 months (54% incidence of PCS in those who received CBT versus 91% in those without).[247] Two other studies also showed promise of CBT following injury but were performed in patients with mild to severe TBI.[248,249]

Tricyclic antidepressants, selective serotonin reuptake inhibitors, and bupropion have all been suggested as pharmacological therapies for depression following a TBI based on their effectiveness in depression[106,175,183,189,223,224,250–252] (Table 5.5).[175] Studies in clinical efficacy for which specific agent is most effective in depression following a *concussion* are lacking and therefore strict recommendations are limited.[253] The two most commonly recommended SSRIs for treatment of depression have been citalopram and sertraline based on literature regarding TBI, but not specific to concussion.[11,184,186,188,189,220] In studies analyzing TBI patients with major depression, citalopram has shown either limited efficacy in comparison to placebo or had a poor response rate among participants.[254,255] Sertraline, on the other hand, has demonstrated improved performance in both a nonrandomized and randomized clinical study, but the results are speculative due to the lack of a placebo control arm.[256,257]

Exercise therapy

All clinical interventions for PCS, discussed throughout this chapter, each have their own specific symptom targets. One noninvasive therapy that potentially mitigates somatic, cognitive, and effective symptoms is exercise therapy.[220] Exercise therapy is cardiovascular activity, walking, jogging, or running on a treadmill, in which the speed/tempo is dictated by symptom development. The goal of further exercise is to maintain one's heart rate below that which cause symptoms.[258] This subthreshold exercise has been recommended in athletes after at least 1 month from injury who demands persistent symptoms.[259] Importantly, this intervention must be gradual in nature and under the guidance of a professional in order to prevent any harm to the athlete.

Not only does exercise promote increased cerebral blood flow and improvements in vascular reactivity, a physiological benefit, it likely also has a psychological benefit in the postinjury sedentary athlete.[171,258] Studies in the use of exercise therapy have demonstrated improvement in depression/effective symptoms, sleep difficulties, cognitive impairments, fatigue, cognition, and exercise tolerance.[258,260–263] Baker et. al. prospectively reviewed patients with PCS who were offered an exercise rehabilitation program. In this study, 77% (27 of 35 patients) that elected to be in the exercise group had complete return to daily activities while only 20% (1 of 5 patients) who refused the program had complete return to daily activities.[264] Though there is inherent bias between the two cohorts due to the lack of randomization and power, this study suggests a potential benefit of exercise therapy in those with protracted recovery from concussion. Leddy et al. similarly studied the role of exercise therapy following concussion where eight athletes following injury were instructed to either perform exercise therapy (intervention group) or stretching (placebo group) and were compared to four healthy controls.[265] All athletes following a concussive injury demonstrated changes in fMRI imaging in comparison to controls but only those that received the exercise therapy program showed neuroimaging improvements with time. The extent of benefits from exercise therapy in postconcussive symptoms can only be elucidated once blinded randomized studies are completed.[266]

Table 5.5 Pharmacotherapy for Depression

Symptom	Class	Medication	Brand Names	Dosing	Side Effects
Depression	Tricyclic antidepressants	Amitriptyline	Elavil, Endep, Vanatrip	10–25 mg QHS; titrate up for effect (usually doses of # 150 mg)	Nausea, GI upset, weakness, blurred vision, changes in appetite, drowsiness, dizziness, arrhythmia, motor tics, seizures, hallucination, unusual bleeding
		Nortriptyline	Aventyl, Pamelor	10–25 mg QHS; titrate as above	
	Selective serotonin reuptake inhibitors	Sertraline	Zoloft	25 mg daily; can increase weekly in 25-mg increments (maximum daily dose, 200 mg)	Aggressiveness, strange changes in behavior, suicidal thoughts/behavior, extreme changes in mood, insomnia, nausea, dry mouth, decreased libido, dizziness, diarrhea
		Citalopram	Celexa	10 mg daily; can titrate dose up for effect (maximum daily dose, 80 mg)	Constipation, decreased sexual desire or ability, diarrhea, dizziness, drowsiness, dry mouth, increased sweating, lightheadedness
		Escitalopram	Lexapro	10–20 mg daily	Nausea, dizziness, GI upset, increased appetite, hallucination, arrhythmia
		Paroxetine	Paxil	20 mg daily; can titrate dose up for effect (maximum daily dose, 50 mg)	Anxiety, blurred vision, constipation, decreased sexual desire or ability, diarrhea, dizziness, drowsiness, dry mouth, loss of appetite, nausea, nervousness, stomach upset
		Fluoxetine	Prozac	20 mg daily; can increase maintenance dose up to 80 mg daily	Anxiety, nausea, motor tics, decreased appetite, weakness
	Other anti-depressants	Bupropion	Wellbutrin, Zyban	Dose depends on if immediate release vs sustained release vs extended release; (maximum daily dose, 450 mg)	Seizures, delirium, hallucinations

Note: GI, gastrointestinal; QHS, at bedtime.
Source: Petraglia AL, Maroon JC, Bailes JE. From the field of play to the field of combat: a review of the pharmacological management of concussion. *Neurosurgery.* 2012 Jun;70(6):1520–33.

Prolonged postconcussive disorder

Prolonged postconcussive disorder, or PPCS, are athletes that suffer with PCS lasting greater than 6 months.[175] These are incredibly challenging patients and therefore should be managed through a multidisciplinary approach at a specialized concussion clinic, if available. Similar to managing PCS, a patient with PPCS should continue to receive objective measures of clinical progress like neuropsychological testing and symptom checklists. It is always important to reassess the patient frequently with a thorough history, addressing the different domains of PCS like cognitive, somatic, and effective symptoms. The athlete's symptomatology may change as certain aspects are better managed, and therefore, may warrant a different approach. Also, repeated neurological exams are recommended because they may elicit new vestibular, visual, or cervical issues requiring further evaluation, imaging, or management strategies. Continuous assessment of psychosocial issues like stress, anxiety, and depression is paramount as the athlete finds himself/herself further from returning to play. Lastly, for those athletes that have persistent symptoms beyond 6 months to 1 year, the likelihood of the athlete becoming symptom free is rather unlikely and management should be focused on daily functioning rather than complete resolution.

It is also important to recognize the many confounders that may prevent an athlete from ever becoming "asymptomatic." First, many nonconcussed, healthy athletes are found to be "symptomatic" on formal objective testing.[33] Secondly, many athletes at baseline may have symptoms that have now become exacerbated due to the concussion. Though the athlete has returned to their baseline symptom level, they may subjectively feel that they have not gotten "back to what they used to be." This has been termed as the "good-old-days" bias.[267] Lastly, social factors such as litigation, workman's compensation, academic absence, or loss of interest in sport may cause a malingering propensity in the athlete.

Conclusion

Though a majority of athletes recover from concussion within the acute window, there are an unfortunate few that develop persistent symptoms warranting the diagnosis of PCS. As detailed, proper management involves risk factor recognition, symptom management, and persistent medical supervision and reevaluation. It is important to recognize not only the strong psychological factors involved in PCS, but also the structural injury that has occurred leading to symptom development.

References

1. Mayers LB. Outcomes of sport-related concussion among college athletes. *The Journal of Neuropsychiatry and Clinical Neurosciences.* 2013; 25(2): 115–119.

2. Lovell MR, Collins MW, Iverson GL et al. Recovery from mild concussion in high school athletes. *Journal of Neurosurgery.* 2003; 98(2): 296–301.

3. McCrory P, Meeuwisse W, Aubry M et al. Consensus statement on concussion in sport— The 4th International Conference on Concussion in Sport held in Zurich, November 2012. *Physical Therapy in Sport.* 2013; 14(2): e1–e13.

4. Cancelliere C, Hincapie CA, Keightley M et al. Systematic review of prognosis and return to play after sport concussion: results of the International Collaboration on Mild Traumatic Brain Injury Prognosis. *Archives of Physical Medicine and Rehabilitation.* 2014; 95(3 Suppl): S210–229.

5. Jotwani V, Harmon KG. Postconcussion syndrome in athletes. *Current Sports Medicine Reports.* 2010; 9(1): 21–26.

6. Boake C, McCauley SR, Levin HS et al. Diagnostic criteria for postconcussional syndrome after mild to moderate traumatic brain injury. *The Journal of Neuropsychiatry and Clinical Neurosciences.* 2005; 17(3): 350–356.

7. World Heatlh Organization: ICD 10 Classification of Mental and Behavioral Disorders: Diagnostic Criteria for Research. *Geneva: World Health Organization.*

8. Neurocognitive Disorders. *Diagnostic and Statistical Manual of Mental Disorders.*

9. Tator CH, Davis HS, Dufort PA et al. Postconcussion syndrome: demographics and predictors in 221 patients. *Journal of Neurosurgery.* 2016: 1–11.

10. Purcell L, Kissick J, Rizos J. Concussion. *Canadian Medical Association Journal.* 2013; 185(11): 981.

11. Barlow KM. Postconcussion syndrome: a review. *Journal of Child Neurology.* 2014.

12. Laborey M, Masson F, Ribereau-Gayon R, Zongo D, Salmi LR, Lagarde E. Specificity of postconcussion symptoms at 3 months after mild traumatic brain injury: results from a comparative cohort study. *The Journal of Head Trauma Rehabilitation.* 2014; 29(1): E28–36.

13. Rose SC, Fischer AN, Heyer GL. How long is too long? The lack of consensus regarding the post-concussion syndrome diagnosis. *Brain Injury.* 2015; 29(7–8): 798–803.

14. Leddy JJ, Sandhu H, Sodhi V, Baker JG, Willer B. Rehabilitation of concussion and post-concussion syndrome. *Sports Health*. 2012; 4(2): 147–154.

15. Prigatano GP, Gale SD. The current status of postconcussion syndrome. *Current Opinion in Psychiatry*. 2011; 24(3): 243–250.

16. Grubenhoff JA, Deakyne SJ, Comstock RD, Kirkwood MW, Bajaj L. Outpatient follow-up and return to school after emergency department evaluation among children with persistent post-concussion symptoms. *Brain Injury*. 2015: 1–6.

17. Eisenberg MA, Andrea J, Meehan W, Mannix R. Time interval between concussions and symptom duration. *Pediatrics*. 2013; 132(1): 8–17.

18. Harmon KG, Drezner J, Gammons M et al. American Medical Society for Sports Medicine position statement: concussion in sport. *Clinical Journal of Sport Medicine*. 2013; 23(1): 1–18.

19. Harmon KG, Drezner JA, Gammons M et al. American Medical Society for Sports Medicine position statement: concussion in sport. *British Journal of Sports Medicine*. 2013; 47(1): 15–26.

20. Ingebrigtsen T, Waterloo K, Marup-Jensen S, Attner E, Romner B. Quantification of post-concussion symptoms 3 months after minor head injury in 100 consecutive patients. *Journal of Neurology*. 1998; 245(9): 609–612.

21. Bazarian JJ, Wong T, Harris M, Leahey N, Mookerjee S, Dombovy M. Epidemiology and predictors of post-concussive syndrome after minor head injury in an emergency population. *Brain Injury*. 1999; 13(3): 173–189.

22. Sigurdardottir S, Andelic N, Roe C, Jerstad T, Schanke AK. Post-concussion symptoms after traumatic brain injury at 3 and 12 months post-injury: a prospective study. *Brain Injury*. 2009; 23(6): 489–497.

23. McMahon P, Hricik A, Yue JK et al. Symptomatology and functional outcome in mild traumatic brain injury: results from the prospective TRACK–TBI study. *Journal of Neurotrauma*. 2014; 31(1): 26–33.

24. Barlow KM, Crawford S, Stevenson A, Sandhu SS, Belanger F, Dewey D. Epidemiology of postconcussion syndrome in pediatric mild traumatic brain injury. *Pediatrics*. 2010; 126(2): e374–381.

25. Hou R, Moss-Morris R, Peveler R, Mogg K, Bradley BP, Belli A. When a minor head injury results in enduring symptoms: a prospective investigation of risk factors for postconcussional syndrome after mild traumatic brain injury. *Journal of Neurology, Neurosurgery, and Psychiatry*. 2012; 83(2): 217–223.

26. Babcock L, Byczkowski T, Wade SL, Ho M, Mookerjee S, Bazarian JJ. Predicting post-concussion syndrome after mild traumatic brain injury in children and adolescents who present to the emergency department. *The Journal of the American Medical Association Pediatrics*. 2013; 167(2): 156–161.

27. Barlow KM, Crawford S, Brooks BL, Turley B, Mikrogianakis A. The incidence of post-concussion syndrome remains stable following mild traumatic brain injury in children. *Pediatric Neurology*. 2015.

28. Iverson GL, Lange RT. Examination of "post-concussion-like" symptoms in a healthy sample. *Applied Neuropsychology*. 2003; 10(3): 137–144.

29. Meares S, Shores EA, Taylor AJ et al. Mild traumatic brain injury does not predict acute postconcussion syndrome. *Journal of Neurology, Neurosurgery, and Psychiatry*. 2008; 79(3): 300–306.

30. Garden N, Sullivan KA. An examination of the base rates of post-concussion symptoms: the influence of demographics and depression. *Applied Neuropsychology*. 2010; 17(1): 1–7.

31. Waljas M, Iverson GL, Lange RT et al. A prospective biopsychosocial study of the persistent post-concussion symptoms following mild traumatic brain injury. *Journal of Neurotrauma*. 2015; 32(8): 534–547.

32. Garden N, Sullivan KA, Lange RT. The relationship between personality characteristics and postconcussion symptoms in a nonclinical sample. *Neuropsychology*. 2010; 24(2): 168–175.

33. Wang Y, Chan RC, Deng Y. Examination of postconcussion-like symptoms in healthy university students: relationships to subjective and objective neuropsychological function performance. *Archives of Clinical Neuropsychology*. 2006; 21(4): 339–347.

34. Iverson GL, Silverberg ND, Mannix R et al. Factors associated with concussion-like symptom reporting in high school athletes. *The Journal of the American Medical Association Pediatrics*. 2015: 1–9.

35. Guinto G, Guinto-Nishimura Y. Postconcussion syndrome: a complex and underdiagnosed clinical entity. *World Neurosurgery*. 2014; 82(5): 627–628.

36. Reynolds E, Collins MW, Mucha A, Troutman-Ensecki C. Establishing a clinical service for the management of sports-related concussions. *Neurosurgery*. 2014; 75 Suppl 4: S71–81.

37. Abrahams S, Fie SM, Patricios J, Posthumus M, September AV. Risk factors for sports concussion: an evidence-based systematic review. *British Journal of Sports Medicine*. 2014; 48(2): 91–97.

38. Makdissi M, Davis G, Jordan B, Patricios J, Purcell L, Putukian M. Revisiting the modifiers: how should the evaluation and management of acute concussions differ in specific groups? *British Journal of Sports Medicine*. 2013; 47(5): 314–320.

39. Kerr HA. Concussion risk factors and strategies for prevention. *Pediatric Annals*. 2014; 43(12): e309–315.

40. Dessy A, Rasouli J, Gometz A, Choudhri T. A review of modifying factors affecting usage of diagnostic rating scales in concussion management. *Clinical Neurology and Neurosurgery*. 2014; 122: 59–63.

41. Ponsford J, Willmott C, Rothwell A et al. Factors influencing outcome following mild traumatic brain injury in adults. *Journal of the International Neuropsychological Society*. 2000; 6(5): 568–579.

42. Foley C, Gregory A, Solomon G. Young age as a modifying factor in sports concussion management: what is the evidence? *Current Sports Medicine Reports*. 2014; 13(6): 390–394.

43. Giza CC, Kutcher JS, Ashwal S et al. Summary of evidence-based guideline update: evaluation and management of concussion in sports: report of the Guideline Development Subcommittee of the American Academy of Neurology. *Neurology*. 2013; 80(24): 2250–2257.

44. Kontos AP, Braithwaite R, Dakan S, Elbin RJ. Computerized neurocognitive testing within 1 week of sport-related concussion: meta-analytic review and analysis of moderating factors. *Journal of the International Neuropsychological Society*. 2014; 20(3): 324–332.

45. Pellman EJ, Lovell MR, Viano DC, Casson IR. Concussion in professional football: recovery of NFL and high school athletes assessed by computerized neuropsychological testing—Part 12. *Neurosurgery*. 2006; 58(2): 263–274.

46. Pellman EJ, Lovell MR, Viano DC, Casson IR, Tucker AM. Concussion in professional football: neuropsychological testing—part 6. *Neurosurgery*. 2004; 55(6): 1290–1303.

47. Iverson GL, Brooks BL, Collins MW, Lovell MR. Tracking neuropsychological recovery following concussion in sport. *Brain Injury*. 2006; 20(3): 245–252.

48. Dougan BK, Horswill MS, Geffen GM. Athletes' age, sex, and years of education moderate the acute neuropsychological impact of sports-related concussion: a meta-analysis. *Journal of the International Neuropsychological Society*. 2014; 20(1): 64–80.

49. Collins MW, Field M, Lovell MR et al. Relationship between postconcussion headache and neuropsychological test performance in high school athletes. *The American Journal of Sports Medicine*. 2003; 31(2): 168–173.

50. Gessel LM, Fields SK, Collins CL, Dick RW, Comstock RD. Concussions among United States high school and collegiate athletes. *Journal of Athletic Training*. 2007; 42(4): 495–503.

51. Field M, Collins MW, Lovell MR, Maroon J. Does age play a role in recovery from sports-related concussion? A comparison of high school and collegiate athletes. *The Journal of Pediatrics*. 2003; 142(5): 546–553.

52. Howell DR, Osternig LR, Chou LS. Adolescents demonstrate greater gait balance control deficits after concussion than young adults. *The American Journal of Sports Medicine*. 2015; 43(3): 625–632.

53. Williams RM, Puetz TW, Giza CC, Broglio SP. Concussion recovery time among high school and collegiate athletes: a systematic review and meta-analysis. *Sports Medicine*. 2015; 45(6): 893–903.

54. Zuckerman SL, Lee YM, Odom MJ, Solomon GS, Forbes JA, Sills AK. Recovery from sports-related concussion: Days to return to neurocognitive baseline in adolescents versus young adults. *Surgical Neurology International*. 2012; 3: 130.

55. Lee YM, Odom MJ, Zuckerman SL, Solomon GS, Sills AK. Does age affect symptom recovery after sports-related concussion? A study of high school and college athletes. *Journal of Neurosurgery Pediatrics*. 2013; 12(6): 537–544.

56. Karlin AM. Concussion in the pediatric and adolescent population: "Different population, different concerns." *PM & R: the Journal of Injury, Function, and Rehabilitation*. 2011; 3(10 Suppl 2): S369–379.

57. Meehan WP, 3rd, Taylor AM, Proctor M. The pediatric athlete: younger athletes with sport-related concussion. *Clinics in Sports Medicine*. 2011; 30(1): 133–144, x.

58. Theye F, Mueller KA. "Heads up": concussions in high school sports. *Clinical Medicine and Research*. 2004; 2(3): 165–171.

59. Charleswell C, Ross B, Tran T, Walsh E. Traumatic brain injury: considering collaborative strategies for early detection and interventional research. *Journal of Epidemiology and Community Health*. 2015; 69(3): 290–292.

60. Caskey RC, Nance ML. Management of pediatric mild traumatic brain injury. *Advances in Pediatrics*. 2014; 61(1): 271–286.

61. Bauer R, Fritz H. Pathophysiology of traumatic injury in the developing brain: an introduction and short update. *Experimental and Toxicologic Pathology*. 2004; 56(1–2): 65–73.

62. Lannsjo M, Backheden M, Johansson U, Af Geijerstam JL, Borg J. Does head CT scan pathology predict outcome after mild traumatic brain injury? *European Journal of Neurology*. 2013; 20(1): 124–129.

63. King NS. A systematic review of age and gender factors in prolonged post-concussion symptoms after mild head injury. *Brain Injury*. 2014; 28(13–14): 1639–1645.

64. Scholten AC, Haagsma JA, Andriessen TM et al. Health-related quality of life after mild, moderate and severe traumatic brain injury: patterns and predictors of suboptimal functioning during the first year after injury. *Injury*. 2015; 46(4): 616–624.

65. Lingsma HF, Yue JK, Maas AI et al. Outcome prediction after mild and complicated mild traumatic brain injury: external validation of existing models and identification of new predictors using the TRACK-TBI pilot study. *Journal of Neurotrauma*. 2015; 32(2): 83–94.

66. King N. Permanent post-concussion symptoms after mild head injury: a systematic review of age and gender factors. *NeuroRehabilitation*. 2014; 34(4): 741–748.

67. King NS, Kirwilliam S. Permanent post-concussion symptoms after mild head injury. *Brain Injury*. 2011; 25(5): 462–470.

68. Benedict PA, Baner NV, Harrold GK et al. Gender and age predict outcomes of cognitive, balance and vision testing in a multidisciplinary concussion center. *Journal of the Neurological Sciences*. 2015; 353(1–2): 111–115.

69. Covassin T, Swanik CB, Sachs ML. Sex differences and the incidence of concussions among collegiate athletes. *Journal of Athletic Training*. 2003; 38(3): 238–244.

70. Dick RW. Is there a gender difference in concussion incidence and outcomes? *British Journal of Sports Medicine*. 2009; 43 Suppl 1: i46–50.

71. Zuckerman SL, Apple RP, Odom MJ, Lee YM, Solomon GS, Sills AK. Effect of sex on symptoms and return to baseline in sport-related concussion. *Journal of Neurosurgery Pediatrics*. 2014; 13(1): 72–81.

72. Covassin T, Elbin RJ. The female athlete: the role of gender in the assessment and management of sport-related concussion. *Clinics in Sports Medicine*. 2011; 30(1): 125–131, x.

73. McCauley SR, Boake C, Levin HS, Contant CF, Song JX. Postconcussional disorder following mild to moderate traumatic brain injury: anxiety, depression, and social support as risk factors and comorbidities. *Journal of Clinical and Experimental Neuropsychology*. 2001; 23(6): 792–808.

74. Meares S, Shores EA, Taylor AJ et al. The prospective course of postconcussion syndrome: the role of mild traumatic brain injury. *Neuropsychology*. 2011; 25(4): 454–465.

75. Silverberg ND, Gardner AJ, Brubacher JR, Panenka WJ, Li JJ, Iverson GL. Systematic review of multivariable prognostic models for mild traumatic brain injury. *Journal of Neurotrauma*. 2015; 32(8): 517–526.

76. Farace E, Alves WM. Do women fare worse? A metaanalysis of gender differences in outcome after traumatic brain injury. *Neurosurgical Focus*. 2000; 8(1): e6.

77. Kostyun RO, Hafeez I. Protracted recovery from a concussion: a focus on gender and treatment interventions in an adolescent population. *Sports Health*. 2015; 7(1): 52–57.

78. Preiss-Farzanegan SJ, Chapman B, Wong TM, Wu J, Bazarian JJ. The relationship between gender and postconcussion symptoms after sport-related mild traumatic brain injury. *PM & R*. 2009; 1(3): 245–253.

79. Covassin T, Schatz P, Swanik CB. Sex differences in neuropsychological function and post-concussion symptoms of concussed collegiate athletes. *Neurosurgery*. 2007; 61(2): 345–350.

80. Covassin T, Elbin RJ, Bleecker A, Lipchik A, Kontos AP. Are there differences in neurocognitive function and symptoms between male and female soccer players after concussions? *The American Journal of Sports Medicine*. 2013; 41(12): 2890–2895.

81. Covassin T, Elbin RJ, Harris W, Parker T, Kontos A. The role of age and sex in symptoms, neurocognitive performance, and postural stability in athletes after concussion. *The American Journal of Sports Medicine*. 2012; 40(6): 1303–1312.

82. Baker JG, Leddy JJ, Darling SR, Shucard J, Makdissi M, Willer BS. Gender differences in recovery from sports-related concussion in adolescents. *Clinical Pediatrics*. 2015.

83. Kutcher JS, Eckner JT. At-risk populations in sports-related concussion. *Current Sports Medicine Reports*. 2010; 9(1): 16–20.

84. Bock S, Grim R, Barron TF et al. Factors associated with delayed recovery in athletes with concussion treated at a pediatric neurology concussion clinic. *ChNS*. 2015; 31(11): 2111–2116.

85. Broshek DK, Kaushik T, Freeman JR, Erlanger D, Webbe F, Barth JT. Sex differences in outcome following sports-related concussion. *Journal of Neurosurgery*. 2005; 102(5): 856–863.

86. Colvin AC, Mullen J, Lovell MR, West RV, Collins MW, Groh M. The role of concussion history and gender in recovery from soccer-related concussion. *The American Journal of Sports Medicine*. 2009; 37(9): 1699–1704.

87. Stulemeijer M, van der Werf S, Borm GF, Vos PE. Early prediction of favourable recovery 6 months after mild traumatic brain injury. *Journal of Neurology, Neurosurgery, and Psychiatry*. 2008; 79(8): 936–942.

88. Frommer LJ, Gurka KK, Cross KM, Ingersoll CD, Comstock RD, Saliba SA. Sex differences in concussion symptoms of high school athletes. *Journal of Athletic Training*. 2011; 46(1): 76–84.

89. Brown DA, Elsass JA, Miller AJ, Reed LE, Reneker JC. Differences in symptom reporting between males and females at baseline and after a sports-related concussion: a systematic review and meta-analysis. *Sports Medicine*. 2015; 45(7): 1027–1040.

90. Wunderle K, Hoeger KM, Wasserman E, Bazarian JJ. Menstrual phase as predictor of outcome after mild traumatic brain injury in women. *The Journal of Head Trauma Rehabilitation*. 2014; 29(5): E1–8.

91. Mannix R, Iverson GL, Maxwell B, Atkins JE, Zafonte R, Berkner PD. Multiple prior concussions are associated with symptoms in high school athletes. *Annals of Clinical and Translational Neurology*. 2014; 1(6): 433–438.

92. Guskiewicz KM, McCrea M, Marshall SW et al. Cumulative effects associated with recurrent concussion in collegiate football players: the NCAA Concussion Study. *The Journal of the American Medical Association*. 2003; 290(19): 2549–2555.

93. Schatz P, Moser RS, Covassin T, Karpf R. Early indicators of enduring symptoms in high school athletes with multiple previous concussions. *Neurosurgery*. 2011; 68(6): 1562–1567.

94. Valovich McLeod TC, Bay RC, Lam KC, Chhabra A. Representative baseline values on the Sport Concussion Assessment Tool 2 (SCAT2) in adolescent athletes vary by gender, grade, and concussion history. *The American Journal of Sports Medicine*. 2012; 40(4): 927–933.

95. Covassin T, Moran R, Wilhelm K. Concussion symptoms and neurocognitive performance of high school and college athletes who incur multiple concussions. *The American Journal of Sports Medicine*. 2013; 41(12): 2885–2889.

96. Tator CH, Davis H. The postconcussion syndrome in sports and recreation: clinical features and demography in 138 athletes. *Neurosurgery*. 2014; 75 Suppl 4: S106–112.

97. Morgan CD, Zuckerman SL, Lee YM et al. Predictors of postconcussion syndrome after sports-related concussion in young athletes: a matched case-control study. *Journal of Neurosurgery Pediatrics*. 2015; 15(6): 589–598.

98. Wasserman EB, Kerr ZY, Zuckerman SL, Covassin T. Epidemiology of sports-related concussions in national collegiate athletic association athletes from 2009–2010 to 2013–2014: symptom prevalence, symptom resolution time, and return-to-play time. *The American Journal of Sports Medicine*. 2015.

99. Corwin DJ, Zonfrillo MR, Master CL et al. Characteristics of prolonged concussion recovery in a pediatric subspecialty referral population. *The Journal of Pediatrics*. 2014; 165(6): 1207–1215.

100. Delaney JS, Al-Kashmiri A, Correa JA. Mechanisms of injury for concussions in university football, ice hockey, and soccer. *Clinical Journal of Sport Medicine*. 2014; 24(3): 233–237.

101. Ellis MJ, Ritchie LJ, Koltek M et al. Psychiatric outcomes after pediatric sports-related concussion. *Journal of Neurosurgery Pediatrics*. 2015: 1–10.

102. Olsson KA, Lloyd OT, Lebrocque RM, McKinlay L, Anderson VA, Kenardy JA. Predictors of child post-concussion symptoms at 6 and 18 months following mild traumatic brain injury. *Brain Injury*. 2013; 27(2): 145–157.

103. Babikian T, McArthur D, Asarnow RF. Predictors of 1-month and 1-year neuro-cognitive functioning from the UCLA longitudinal mild, uncomplicated, pediatric traumatic brain injury study. *Journal of the International Neuropsychological Society.* 2013; 19(2): 145–154.

104. Broshek DK, De Marco AP, Freeman JR. A review of post-concussion syndrome and psychological factors associated with concussion. *Brain Injury.* 2015; 29(2): 228–237.

105. Al-Ozairi A, McCullagh S, Feinstein A. Predicting posttraumatic stress symptoms following mild, moderate, and severe traumatic brain injury: the role of posttraumatic amnesia. *The Journal of Head Trauma Rehabilitation.* 2015; 30(4): 283–289.

106. Wood RL, O'Hagan G, Williams C, McCabe M, Chadwick N. Anxiety sensitivity and alexithymia as mediators of postconcussion syndrome following mild traumatic brain injury. *The Journal of Head Trauma Rehabilitation.* 2014; 29(1): E9–e17.

107. Waldron-Perrine B, Hennrick H, Spencer RJ, Pangilinan PH, Bieliauskas LA. Postconcussive symptom report in polytrauma: influence of mild traumatic brain injury and psychiatric distress. *Military Medicine.* 2014; 179(8): 856–864.

108. Yang J, Peek-Asa C, Covassin T, Torner JC. Post-concussion symptoms of depression and anxiety in division I collegiate athletes. *Developmental Neuropsychology.* 2015; 40(1): 18–23.

109. Motzkin JC, Koenigs MR. Post-traumatic stress disorder and traumatic brain injury. *Handbook of Clinical Neurology.* 2015; 128: 633–648.

110. Wang X, Wei XE, Li MH et al. Microbleeds on susceptibility-weighted MRI in depressive and non-depressive patients after mild traumatic brain injury. *Neurological Sciences.* 2014; 35(10): 1533–1539.

111. Maller JJ, Thomson RH, Pannek K, Bailey N, Lewis PM, Fitzgerald PB. Volumetrics relate to the development of depression after traumatic brain injury. *Behavioural Brain Research.* 2014; 271: 147–153.

112. Chen JK, Johnston KM, Petrides M, Ptito A. Neural substrates of symptoms of depression following concussion in male athletes with persisting postconcussion symptoms. *Archives of General Psychiatry.* 2008; 65(1): 81–89.

113. Ponsford J, Willmott C, Rothwell A et al. Impact of early intervention on outcome after mild traumatic brain injury in children. *Pediatrics.* 2001; 108(6): 1297–1303.

114. Merritt VC, Arnett PA. Premorbid predictors of postconcussion symptoms in collegiate athletes. *Journal of Clinical and Experimental Neuropsychology.* 2014; 36(10): 1098–1111.

115. Adeyemo BO, Biederman J, Zafonte R et al. Mild traumatic brain injury and ADHD: a systematic review of the literature and meta-analysis. *Journal of Attention Disorders.* 2014; 18(7): 576–584.

116. Bonfield CM, Lam S, Lin Y, Greene S. The impact of attention deficit hyperactivity disorder on recovery from mild traumatic brain injury. *Journal of Neurosurgery Pediatrics.* 2013; 12(2): 97–102.

117. Choe MC, Giza CC. Diagnosis and management of acute concussion. *Seminars in Neurology.* 2015; 35(1): 29–41.

118. Pineau H, Marchand A, Guay S. Objective neuropsychological deficits in post-traumatic stress disorder and mild traumatic brain injury: what remains beyond symptom similarity? *Behavioral Sciences.* 2014; 4(4): 471–486.

119. Shandera-Ochsner AL, Berry DT, Harp JP et al. Neuropsychological effects of self-reported deployment-related mild TBI and current PTSD in OIF/OEF veterans. *The Clinical Neuropsychologist.* 2013; 27(6): 881–907.

120. Nelson LD, Guskiewicz KM, Marshall SW et al. Multiple self-reported concussions are more prevalent in athletes with ADHD and learning disability. *Clinical Journal of Sport Medicine*. 2015.

121. Mautner K, Sussman WI, Axtman M, Al-Farsi Y, Al-Adawi S. Relationship of attention deficit hyperactivity disorder and postconcussion recovery in youth athletes. *Clinical Journal of Sport Medicine*. 2015; 25(4): 355–360.

122. Ganti L, Khalid H, Patel PS, Daneshvar Y, Bodhit AN, Peters KR. Who gets post-concussion syndrome? An emergency department-based prospective analysis. *International Journal of Emergency Medicine*. 2014; 7: 31.

123. Dougan BK, Horswill MS, Geffen GM. Do injury characteristics predict the severity of acute neuropsychological deficits following sports-related concussion? A meta-analysis. *Journal of the International Neuropsychological Society*. 2014; 20(1): 81–87.

124. McCrea M, Guskiewicz K, Randolph C et al. Incidence, clinical course, and predictors of prolonged recovery time following sport-related concussion in high school and college athletes. *Journal of the International Neuropsychological Society*. 2013; 19(1): 22–33.

125. Register-Mihalik JK, De Maio VJ, Tibbo-Valeriote HL, Wooten JD. Characteristics of pediatric and adolescent concussion clinic patients with postconcussion amnesia. *Clinical Journal of Sport Medicine*. 2014.

126. Scopaz KA, Hatzenbuehler JR. Risk modifiers for concussion and prolonged recovery. *Sports Health*. 2013; 5(6): 537–541.

127. Merritt VC, Rabinowitz AR, Arnett PA. Injury-related predictors of symptom severity following sports-related concussion. *Journal of Clinical and Experimental Neuropsychology*. 2015; 37(3): 265–275.

128. Heidari K, Asadollahi S, Jamshidian M, Abrishamchi SN, Nouroozi M. Prediction of neuropsychological outcome after mild traumatic brain injury using clinical parameters, serum S100B protein and findings on computed tomography. *Brain Injury*. 2015; 29(1): 33–40.

129. Wolf H, Frantal S, Pajenda G, Leitgeb J, Sarahrudi K, Hajdu S. Analysis of S100 calcium binding protein B serum levels in different types of traumatic intracranial lesions. *Journal of Neurotrauma*. 2015; 32(1): 23–27.

130. Papa L, Silvestri S, Brophy GM et al. GFAP out-performs S100beta in detecting traumatic intracranial lesions on computed tomography in trauma patients with mild traumatic brain injury and those with extracranial lesions. *Journal of Neurotrauma*. 2014; 31(22): 1815–1822.

131. Wolf H, Frantal S, Pajenda GS et al. Predictive value of neuromarkers supported by a set of clinical criteria in patients with mild traumatic brain injury: S100B protein and neuron-specific enolase on trial: clinical article. *Journal of Neurosurgery*. 2013; 118(6): 1298–1303.

132. Mussack T, Biberthaler P, Kanz KG et al. Immediate S-100B and neuron-specific enolase plasma measurements for rapid evaluation of primary brain damage in alcohol-intoxicated, minor head-injured patients. *Shock*. 2002; 18(5): 395–400.

133. Kulbe JR, Geddes JW. Current status of fluid biomarkers in mild traumatic brain injury. *Experimental Neurology*. 2015.

134. Bazarian JJ, Blyth BJ, He H et al. Classification accuracy of serum Apo A-I and S100B for the diagnosis of mild traumatic brain injury and prediction of abnormal initial head computed tomography scan. *Journal of Neurotrauma*. 2013; 30(20): 1747–1754.

135. Grubenhoff JA, Deakyne SJ, Brou L, Bajaj L, Comstock RD, Kirkwood MW. Acute concussion symptom severity and delayed symptom resolution. *Pediatrics*. 2014; 134(1): 54–62.

136. Subbian V, Meunier JM, Korfhagen JJ, Ratcliff JJ, Shaw GJ, Beyette FR, Jr. Quantitative assessment of post-concussion syndrome following mild traumatic brain injury using robotic technology. *Conference Proceedings*. 2014; 2014: 5353–5356.

137. Lau BC, Collins MW, Lovell MR. Cutoff scores in neurocognitive testing and symptom clusters that predict protracted recovery from concussions in high school athletes. *Neurosurgery*. 2012; 70(2): 371–379.

138. Lau BC, Kontos AP, Collins MW, Mucha A, Lovell MR. Which on-field signs/symptoms predict protracted recovery from sport-related concussion among high school football players? *The American Journal of Sports Medicine*. 2011; 39(11): 2311–2318.

139. Colloca L, Finniss D. Nocebo effects, patient-clinician communication, and therapeutic outcomes. *The Journal of the American Medical Association*. 2012; 307(6): 567–568.

140. Snell DL, Hay-Smith EJ, Surgenor LJ, Siegert RJ. Examination of outcome after mild traumatic brain injury: the contribution of injury beliefs and Leventhal's common sense model. *Neuropsychological Rehabilitation*. 2013; 23(3): 333–362.

141. Snell DL, Surgenor LJ, Hay-Smith EJ, Williman J, Siegert RJ. The contribution of psychological factors to recovery after mild traumatic brain injury: is cluster analysis a useful approach? *Brain Injury*. 2015; 29(3): 291–299.

142. Araujo GC, Antonini TN, Monahan K et al. The relationship between suboptimal effort and post-concussion symptoms in children and adolescents with mild traumatic brain injury. *The Clinical Neuropsychologist*. 2014; 28(5): 786–801.

143. Whittaker R, Kemp S, House A. Illness perceptions and outcome in mild head injury: a longitudinal study. *Journal of Neurology, Neurosurgery, and Psychiatry*. 2007; 78(6): 644–646.

144. Snell DL, Siegert RJ, Hay-Smith EJ, Surgenor LJ. Associations between illness perceptions, coping styles and outcome after mild traumatic brain injury: preliminary results from a cohort study. *Brain Injury*. 2011; 25(11): 1126–1138.

145. Sullivan KA, Edmed SL, Allan AC, Smith SS, Karlsson LJ. The role of psychological resilience and mTBI as predictors of postconcussional syndrome symptomatology. *Rehabilitation Psychology*. 2015; 60(2): 147–154.

146. McCauley SR, Wilde EA, Miller ER et al. Preinjury resilience and mood as predictors of early outcome following mild traumatic brain injury. *Journal of Neurotrauma*. 2013; 30(8): 642–652.

147. Maestas KL, Sander AM, Clark AN et al. Preinjury coping, emotional functioning, and quality of life following uncomplicated and complicated mild traumatic brain injury. *The Journal of Head Trauma Rehabilitation*. 2014; 29(5): 407–417.

148. Belanger HG, Curtiss G, Demery JA, Lebowitz BK, Vanderploeg RD. Factors moderating neuropsychological outcomes following mild traumatic brain injury: a meta-analysis. *Journal of the International Neuropsychological Society*. 2005; 11(3): 215–227.

149. Lees-Haley PR, Brown RS. Neuropsychological complaint base rates of 170 personal injury claimants. *Archives of Clinical Neuropsychology*. 1993; 8(3): 203–209.

150. Wood RL. Understanding the 'miserable minority': a diasthesis-stress paradigm for post-concussional syndrome. *Brain Injury*. 2004; 18(11): 1135–1153.

151. Sandy Macleod AD. Post-concussion syndrome: the attraction of the psychological by the organic. *Medical Hypotheses*. 2010; 74(6): 1033–1035.

152. Lagarde E, Salmi LR, Holm LW et al. Association of symptoms following mild traumatic brain injury with posttraumatic stress disorder vs. postconcussion syndrome. *The Journal of the American Medical Association Psychiatry*. 2014; 71(9): 1032–1040.

153. King NS. Post-concussion syndrome: Clarity amid the controversy? *The British Journal of Psychiatry*. 2003; 183: 276–278.

154. Gaetz M, Weinberg H. Electrophysiological indices of persistent post-concussion symptoms. *Brain Injury*. 2000; 14(9): 815–832.

155. Dupuis F, Johnston KM, Lavoie M, Lepore F, Lassonde M. Concussions in athletes produce brain dysfunction as revealed by event-related potentials. *Neuroreport*. 2000; 11(18): 4087–4092.

156. Dean PJ, Sato JR, Vieira G, McNamara A, Sterr A. Long-term structural changes after mTBI and their relation to post-concussion symptoms. *Brain Injury*. 2015; 1–8.

157. Messe A, Caplain S, Pelegrini-Issac M et al. Specific and evolving resting-state network alterations in post-concussion syndrome following mild traumatic brain injury. *PLoS One*. 2013; 8(6): e65470.

158. Lovell MR, Pardini JE, Welling J et al. Functional brain abnormalities are related to clinical recovery and time to return-to-play in athletes. *Neurosurgery*. 2007; 61(2): 352–359.

159. Smits M, Houston GC, Dippel DW et al. Microstructural brain injury in post-concussion syndrome after minor head injury. *Neuroradiology*. 2011; 53(8): 553–563.

160. Oeur RA, Karton C, Post-A et al. A comparison of head dynamic response and brain tissue stress and strain using accident reconstructions for concussion, concussion with persistent postconcussive symptoms, and subdural hematoma. *Journal of Neurosurgery*. 2015; 123(2): 415–422.

161. Post A, Kendall M, Koncan D et al. Characterization of persistent concussive syndrome using injury reconstruction and finite element modelling. *Journal of the Mechanical Behavior of Biomedical Materials*. 2015; 41: 325–335.

162. Rathbone AT, Tharmaradinam S, Jiang S, Rathbone MP, Kumbhare DA. A review of the neuro- and systemic inflammatory responses in post-concussion symptoms: Introduction of the "post-inflammatory brain syndrome" PIBS. *Brain, Behavior, and Immunity*. 2015; 46: 1–16.

163. Zasler ND. Sports concussion headache. *Brain Injury*. 2015; 29(2): 207–220.

164. Mayer CL, Huber BR, Peskind E. Traumatic brain injury, neuroinflammation, and post-traumatic headaches. *Headache*. 2013; 53(9): 1523–1530.

165. Benromano T, Defrin R, Ahn AH, Zhao J, Pick CG, Levy D. Mild closed head injury promotes a selective trigeminal hyperno-ciception: implications for the acute emergence of post-traumatic headache. *European Journal of Pain*. 2015; 19(5): 621–628.

166. Gardner AJ, Tan CO, Ainslie PN et al. Cerebrovascular reactivity assessed by transcranial Doppler ultrasound in sport-related concussion: A systematic review. *British Journal of Sports Medicine*. 2015; 49(16): 1050–1055.

167. Militana AR, Donahue MJ, Sills AK et al. Alterations in default-mode network connectivity may be influenced by cerebrovascular changes within 1 week of sports related concussion in college varsity athletes: a pilot study. *Brain Imaging and Behavior*. 2015.

168. Newberg AB, Serruya M, Gepty A et al. Clinical comparison of 99mTc exametazime and 123I Ioflupane SPECT in patients with chronic mild traumatic brain injury. *PLoS One*. 2014; 9(1): e87009.

169. Astafiev SV, Shulman GL, Metcalf NV et al. Abnormal white matter blood-oxygen-level-dependent signals in chronic mild traumatic brain injury. *Journal of Neurotrauma*. 2015; 32(16): 1254–1271.

170. Agrawal D, Gowda NK, Bal CS, Pant M, Mahapatra AK. Is medial temporal injury responsible for pediatric postconcussion syndrome? A prospective controlled study with single-photon emission computerized tomography. *Journal of Neurosurgery*. 2005; 102(2 Suppl): 167–171.

171. Clausen M, Pendergast DR, Willer B, Leddy J. Cerebral blood flow during treadmill exercise is a marker of physiological postconcussion syndrome in female athletes. *The Journal of Head Trauma Rehabilitation*. 2015.

172. Chen SH, Kareken DA, Fastenau PS, Trexler LE, Hutchins GD. A study of persistent postconcussion symptoms in mild head trauma using positron emission tomography. *Journal of Neurology, Neurosurgery, and Psychiatry*. 2003; 74(3): 326–332.

173. Daneshvar DH, Riley DO, Nowinski CJ, McKee AC, Stern RA, Cantu RC. Long-term consequences: effects on normal development profile after concussion. *Physical Medicine and Rehabilitation Clinics of North America*. 2011; 22(4): 683–700, ix.

174. Silverberg ND, Iverson GL. Etiology of the post-concussion syndrome: Physiogenesis and Psychogenesis revisited. *NeuroRehabilitation*. 2011; 29(4): 317–329.

175. Petraglia AL, Maroon JC, Bailes JE. From the field of play to the field of combat: a review of the pharmacological management of concussion. *Neurosurgery*. 2012; 70(6): 1520–1533.

176. McCrory P, Meeuwisse WH, Aubry M et al. Consensus statement on concussion in sport: the 4th International Conference on Concussion in Sport, Zurich, November 2012. *Journal of Athletic Training*. 2013; 48(4): 554–575.

177. Snell DL, Surgenor LJ, Hay-Smith EJ, Siegert RJ. A systematic review of psychological treatments for mild traumatic brain injury: an update on the evidence. *Journal of Clinical and Experimental Neuropsychology*. 2009; 31(1): 20–38.

178. Iverson GL. Misdiagnosis of the persistent postconcussion syndrome in patients with depression. *Archives of Clinical Neuropsychology*. 2006; 21(4): 303–310.

179. De Marco AP, Broshek DK. Computerized cognitive testing in the management of youth sports-related concussion. *Journal of Child Neurology*. 2014; 31(1): 68–75.

180. Bramley H, Heverley S, Lewis MM, Kong L, Rivera R, Silvis M. Demographics and treatment of adolescent posttraumatic headache in a regional concussion clinic. *Pediatric Neurology*. 2015; 52(5): 493–498.

181. Seifert TD. Sports concussion and associated post-traumatic headache. *Headache*. 2013; 53(5): 726–736.

182. Heyer GL, Young JA, Rose SC, McNally KA, Fischer AN. Post-traumatic headaches correlate with migraine symptoms in youth with concussion. *Cephalalgia*. 2015.

183. Ropper AH, Gorson KC. Clinical practice. Concussion. *The New England Journal of Medicine*. 2007; 356(2): 166–172.

184. Meehan WP, 3rd. Medical therapies for concussion. *Clinics in Sports Medicine*. 2011; 30(1): 115–124, ix.

185. Pinchefsky E, Dubrovsky AS, Friedman D, Shevell M. Part II—Management of pediatric post-traumatic headaches. *Pediatric Neurology*. 2015; 52(3): 270–280.

186. Reddy CC. Postconcussion syndrome: a physiatrist's approach. *PM & R*. 2011; 3(10 Suppl 2): S396–405.

187. Kernick DP, Goadsby PJ. Guidance for the management of headache in sport on behalf of The Royal College of General Practitioners and The British Association for the Study of Headache. *Cephalalgia*. 2011; 31(1): 106–111.

188. Comper P, Bisschop SM, Carnide N, Tricco A. A systematic review of treatments for mild traumatic brain injury. *Brain Injury*. 2005; 19(11): 863–880.

189. Willer B, Leddy JJ. Management of concussion and post-concussion syndrome. *Current Treatment Options in Neurology*. 2006; 8(5): 415–426.

190. Blume HK. Headaches after concussion in pediatrics: a review. *Current Pain and Headache Reports*. 2015; 19(9): 42.

191. Pasek TA, Locasto LW, Reichard J, Fazio Sumrok VC, Johnson EW, Kontos AP. The headache electronic diary for children with concussion. *Clinical Nurse Specialist CNS*. 2015; 29(2): 80–88.

192. Leddy JJ, Baker JG, Merchant A et al. Brain or strain? Symptoms alone do not distinguish physiologic concussion from cervical/vestibular injury. *Clinical Journal of Sport Medicine*. 2015; 25(3): 237–242.

193. Fredriksen TA, Antonaci F, Sjaastad O. Cervicogenic headache: too important to be left un-diagnosed. *The Journal of Headache and Pain*. 2015; 16(1): 6.

194. Khusid MA. Clinical indications for acupuncture in chronic post-traumatic headache management. *Military Medicine*. 2015; 180(2): 132–136.

195. Burns SL. Concussion treatment using massage techniques: a case study. *International Journal of Therapeutic Massage & Bodywork*. 2015; 8(2): 12–17.

196. Zaremski JL, Herman DC, Clugston JR, Hurley RW, Ahn AH. Occipital neuralgia as a sequela of sports concussion: a case series and review of the literature. *Current Sports Medicine Reports*. 2015; 14(1): 16–19.

197. Ducic I, Sinkin JC, Crutchfield KE. Interdisciplinary treatment of post-concussion and post-traumatic headaches. *Microsurgery*. 2015.

198. Orff HJ, Ayalon L, Drummond SP. Traumatic brain injury and sleep disturbance: a review of current research. *The Journal of Head Trauma Rehabilitation*. 2009; 24(3): 155–165.

199. Gronwall D, Wrightson P. Delayed recovery of intellectual function after minor head injury. *Lancet*. 1974; 2(7881): 605–609.

200. Sabir M, Gaudreault PO, Freyburger M et al. Impact of traumatic brain injury on sleep structure, electrocorticographic activity and transcriptome in mice. *Brain, Behavior, and Immunity*. 2015; 47: 118–130.

201. Rowe RK, Striz M, Bachstetter AD et al. Diffuse brain injury induces acute post-traumatic sleep. *PLoS One*. 2014; 9(1): e82507.

202. Jaffee MS, Winter WC, Jones CC, Ling G. Sleep disturbances in athletic concussion. *Brain Injury*. 2015; 29(2): 221–227.

203. Chiu HY, Lo WC, Chiang YH, Tsai PS. The effects of sleep on the relationship between brain injury severity and recovery of cognitive function: a prospective study. *International Journal of Nursing Studies*. 2014; 51(6): 892–899.

204. Ponsford JL, Parcell DL, Sinclair KL, Roper M, Rajaratnam SM. Changes in sleep patterns following traumatic brain injury: a controlled study. *Neurorehabilitation and Neural Repair*. 2013; 27(7): 613–621.

205. Tham SW, Fales J, Palermo TM. Subjective and objective assessment of sleep in adolescents with mild traumatic brain injury. *Journal of Neurotrauma*. 2015; 32(11): 847–852.

206. Sullivan KA, Edmed SL, Allan AC, Karlsson LJ, Smith SS. Characterizing self-reported sleep disturbance after mild traumatic brain injury. *Journal of Neurotrauma*. 2015; 32(7): 474–486.

207. Huang TY, Ma HP, Tsai SH, Chiang YH, Hu CJ, Ou J. Sleep duration and sleep quality following acute mild traumatic brain injury: a propensity score analysis. *Behavioural Neurology*. 2015; 2015: 378726.

208. Sufrinko A, Pearce K, Elbin RJ et al. The effect of preinjury sleep difficulties on neurocognitive impairment and symptoms after sport-related concussion. *The American Journal of Sports Medicine.* 2015; 43(4): 830–838.

209. Kostyun RO, Milewski MD, Hafeez I. Sleep disturbance and neurocognitive function during the recovery from a sport-related concussion in adolescents. *The American Journal of Sports Medicine.* 2015; 43(3): 633–640.

210. Kallestad H, Jacobsen HB, Landro NI, Borchgrevink PC, Stiles TC. The role of insomnia in the treatment of chronic fatigue. *Journal of Psychosomatic Research.* 2015; 78(5): 427–432.

211. Mihalik JP, Lengas E, Register-Mihalik JK, Oyama S, Begalle RL, Guskiewicz KM. The effects of sleep quality and sleep quantity on concussion baseline assessment. *Clinical Journal of Sport Medicine.* 2013; 23(5): 343–348.

212. McClure DJ, Zuckerman SL, Kutscher SJ, Gregory AJ, Solomon GS. Baseline neurocognitive testing in sports-related concussions: the importance of a prior night's sleep. *The American Journal of Sports Medicine.* 2014; 42(2): 472–478.

213. Hou L, Han X, Sheng P et al. Risk factors associated with sleep disturbance following traumatic brain injury: clinical findings and questionnaire based study. *PLoS One.* 2013; 8(10): e76087.

214. Bryan CJ. Repetitive traumatic brain injury (or concussion) increases severity of sleep disturbance among deployed military personnel. *Sleep.* 2013; 36(6): 941–946.

215. Elbin RJ, Schatz P, Lowder HB, Kontos AP. An empirical review of treatment and rehabilitation approaches used in the acute, sub-acute, and chronic phases of recovery following sports-related concussion. *Current Treatment Options in Neurology.* 2014; 16(11): 320.

216. Al Sayegh A, Sandford D, Carson AJ. Psychological approaches to treatment of postconcussion syndrome: a systematic review. *Journal of Neurology, Neurosurgery, and Psychiatry.* 2010; 81(10): 1128–1134.

217. Menn SJ, Yang R, Lankford A. Armodafinil for the treatment of excessive sleepiness associated with mild or moderate closed traumatic brain injury: a 12-week, randomized, double-blind study followed by a 12-month open-label extension. *Journal of Clinical Sleep Medicine.* 2014; 10(11): 1181–1191.

218. Kaiser PR, Valko PO, Werth E et al. Modafinil ameliorates excessive daytime sleepiness after traumatic brain injury. *Neurology.* 2010; 75(20): 1780–1785.

219. Jha A, Weintraub A, Allshouse A et al. A randomized trial of modafinil for the treatment of fatigue and excessive daytime sleepiness in individuals with chronic traumatic brain injury. *The Journal of Head Trauma Rehabilitation.* 2008; 23(1): 52–63.

220. Makdissi M, Cantu RC, Johnston KM, McCrory P, Meeuwisse WH. The difficult concussion patient: what is the best approach to investigation and management of persistent (>10 days) postconcussive symptoms? *British Journal of Sports Medicine.* 2013; 47(5): 308–313.

221. Reddy CC, Collins M, Lovell M, Kontos AP. Efficacy of amantadine treatment on symptoms and neurocognitive performance among adolescents following sports-related concussion. *The Journal of Head Trauma Rehabilitation.* 2013; 28(4): 260–265.

222. Sawyer E, Mauro LS, Ohlinger MJ. Amantadine enhancement of arousal and cognition after traumatic brain injury. *The Annals of Pharmacotherapy.* 2008; 42(2): 247–252.

223. Wang X, Zhao X, Mao ZY, Wang XM, Liu ZL. Neuroprotective effect of docosahexaenoic acid on glutamate-induced cytotoxicity in rat hippocampal cultures. *Neuroreport.* 2003; 14(18): 2457–2461.

224. Chew E, Zafonte RD. Pharmacological management of neurobehavioral disorders following traumatic brain injury—a state-of-the-art review. *Journal of Rehabilitation Research and Development*. 2009; 46(6): 851–879.

225. Whyte J, Hart T, Vaccaro M et al. Effects of methylphenidate on attention deficits after traumatic brain injury: a multidimensional, randomized, controlled trial. *American Journal of Physical Medicine & Rehabilitation*. 2004; 83(6): 401–420.

226. Whyte J, Hart T, Schuster K, Fleming M, Polansky M, Coslett HB. Effects of methylphenidate on attentional function after traumatic brain injury. A randomized, placebo-controlled trial. *American Journal of Physical Medicine and Rehabilitation*. 1997; 76(6): 440–450.

227. Whelan FJ, Walker MS, Schultz SK. Donepezil in the treatment of cognitive dysfunction associated with traumatic brain injury. *Annals of Clinical Psychiatry*. 2000; 12(3): 131–135.

228. Flanagan SR, Greenwald B, Wieber S. Pharmacological treatment of insomnia for individuals with brain injury. *The Journal of Head Trauma Rehabilitation*. 2007; 22(1): 67–70.

229. Samantaray S, Das A, Thakore NP et al. Therapeutic potential of melatonin in traumatic central nervous system injury. *Journal of Pineal Research*. 2009; 47(2): 134–142.

230. Buscemi N, Vandermeer B, Hooton N et al. Efficacy and safety of exogenous melatonin for secondary sleep disorders and sleep disorders accompanying sleep restriction: meta-analysis. *British Medical Journal*. 2006; 332(7538): 385–393.

231. Maldonado MD, Murillo-Cabezas F, Terron MP et al. The potential of melatonin in reducing morbidity-mortality after craniocerebral trauma. *Journal of Pineal Research*. 2007; 42(1): 1–11.

232. Barlow KM, Brooks BL, MacMaster FP et al. A double-blind, placebo-controlled intervention trial of 3 and 10 mg sublingual melatonin for post-concussion syndrome in youths (PLAYGAME): study protocol for a randomized controlled trial. *Trials*. 2014; 15: 271.

233. Iverson GL, Atkins JE, Zafonte R, Berkner PD. Concussion history in adolescent athletes with attention-deficit hyperactivity disorder. *Journal of Neurotrauma*. 2014.

234. Chrisman SP, Richardson LP. Prevalence of diagnosed depression in adolescents with history of concussion. *The Journal of Adolescent Health*. 2014; 54(5): 582–586.

235. Vargas G, Rabinowitz A, Meyer J, Arnett PA. Predictors and prevalence of postconcussion depression symptoms in collegiate athletes. *Journal of Athletic Training*. 2015; 50(3): 250–255.

236. Haagsma JA, Scholten AC, Andriessen TM, Vos PE, Van Beeck EF, Polinder S. Impact of depression and post-traumatic stress disorder on functional outcome and health-related quality of life of patients with mild traumatic brain injury. *Journal of Neurotrauma*. 2015; 32(11): 853–862.

237. Kerr ZY, Marshall SW, Harding HP, Jr., Guskiewicz KM. Nine-year risk of depression diagnosis increases with increasing self-reported concussions in retired professional football players. *The American Journal of Sports Medicine*. 2012; 40(10): 2206–2212.

238. Guskiewicz KM, Marshall SW, Bailes J et al. Recurrent concussion and risk of depression in retired professional football players. *Medicine and Science in Sports and Exercise*. 2007; 39(6): 903–909.

239. Max JE, Schachar RJ, Landis J et al. Psychiatric disorders in children and adolescents in the first six months after mild traumatic brain injury. *The Journal of Neuropsychiatry and Clinical Neurosciences*. 2013; 25(3): 187–197.

240. Max JE, Pardo D, Hanten G et al. Psychiatric disorders in children and adolescents six-to-twelve months after mild traumatic

brain injury. *The Journal of Neuropsychiatry and Clinical Neurosciences.* 2013; 25(4): 272–282.

241. Silver JM. Neuropsychiatry of persistent symptoms after concussion. *The Psychiatric Clinics of North America.* 2014; 37(1): 91–102.

242. Conder R, Conder AA. Neuropsychological and psychological rehabilitation interventions in refractory sport-related postconcussive syndrome. *Brain Injury.* 2015; 29(2): 249–262.

243. Kontos AP, Elbin RJ, Newcomer Appaneal R, Covassin T, Collins MW. A comparison of coping responses among high school and college athletes with concussion, orthopedic injuries, and healthy controls. *Research in Sports Medicine (Print).* 2013; 21(4): 367–379.

244. Nelson Sheese AL, Hammeke TA. Rehabilitation from postconcussion syndrome: nonpharmacological treatment. *Progress in Neurological Surgery.* 2014; 28: 149–160.

245. Van Vleet TM, Chen A, Vernon A, Novakovic-Agopian T, D'Esposito MT. Tonic and phasic alertness training: a novel treatment for executive control dysfunction following mild traumatic brain injury. *Neurocase.* 2015; 21(4): 489–498.

246. Potter S, Brown RG. Cognitive behavioural therapy and persistent post-concussional symptoms: Integrating conceptual issues and practical aspects in treatment. *Neuropsychological Rehabilitation.* 2012; 22(1): 1–25.

247. Silverberg ND, Hallam BJ, Rose A et al. Cognitive-behavioral prevention of postconcussion syndrome in at-risk patients: a pilot randomized controlled trial. *The Journal of Head Trauma Rehabilitation.* 2013; 28(4): 313–322.

248. Fann JR, Bombardier CH, Vannoy S et al. Telephone and in-person cognitive behavioral therapy for major depression after traumatic brain injury: a randomized controlled trial. *Journal of Neurotrauma.* 2015; 32(1): 45–57.

249. Bradbury CL, Christensen BK, Lau MA, Ruttan LA, Arundine AL, Green RE. The efficacy of cognitive behavior therapy in the treatment of emotional distress after acquired brain injury. *Archives of Physical Medicine and Rehabilitation.* 2008; 89(12 Suppl): S61–68.

250. Tenovuo O. Pharmacological enhancement of cognitive and behavioral deficits after traumatic brain injury. *Current Opinion in Neurology.* 2006; 19(6): 528–533.

251. Silver JM, McAllister TW, Arciniegas DB. Depression and cognitive complaints following mild traumatic brain injury. *The American Journal of Psychiatry.* 2009; 166(6): 653–661.

252. Moran B, Tadikonda P, Sneed KB, Hummel M, Guiteau S, Coris EE. Postconcussive syndrome following sports-related concussion: a treatment overview for primary care physicians. *Southern Medical Journal.* 2015; 108(9): 553–558.

253. Barker-Collo S, Starkey N, Theadom A. Treatment for depression following mild traumatic brain injury in adults: a meta-analysis. *Brain Injury.* 2013; 27(10): 1124–1133.

254. Rapoport MJ, Mitchell RA, McCullagh S et al. A randomized controlled trial of antidepressant continuation for major depression following traumatic brain injury. *The Journal of Clinical Psychiatry.* 2010; 71(9): 1125–1130.

255. Rapoport MJ, Chan F, Lanctot K, Herrmann N, McCullagh S, Feinstein A. An open-label study of citalopram for major depression following traumatic brain injury. *Journal of Psychopharmacology.* 2008; 22(8): 860–864.

256. Ansari A, Jain A, Sharma A, Mittal RS, Gupta ID. Role of sertraline in posttraumatic brain injury depression and quality-of-life in TBI. *Asian Journal of Neurosurgery.* 2014; 9(4): 182–188.

257. Borg J, Holm L, Peloso PM et al. Non-surgical intervention and cost for mild traumatic brain injury: results of the WHO Collaborating Centre Task Force on Mild Traumatic Brain Injury. *Journal of Rehabilitation Medicine.* 2004(43 Suppl): 76–83.

258. Leddy JJ, Kozlowski K, Fung M, Pendergast DR, Willer B. Regulatory and autoregulatory physiological dysfunction as a primary characteristic of post-concussion syndrome: implications for treatment. *NeuroRehabilitation*. 2007; 22(3): 199–205.

259. Gagnon I, Galli C, Friedman D, Grilli L, Iverson GL. Active rehabilitation for children who are slow to recover following sport-related concussion. *Brain Injury*. 2009; 23(12): 956–964.

260. Leddy JJ, Kozlowski K, Donnelly JP, Pendergast DR, Epstein LH, Willer B. A preliminary study of subsymptom threshold exercise training for refractory post-concussion syndrome. *Clinical Journal of Sport Medicine*. 2010; 20(1): 21–27.

261. Gagnon I, Grilli L, Friedman D, Iverson GL. A pilot study of active rehabilitation for adolescents who are slow to recover from sport-related concussion. *Scandinavian Journal of Medicine and Science in Sports*. 2015.

262. Chin LM, Keyser RE, Dsurney J, Chan L. Improved cognitive performance following aerobic exercise training in people with traumatic brain injury. *Archives of Physical Medicine and Rehabilitation*. 2015; 96(4): 754–759.

263. Chin LM, Chan L, Woolstenhulme JG, Christensen EJ, Shenouda CN, Keyser RE. Improved cardiorespiratory fitness with aerobic exercise training in individuals with traumatic brain injury. *The Journal of Head Trauma Rehabilitation*. 2014.

264. Baker JG, Freitas MS, Leddy JJ, Kozlowski KF, Willer BS. Return to full functioning after graded exercise assessment and progressive exercise treatment of postconcussion syndrome. *Rehabilitation Research and Practice*. 2012; 2012: 705309.

265. Leddy JJ, Cox JL, Baker JG et al. Exercise treatment for postconcussion syndrome: a pilot study of changes in functional magnetic resonance imaging activation, physiology, and symptoms. *The Journal of Head Trauma Rehabilitation*. 2013; 28(4): 241–249.

266. Reed N, Greenspoon D, Iverson GL et al. Management of persistent postconcussion symptoms in youth: a randomised control trial protocol. *British Medical Journal Open*. 2015; 5(7): e008468.

267. Lange RT, Iverson GL, Rose A. Post-concussion symptom reporting and the "good-old-days" bias following mild traumatic brain injury. *Archives of Clinical Neuropsychology*. 2010; 25(5): 442–450.

Outpatient care of the concussed athlete: Gauging recovery to tailor rehabilitative needs

With Elizabeth M. Pieroth, Psy.D.

Introduction

The complex pathophysiology of injury and recovery of the nervous system emulates the diverse presentation, symptomatology, and challenges to diagnosis of concussion. As science continues to unfold the nature of the critical window period of recovery following injury, it is imperative that accurate tools to evaluate the injured athlete during this period are developed and researched. Only through proper assessment, including monitoring of the patient's subjective symptoms and use of validated objective measures, can clinicians attempt to determine when the brain is recovered from injury without concerns of exacerbating symptoms or perpetuating long-term harm. Similarly to the multimodal nature in the acute assessment of concussion diagnosis (symptom checklists, neurocognitive assessment, balance/coordination/ocular testing), observation and quantification of recovery employs a similar approach.[1] This multimodal approach is comprised of continual clinical history and exams, neurocognitive testing (in the form of sideline assessment tools), symptom checklists (as discussed in Chapter 3), psychiatric evaluation (as discussed in Chapter 5), and most importantly, neuropsychological testing and other complimentary modalities like oculomotor, vestibular, gait/balance, and electrophysiological evaluations.[2] A survey, completed by 610 NCAA athletic trainers in 2014, stated that a total of 71.2%, 79.2%, and 66.9% athletic trainers employed at least three techniques to: obtain an athletes' baseline neurological status, acutely assess postconcussion, and to determine appropriate return to play.[3] The likelihood of receiving multimodal techniques for assessment is highly influenced by the available resources at that institution. Therefore, these techniques may differ versus those used at a high school setting a Division I university.

Though this multimodal approach is laborious, it is necessary due to the heterogeneous clinical picture post-injury for each athlete composed of various symptoms on deficits, and also their recovery pattern. Athletes may present with profound symptoms and neurological findings on balance, oculomotor, and neuropsychological assessments, that recover at different periods. Multiple studies have attempted to characterize this process demonstrating that posture, balance, and vestibular/ocular deficits usually present early with improvement by 3–5 days post injury, while subjective symptoms tend to last longer, resolving by 3–14 days post injury. Neurocognitive deficits, on the other hand, have been shown to persist longer with recovery from 1 to 4 weeks after injury.[4–13] These time frames are not set rules but do give an appreciation to the varying recovery period exposed by the specific assessment tool that is used.[14] Also, depending on the nature or severity of the injury, athletes may present only with one neurological deficit (for example balance issues) without the myriad of other symptoms or cognitive changes on neuropsychological testing.[15] This undoubtedly highlights the importance for a multimodal approach with many clinical tools, and emphasizes the need to repeatedly assess the athlete following injury in order to correctly identify those that have recovered from their brain injury, versus those that require a prolonged gradation of return to activity.

Due to the varying neurological deficits following a concussive injury and the many limitations to each modality, the repeated use of a multimodal testing protocol will improve the sensitivity in formulating a broader picture of neurological recovery of the athlete.[1] This will not only determine which athletes are suited to return to play, but will also allow a more individualized approach to player rehabilitation. This multimodal approach has been adopted and applied to clinics geared towards the management of the concussed athlete. For instance, a model proposed by the University of Pittsburgh Medical Center Sports Concussion Program incorporates the clinical interview, symptom and neurocognitive testing, and vestibular-ocular screening in order to obtain a holistic neurological assessment of the concussed athlete.[16,17] This information is then used to develop an individualized treatment regimen with rehabilitative services based on the needs of the patient (vestibular, cognitive, ocular, balance, gait, etc.) and also the many referrals the athlete requires to assist in further evaluation and treatment (Figure 6.1).[18] This approach allows a more detailed treatment with specific cognitive and physical restrictions and rehabilitation schedule for the athlete based on their particular deficits.

The intricate nature of concussive injury, presentation, and recovery, requires a comprehensive method in the outpatient setting to gauge recovery and improve return to activity recommendations. The continued assessment following injury should entail a combination of clinical history/exam, sideline or other neurocognitive testing, symptom checklists, neuropsychological testing (if accessible), and other modalities like oculomotor, vestibular, gait, and electrophysiological evaluations. In this chapter, we will discuss these sensitive assessments, and their shortcomings, that are used in the concussed athlete to measure their neurological deficit and monitor their recovery. Through proper identification of these deficits, specific rehabilitative recommendations can be made to individually tailor the athlete's road to recovery.

Neuropsychological testing

"The application of neuropsychological testing in concussion has been shown to be of clinical value and contributes significant information in concussion evaluation. Although in most cases cognitive recovery largely overlaps with the time course of symptom recovery, it has been demonstrated that cognitive recovery may occasionally precede or more commonly follow clinical

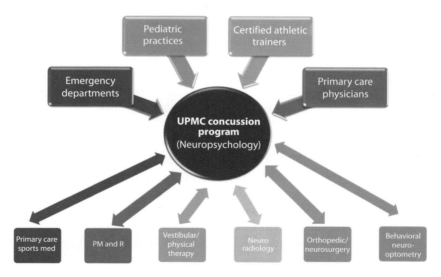

Figure 6.1   Schematic diagram of University of Pittsburgh Medical Center Sports Concussion Program. Primary referral is through emergency departments, primary care physicians, and athletic trainers. A comprehensive evaluation is performed by a neuropsychologist to determine rehabilitative needs and need for referrals to other medical professionals. (From Reynolds E et al., Establishing a Clinical Service for the Management of Sports-Related Concussions. *Neurosurgery* v75, 2014. Wolters Kluwer Health, Inc. With permission.)

symptom resolution…it must be emphasized, however, that neuropsychological assessment should not be the sole basis of management decision. Rather, it should be seen as an aid to the clinical decision-making process in conjunction with a range of assessments of different clinical domains and investigational results… At present, there is insufficient evidence to recommend the widespread routine use of baseline NP testing".[19] Reflective of this encompassing stance of neuropsychological testing (NPT) taken by the 2013 Zurich Guidelines, we will further introduce NPT, along with the benefits, limitations, and recommendations for the use of NPT. We hope that this will relay to the reader why NPT has been so actively adopted for use in return to activity decisions, specifically in athletes experiencing a challenging postinjury course, in either high school, collegiate (NCAA), or professional sporting arenas (NFL, NHL, MLS, NBA).[20,21]

Types of neuropsychological testing

Neuropsychological tests (NPTs) are written or computerized tests that measure cognitive abilities like attention/concentration, memory acquisition, verbal and visual memory, executive functioning, psychomotor reaction time, and global cognitive abilities.[22–25] A clinician can then compare postinjury NPT scores to either age-matched normative values and/or preinjury baseline scores to objectively measure the postinjury neurological/cognitive deficit and make suggestions for the player's recovery/rehabilitative process.[26] Many have advocated for this "return to baseline" approach for the decision process of return to activity.[27] It should be emphasized that NPT is not intended to be used diagnostically, but as an objective measure of neurological sequelae and recovery following concussive injury.[1,19,24,25]

There are numerous written (paper-pencil) cognitive tests that can be used in concussion assessment. The choice of tests is made by the examiner, as there is no specific battery of paper-pencil tests for concussion assessment. One of the disadvantages of paper-pencil cognitive tests is the lack of alternative forms available for repeat testing. The test–retest reliability of many commonly used paper-pencil tests may be poor and there are concerns about practice effects with

repeated exposure to a test.[28,29] That is, the athlete's improved score on repeat tests may not necessarily be as a result of improvement in symptoms, but rather, their familiarity with the test on repeat attempts. Additionally, traditional written tests do not appear to be sensitive to the subtle changes seen in reaction time postconcussion.[30] Finally, the administration, scoring, and interpretation of paper-pencil tests are significantly longer and require a properly trained neuropsychologist.

Examples of commercially available computer based NPTs are: HeadMinder, Automated Neuropsychological Assessment Metrics (ANAM), Immediate Post Concussion Assessment and Cognitive Battery (ImPACT), CogSport or Axon Sports Computerized Cognitive Assessment tool, Multimodal Assessment of Cognition and Symptoms for Children (MACE).[31–35] The benefits of the computerized method are that they are quicker than the paper-pencil tests, which must be administered by a neuropsychologist or trained psychometrist, therefore allowing greater ease in obtaining baseline and repeated testing following injury. The computerized interface also allows administration to multiple athletes at one time, more precise testing of reaction time, a consistent testing atmosphere, use of multiple alternative forms for serial testing, and provides immediate results.[32,36,37]

However, legitimate concerns have been raised about the use of computerized testing in neuropsychological assessment. The National Academy of Neuropsychology and the American Academy of Neuropsychology published a joint statement addressing the use of computerized neuropsychological assessment devices (CNAD).[38] The concerns in the paper were not specific to concussion assessment tools but rather the concerns about interpretation of CNADs, technical hardware/software issues, privacy and data security, psychometric development issues, and the reliability/validity of commercially available tests.

ImPACT is the most commonly used computerized NPT; one study states that 93% of high schools specifically use this tool.[39] The test is composed of six modules that assess verbal and visual memory, processing speed, reaction time, and impulse control.[36] Additionally, the computerized nature of this test allows the ability to measure reaction time more precisely, which is a sensitive marker of injury that persists beyond symptom resolution.[40] There is also a 20-question symptom checklist that asks the examinee to rate their subjective physical and cognitive symptoms. A benefit to its use is that ImPACT does have age matched reference values if baseline testing is not available.[41] ImPACT has been extensively validated and shown to have a specificity of 69%–97% and a sensitivity of 82%–95%.[42–46] However, other researchers have questioned the retest reliability of ImPACT.[47,48]

The CogSport is another NPT that is less time intensive (10 min) than the ImPACT (20–30 min). This computerized NPT reduced issues with language barriers by using playing cards that test reaction time, working/sustained memory, and new learning.[38] Also, the CogSport (now commercially available as Axon Sports; www.axonsports .com) has shown strong retest reliability in comparison to ImPACT but only limited research has been performed.[49]

Lastly, the MACE is a computerized NPT for the assessment of children ages 5–12.[50] It similarly tests learning, memory, reaction time, and processing speed and produces two composite scores: response speed and learning memory accuracy. Due to the progression through cognitive milestones from youth to high school age, repeated baseline testing is recommended, which can be used then after injury.

There are additional tests available for purchase, which are not widely used. The Automated Neuropsychological Assessment Metrics (ANAM) was originally developed for the Department of Defense.[51–53] Other instruments, new to the market, such as Concussion Vital Signs (www.concus sionvitalsigns.com) and C3 Loxic (www.c3logix .com), have limited research to date supporting their use.

Value of neuropsychological testing

NPT is used during the course of recovery because of its ability to detect cognitive deficits, even after symptom resolution. In general, neurocognitive deficits have been shown to develop acutely (<24–28 h from injury)[54–58] and persist till around 5–14 days.[4–9,23] One specific study of concussed collegiate athletes demonstrated that 42% returned to baseline NPT score within 2 days, and 70% returned to baseline by 8 days.[59] NPT is also sensitive in detecting deficits following repeat concussion. Pedersen et al. reviewed a cohort of collegiate hockey players that had impairment in word recall, as measured by ImPACT, after the first concussion and then exhibited significant visual motor speed deficits following a second concussion.[60]

It was previously assumed that symptom resolution denoted complete recovery from brain injury. However, research has shown that changes in NPT persist in 35% of concussed athletes 2–3 days beyond symptom resolution.[8,10] Another study reviewed 122 concussed high school and collegiate athletes and compared them to 70 uninjured athletes. The authors found that while 64% of concussed patients had an increase from baseline symptomatology, up to 83% had reduced neurocognitive performance.[61] Therefore, neurocognitive testing, in addition to symptom checklists, increased the sensitivity for identifying concussed athletes by 19%. A similar study of 108 concussed high school football players performed by Lau et al. demonstrated that with the addition of both a symptom checklist and neurocognitive testing, athletes were not only better identified, but also predicted those who would have a protracted (>14 days) recovery.[62] Meehan et al. found that NPT testing of athletes, along with standard symptom assessment, increased the sensitivity for detecting postconcussive deficits, and were less likely to return to sport within 7–10 days from injury.[39,63] These studies illustrate that without a multimodal approach, we would likely miss persistent deficits and return an athlete prematurely into play.[39,63]

Additionally, any objective test that measures recovery must have its numerical score correlated to clinical outcomes. The use of NPT as a measure of recovery from concussion has been extensively validated proving that poor scores following injury do predict worse outcomes and delayed recovery. In a cohort of 108 male high school football athletes, Lau et al. demonstrated specific values within visual memory and processing speed that correlated with a protracted (>14 days) recovery.[64] Similarly, Erlanger et al.

determined that reduced performance on NPT correlated with more symptoms and also lengthened recovery.[54] Interestingly, the study observed that a history of prior concussion or the presence of loss of consciousness at time of injury did not have an effect on recovery. Additionally, neuropsychological testing can assess other comorbid conditions that may contribute to the persistent symptom profile. This includes affective disturbance, such as anxiety or depression, or other psychiatric disorders. A thorough evaluation by a neuropsychologist may also uncover other neurological or developmental conditions that impact cognitive functioning, such as Attention Deficit Disorder.

In summary, NPT has been shown to be sensitive following acute and chronic time points after concussion and after repeat concussion. It is sensitive not only for cognitive deficits in the absence of symptoms, but most importantly, it has been validated to predict outcomes.

Limitations with the use of neuropsychological testing

The use of NPT, in theory, would be a successful cornerstone to determining return to activity for an athlete, but there are multiple aspects to NPT that limit their ability to be used as the sole determinant. First, not all facilities have access to NPT. Though dated, a survey in 2006 of primary care physicians stated that only 16% had access to NPT for patients with concussion.[65] There likely is a great inequality in access to this resource between professional or Division I collegiate sports and smaller universities and high schools. Secondly, athletes may present with positive findings in one modality only, not always being NPT.[15] Concussed athletes, in a study by Tsushima et al., had persistent symptoms at 7 days but did not show different ImPACT scores compared to nonconcussed athletes.[10] Lastly, NPT is greatly influenced by numerous environmental factors that may cause false negative or positive results (e.g., computer malfunctioning, distractions in the testing environment). For these reasons, NPT testing is not a stand-alone test and should always be used in concordance with other clinical tools to assist measuring the athlete's recovery.[19,24,25]

Recommendations for neuropsychological testing administration

Though NPT testing is sensitive during the acute period (24–48 h),[55–58] the presence of symptoms (e.g., headache pain, fatigue) can affect the test results and the process of taking the tests can exacerbate symptoms in some patients.[66,67] Therefore, it is recommended that NPT be performed once the patient is asymptomatic.[68–70] If an athlete has persistent symptoms (>1–2 weeks), NPT can be performed with an abbreviated version to prevent symptom exacerbation.[70,71] Information from this assessment can be utilized for academic or workplace accommodations.

Currently, there are no guidelines, due to limited evidence, specifically recommending which athlete requires NPT testing following concussion.[1,19,72] However, NPT testing should be considered in athletes with a protracted course following concussion, with preexisting factors that make them susceptible to a long recovery (psychiatric condition, repeated concussions, etc.), or consideration for retirement from sport.[36]

Last, with the advent of computerized neuropsychological testing, an objective score is easily and rapidly obtained. For this reason, there is a temptation to remove the neuropsychologist from the evaluation process. However, due to the intricacies of NPT testing, especially in the more challenging cases, only neuropsychologists have the proper training in the administration and interpretation of neurocognitive tests, and should be involved in the decision of return to activity.[72–74]

Neuropsychological testing as a predictor of poor outcome

Research suggests that neurocognitive testing can be utilized to predict which patient may have more a protracted recovery after a concussion. Iverson et al. revealed that patients with impaired scores on three of the four ImPACT composite scores were 94.6% more likely to have a complicated recovery (defined as greater than 10 days).[75] Similarly, Lau et al. found that the neurocognitive testing resulted in an 24.4.1% increase in predicting which patients would have longer recovery times (defined as greater than 14 days in this study).[62,76]

Specific postconcussive symptoms have been shown to predict reduced NPT scores in concussed athletes. A study of 110 high school students with the presence of subjective "fogginess" at 5–10 days following injury were more likely to report increased symptom burden, have slower reaction times, and reduced memory and processed speeds on NPT.[77] Another analysis of 78 high school and collegiate athletes demonstrated that increased symptom burden and reduced performance on NPT was 10 and 4 times more likely in athletes who demonstrated retrograde and anterograde amnesia, respectively.[78]

With the validation of NPT as a predictor of outcome following concussion,[54,64] retrospective review of NPT results have identified demographic factors of those athletes that are more likely to have a delayed recovery, like age, sex, and comorbid medical conditions. The age of the patient may result in a different rate of recovery. There have been several studies demonstrating that high school athletes take longer to recover from a concussion than college athletes.[79–84] Other studies have compared high school athletes to professional athletes and showed slower recovery times in the younger players.[85–89] Based on age, normalization of neuropsychological testing occurs roughly in 10–14 days in high school athletes, 5–7 days in collegiate athletes, and 2–5 days in professional athletes.[79,85–87,90]

The research on the role of gender on recovery after concussion is less clear. Female athletes have greater symptom burden at both the high school and collegiate level.[59,83,84,88] However, Frommer et al. found that female high school athletes reported different types of symptoms than their male counterparts but did not take longer to recover from concussion.[91] Another study did not find gender-specific differences in the symptoms reported or cognitive deficits postconcussion.[91–94]

Other factors, such as the history of a learning disability or Attention Deficit Disorder, previous concussions, preexisting affective disturbance, and premorbid migraines may all delay recovery from concussion.[1,40,93,95–124] Refer to Chapter 5 for a more detailed discussion of this and other predictors of outcome following concussion like repetitive concussions and preexisting psychiatric conditions.

Lastly, the presence of litigation has been shown to reduce NPT results.[125,126] A meta-analysis of 39 studies, totaling 1463 cases of mTBI by Belanger et al. revealed that those patients who were involved in litigation were more likely to have persistent cognitive deficits on NPT beyond 3 months from injury.[125]

Particulars of neuropsychological testing

Baseline testing

Baseline testing has been argued to be of no benefit due to poor reproducibility, lack of evidence to support benefit of use, expense of repeated testing, and concern for practice effects.[21,127,128] Poor retest reliability in nonconcussed athletes, baseline testing indisputably brings to question the "return to baseline" approach.[129–131] In addition, Echemendia et al. reviewed 223 collegiate athletes 3–4 days following concussion and determined that the majority of individuals with cognitive decline on NPT were identified through the use of age appropriate normative data in comparison to the use of an individual athlete's baseline score.[132] Additionally, repeated baseline testing is more time consuming, costly, and may require additional personnel.

But, there still exists an argument that baseline testing truly aids in the evaluation of an athlete with a preexisting medical disorder or a young athlete who is developing appropriately, but at a different rate from his age matched peers. Baseline testing is also strongly recommended in individuals who have a preexisting condition like Attention-Deficit/Hyperactivity Disorder or a learning disability, preventing proper application of age matched normative values.[133] Baseline testing with very bright individuals also improves detection of cognitive changes that may be perceived as normal relative to average peers. Without individualized baseline results, normative values may possibly over or underestimate NPT baseline scores, therefore losing sensitivity following injury.

Register et al. presented significant differences in ImPACT composite scores between uninjured high school and collegiate athletes, emphasizing the variable stages of cognitive neurodevelopment specifically based on an athlete's age.[82] For this reason, baseline testing, if accessible, should be considered in the adolescent to young adult age due to the subtle differences in cognitive development. If administered correctly and analyzed by a properly trained neuropsychologist, baseline testing can only improve the interpretation of postinjury NPT.[134] If baseline testing is not available, age-appropriate normative data can be used to assess neurocognitive deficits after injury, but it is important to recognize their limitations.

Environmental influences

Due to the intricate nature of cognitive assessment through NPT, the environment in which the test is administered can influence the NPT results. We will review the various environmental influences with suggestions in how to improve the accuracy and validity of the NPT.

Distractions during the test can greatly reduce the athletes' ability to concentrate and affect their scores across tests. For this reason, both baseline and postinjury testing should be completed in a quiet room with limited distractions. Also, the language in which the test is administered should remain constant. It has been shown that bilingual athletes, though fluent in both languages, perform better in their primary language on NPT.[135–138] Secondly, it is important there be strict administration rules on how the group testing environment should be established. Some researchers have suggested that group testing, in comparison to individualized, can result in more errors and lower NPT test result because of increased distractions in the group setting.[139]

Since NPT testing may occur in relation to a battery of other testing, it is important to understand that exercise also influences outcomes. Covassin et al. described a reduction in NPT scores when immediately administered following participation in a treadmill stress test.[140] An intriguing study by Patel et al. found reduced outcomes in the ANAM, specifically visual memory and self-reports of fatigue, in athletes who had water restriction.[141] Therefore, in the athletic population it is important to assess for proper hydration and fatigue post-exertion.

Lastly, proper education about concussion recovery can impact the athlete's performance on NPT testing.[142,143] A study by Blaine et al. demonstrated improved NPT performance in athletes who received positive encouragement and reminders of a hopeful recovery prior to NPT.[143]

Effort

The accuracy of NPT is improved when athletes are motivated to perform well on both baseline and postinjury testing. Reduced effort can be from a multitude of reasons: lack of interest/motivation on baseline testing,[144] premorbid psychiatric conditions (anxiety, depression, attention deficit disorder), environmental distractions, personal gain/malingering, or "sandbagging." "Sandbagging" refers to the athlete intentionally choosing the wrong answers and/or slowing his/her response time to falsely lower their scores on baseline testing. Lower scores on postinjury testing, secondary to incomplete recovery from a concussion, may then be reviewed as consistent with baseline testing and the player allowed to return to play (false negative results).[145]

Poor effort on NPT has been shown at all age ranges: child, adolescent, and adults.[146] It has been indicated that 15%–23% of children and 11% of high school athletes underperform in NPT.[147,148] More concerning, Szabo et al. reviewed ImPACT scores of 159 collegiate football players and determined that 17.5% were indicative of "sandbagging."[149] Attempts to flag athletes for lack of effort can be through the incorporation of either individualized or supervised group NPT with instructors specifically tasked to monitoring performance.[21,33,150] Also, addition of conformational tests to the NPT battery aid in assessing for underperformance by exposing athletes who are demonstrating inconsistent results and possible malingering.[151,152] But research has also shown that it is more challenging to "sandbag" baseline testing than athletes may believe. Erdal found that only 11% of athletes were able to successfully lower their scores without detection.[153]

Adjunctive measures of concussion recovery

Due to the limitations of NPT and the diverse presentation of neurological findings, clinicians and scientists have validated complimentary clinical tools to help assess the athlete following concussive injury. These specific clinical tests most often assess the vestibular system, but for completeness of discussion we will also discuss a newer proposed technology in concussion assessment that analyzes the brain's electrical activity, event-related potential (ERP) through electroencephalography (EEG).

Vestibular system and concussion

Balance, coordination, spatial orientation, and eye movements are coordinated through an intricate dialogue between afferent signals from the vestibular organs (utricle, saccule, and semicircular canals within the inner ear), visual system, cerebellum, brainstem, and proprioceptive pathways. Alteration or damage to any of these specific areas or their corresponding connecting white matter tracts dissociates the network integration and causes subjective vestibular complaints ("dizziness," vertigo, etc.), balance/gait difficulties, and problems with smooth oculomotor movements.[154]

It is believed that specifically the vestibular organs are exquisitely sensitive to angular acceleration and make them prone to injury following a concussive force.[155] Therefore, vestibular symptoms and clinical findings appear in the vast majority of concussed patients and correlates with worse neurocognitive scores and protracted recovery.[156–159] Subjective "dizziness" has been found to be present in over 70% of patients following concussion.[158] Corwin et al. performed a retrospective review of pediatric concussions (age 5–18, $n = 247$) and found that 81% had a vestibular deficit on clinical exam which correlated with worse NPT and prolonged recovery following concussion.[159] Similar findings were also demonstrated in a smaller collegiate athlete cohort ($n = 27$) by Honaker et al.[157] In a review of concussed pediatric athletes, Zhou et al. found that 15% of those with vestibular dysfunction also had the presence of significant hearing loss.[155] For this reason, a referral for a complete audiological evaluation should be considered for any athlete with significant vestibular findings.

As discussed in Chapter 3, the acute assessment of a concussed player with a sideline evaluation like the SCAT incorporates balance testing because vestibular deficits are seen acutely, <24 h following a concussion.[19,160,161] In general, vestibular symptoms and deficits resolve within 3–5 days from injury,[4–6,154] but may be present weeks to months,[7,11,162–164] even after symptom resolution, following concussion depending on the extent of

injury.[165] Within a cohort of concussed collegiate athletes, Peterson et al. further stratified specific vestibular deficits and determined that subjective symptoms and vestibular function improved within 3 days, while patients with balance deficits had a more protracted course with significant difficulties still observed at 10 days after injury.[6] Similar to NPT, and important for concussion diagnosis and monitoring after injury, balance and gait problems can persist beyond symptom resolution.[166] For this reason, "postural-stability testing provides a useful tool for objectively assessing the motor domain of neurologic functioning and should be considered a reliable and valid addition to the assessment of athletes" in the initial acute evaluation and outpatient phase to determine recovery from injury.[1,19,167]

Vestibular/balance testing

Due to the complex neurophysiology and multiple components that contribute signals to the brain for balance and gait, many clinical modalities have been developed that evaluate the vestibular sense. Various methods are available for balance testing after a concussion, including the Balance Error Scoring System (BESS), force plate technology, Sensory Organization Test (SOT), and instruments that utilize virtual reality technology. Introduced in Chapter 3, the BESS has become a part of the SCAT3 as a way to assess the acutely concussed athlete following injury.[165,168,169] As demonstrated in Figure 3.9 in Chapter 3, the test assesses balance through scoring an athletes ability to stand on both legs, one leg, or in a tandem stance.[167] This test was incorporated into the SCAT due to its sensitivity immediately following injury even in the absence of symptoms,[58,170] can also be used in the rehabilitation phase to assess recovery, and lastly, it is cheap, easy to administer, and portable for sideline use.[171,172] In a review of 43 concussed adolescent athletes roughly 1 week from injury, it was determined that a score of 21 errors or greater was 60% sensitive and 82% specific for concussion.[173] Limitations to this test is that it has been shown to have reduced validity in children and adolescents in comparison to collegiate athletes, and also has practice effects up to 4 weeks from baseline testing.[5,174–176]

The force plate instrument measures[177,178] different angles of force that are applied to its surface through either an athlete standing or stepping onto its flat surface (see Figure 6.2). Commercially available products include the Biodex stability system and the Advanced Mechanical Technology AccuySway force plate.[154] The SOT is a more sophisticated force plate that alters either visual and/or somatosensory input and scores the athletes, response to it.[177,178] With mild injury to a segment of the vestibular system, the body can compensate and adjust with the remaining intact afferent signals (like visual or proprioception) concealing the neurological deficit. The SOT is able to remove or alter visual or proprioceptive cues in order to provoke and expose a balance deficit

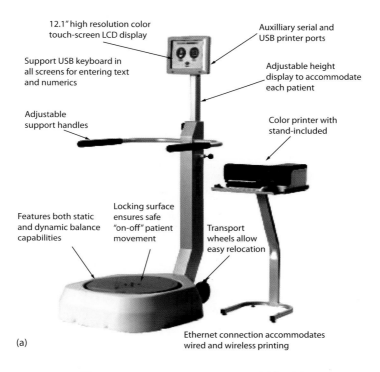

(a)

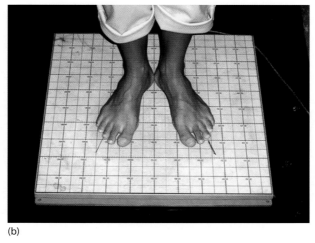

(b)

Figure 6.2 **Commercially available Force Plate Technology systems.** (a) Biodex stability system and (b) Advanced Mechanical Technology AccuySway force plate. (From Rahimi A and Ebrahim Abadi Z, *Journal of Medical Sciences*, 12: 45–50, 2012; Bastos AGD et al., *Revista Brasileira de Otorrinolaringologia*, 71(3): 305–310, 2005.)

(Figure 6.3). Though found to be more sensitive than the BESS, the size, lack of portability, and expense of force plate technology and the SOT, prevents its use as a sideline assessment tool and it is found more typically within the outpatient/rehabilitation field.[5,179]

Similar to the SOT, the use of virtual reality software incites vestibular/balance deficits in the concussed athlete by altering the visual environment.[181] A commercially available virtual reality software, marketed by Head Rehab, provides a portable device with an easy to use interface (Figure 6.4). This newer technology has been validated against the BESS and SOT. Interestingly, athletes have been found to have protracted deficits solely on virtual

reality assessment that are present after symptom recovery and also beyond the return to baseline date determined by the SOT and BESS.[181–185]

Last, vestibular functioning and balance can also be assessed grossly through observing the athlete's gait. It has been demonstrated that gait difficulties are present within the concussed athlete by 48 h and persist 1–4 weeks following injury, even placing the athlete at an increased risk of musculoskeletal injuries up to 6 months from injury.[13,186–189] Powers et al. assessed nine intercollegiate football players following symptom resolution and subsequent return to play, and found persistent gait instability in these athletes.[190] However, this is a small

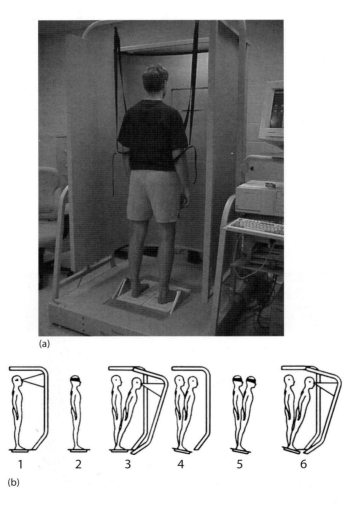

(a)

(b)

Figure 6.3   (a) Sensory Organization Test through the SMART Balance Master System. (b) Six testing conditions for Sensory Organization Test used with NeuroCom's Smart Balance Master System. (From Guskiewicz KM, Ross SE, Marshall SW. Postural Stability and Neuropsychological Deficits After Concussion in Collegiate Athletes. *J Athl Train.* 2001 Sep;36(3):263–273.)

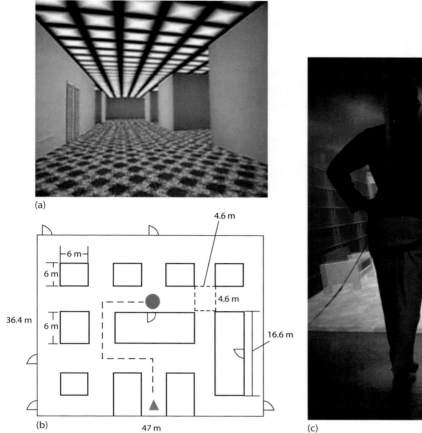

(a)

(b)

4.6 m

6 m

6 m

4.6 m

36.4 m

6 m

16.6 m

47 m

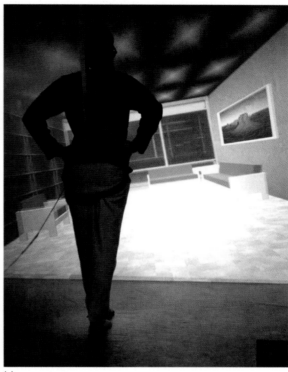

(c)

Figure 6.4 **Head Rehab Virtual Reality for assessment of the concussed athlete.** (a) View of the virtual corridor used for navigation tasks under study. (b) Floor plan, and a sample of the route for one of the runs. (c) Representative example of the VR room tilt (i.e. Roll) while a subject was standing in the heel-to-tow position. Subjects were instructed to look straight and maintain whole body postural stability while being exposed to VR room animation using 2D and 3D options. (From Slobounov SM et al. 2015. Modulation of cortical activity in 2D versus 3D virtual reality environments: An EEG study. *International Journal of Psychophysiology* v95, issue 3. With permission Elsevier.)

study and warrants further investigation. Other studies have specifically examined gait deficits, such as truncal and posture instability, stoppage deficits, and visuomotor navigation around obstacles.[191,192]

Ocular testing

The vestibular system is connected with the visual system and extraocular eye muscles through the brainstem. This relationship allows smooth pursuit of eye movements (saccades) with fixation on a moving object. Damage to the vestibular system following concussion has been shown to impair saccadic eye movements causing multiple pauses

within the pursuit phase.[193–195] Oculomotor deficits have been observed acutely and chronically after concussion.[196–202] These deficits have also demonstrated to predict a prolonged recovery from concussion (40 days versus 21 days, $p = 0.0001$),[203] and correlated with white matter changes seen on diffusion tensor imaging within specific tracts for visuospatial functioning.[204,205]

As discussed in Chapter 3, the King Devick test is a practical, easy to administer side line assessment tool of vestibular ocular deficits.[197–199,206] If obtained immediately following concussion, this simple test can be repeated in the outpatient clinic to monitor for recovery.

Along with oculomotor issues, an athlete can develop reduced visual acuity or depth perception, poor accommodation (making reading difficult), convergence insufficiency, reduced response to visual stimuli (visuospatial attention deficits), nystagmus, or midline shift syndrome (where objects appear at different distances if seen in different visual fields).[207,208] For this reason, any athlete with these specific ocular/visual complaints should be referred to a neuro-ophthalmologist for a comprehensive evaluation.

Electrophysiological testing

The use of an old technology, electroencephalogram (EEG), has more recently been developed as a new application in concussion diagnostics. EEG is obtained through placing electrodes on the athletes' scalp in order to measure their brains' electrical activity. There has been extensive research with regards to the event related to potential P300 wave (electrical activity occurring around 300ms after initiation of a cognitive task) following concussive injury. Changes in electrophysiological parameters, specifically reduction in the ERP P300 amplitude, have been shown experimentally to correlate with TBI severity,[209] injury at acute and chronic time points after concussion,[210–216] repeat concussion exposure,[217] increased postconcussive symptoms,[218] and reduced neurocognitive performance.[219,220] At this time, the use of EEG and ERPs for diagnostic purposes requires continued research and is only for investigational purposes. Therefore, these modalities should not be used as a stand-alone test, but may be considered as an adjunct to the outpatient assessment.[2,221–223]

Rehabilitation of the concussed athlete

The multimodal evaluation and monitoring of the concussed patient exposes specific cognitive, vestibular, and oculomotor deficits in the athlete. This information is imperative to recovery because rehabilitation can be individually catered and focused to their specific need.

If the patient continues to have persistent vestibular symptoms after conservative management, it is appropriate to refer them to a physical therapist that is familiar with managing vestibular deficits.[224–227] Vestibular therapy regimen may consist of gait, balance, and coordination exercises or other modalities depending on the underlying impairment (Table 6.1).[71,228–232] There is limited evidence assessing the outcomes of vestibular rehabilitation therapy, but in a randomized controlled study by Schneider et al., concussed patients 12–30 years old were 3.9 times more likely to return to full activity by 8 weeks if they received vestibular and cervical spine rehab.[228,233–236]

Lastly, any patient with oculomotor deficits may benefit from oculomotor and/or visual rehab.[237] This has been shown to improve reading rate, saccadic eye movements, and accommodation after 6 weeks of therapy.[238–242]

Concussion education

As with any medical condition, a patient's lack of understanding and knowledge of signs and symptoms of a disease can lead to poor recognition and underreporting. Improving clinical outcomes of concussion starts with improving recognition of the injury. Unless all parties involved in youth sports are educated on the signs and symptoms of concussion, development of highly sensitive diagnostic and assessment modalities for concussion will be futile. It appears that many athletes still do not receive specific concussion education. One study stated that 25% of high school football players did not receive concussion education,[243] or had poor retention of the information that what delivered to them.[244]

There has been a push for greater education about concussions with young athletes to increase reporting on injuries, however this has had limited success.[245–247] It has been stated that 40%–50% of concussions are not reported, preventing an athlete from receiving the necessary evaluation and rehabilitation if neurological deficits are present.[248–250] A survey of 496 students demonstrated that though older age was more predictive of greater concussion knowledge, older players were less likely to report a concussion.[251] Education in concussion management appears to focus athletes more on the fact that they will be removed from play rather than the negative long-term effects of repetitive injury.[249,252,253] The barriers to reporting extend beyond the field, in that the athlete may also be concerned with the social

Table 6.1 Diagnosis and Management of Specific causes of Vestibular Deficits including Benign Positional Vertigo, Vestibular Ocular Reflex Impairment, Visual Motion Sensitivity, Impaired Postural Control, Cervicogenic Dizziness, and Exercise-Induced Dizziness

Impairment	Cause	Symptoms	Associated Problems/ Risk Factors	Physical Therapy Treatment
Benign paroxysmal positional vertigo	Mechanical disruption in the vestibular labyrinth (end organ). Otoconia from otoliths become dislodged and displace in semicircular canal	Vertigo with changes in head position	Older age High impact forces	Canalith repositioning maneuvers
VOR impairment	Disrupted function in the VOR pathways, peripherally or centrally	Dizziness	Labyrinthine concussion	Gaze stability training
Visual motion sensitivity	Impaired central processing/integration of vestibular information with visual and other sensory information	Dizziness	Posttraumatic migraine Anxiety	Graded exposure to visually stimulating environments Virtual reality Optokinetic stimulation
Impaired postural control	Disruption/damage to vestibular-spinal reflex pathways, peripherally or centrally	Impaired balance, particularly with: • Vision and/or somatosensation reduced • Cognitive dual/task demand	Common early finding after concussion; typically resolves before other vestibular deficits	Balance rehabilitation strategies Sensory organization training Divided attention training Dynamic balance training
Cervicogenic dizziness	Cervical injury results in abnormal afferent input to CNS; mismatch with other sensory information	Dizziness, related to cervical movement/posture Imbalance Impaired oculomotor control	Cervical pathologic abnormality Cervicogenic headaches	Manual therapy for cervical spine Balance training Oculomotor training
Exercise-induced dizziness	Inadequate central response to cardiovascular and vestibular/ocular demands of exercise	Dizziness with movement-related cardiovascular exercise	• VOR/gaze stability impairment • Visual motion sensitivity • Autonomic dysregulation	

Source: Reprinted from *Clin Sports Med*, Apr;34(2), Broglio SP et al., Current and emerging rehabilitation for concussion: A review of the evidence, 213–31, Copyright 2015, with permission from Elsevier.

implications of being removed from competitions and practices.

Every interaction with the athlete, whether a preparticipation physical, baseline testing, visit with their primary care physician, emergency room assessment, or follow-up care after a concussive injury, is a potential opportunity to develop a relationship with the athlete and educate them about concussions. Education can be provided on a number of issues, including the causes of concussion, the signs and symptoms of the injury, when to seek medical attention after a suspected concussion, behavior modification to reduce concussions, and the limitations to protective equipment.[19,40,69] Other topics following injury should include harm in returning to play the same day of injury, the appropriate level of cognitive and physical rest postinjury, symptom awareness and exacerbating features, and most importantly, emphasis on recovery.[254–257]

Besides the athlete, concussion education should also be directed towards athletic trainers, coaches, school nurses, parents, and other physicians.[258] There have been countless studies emphasizing the poor understanding of concussion by primary care providers, even in the accepted standards of care recommended by concussion guidelines.[259–261] Two surveys revealed that only 28%–36% of doctors who responded recommended cognitive rest (published in 2013),[260,262] and that only 60% advocated for a graduated return to learn (published in 2014),[263] which were then and currently accepted guideline recommendations. The hope is that improved concussion knowledge among all those involved with an athlete may reduce the rate of concussions, increase recognition of the injury, and improve the treatment of athletes.

Conclusion

Every concussion is different, as are the mechanisms causing injury, symptom presentations, neurological deficits, and ultimately, the recoveries. For this reason, the management and monitoring of the concussed athlete requires a multimodal, multifaceted approach. It should be composed of a thorough history, clinical exam, symptom assessment, and neuropsychological testing along with oculomotor, vestibular, gait, and electrophysiological evaluations with empirically validated instruments. Due to the limitations discussed with each modality, it is recommended that clinicians use several to improve accuracy of diagnosis and follow an athlete's recovery to safely determine the time of return to activity.

References

1. Giza CC, Kutcher JS, Ashwal S et al. Summary of evidence-based guideline update: evaluation and management of concussion in sports: report of the Guideline Development Subcommittee of the American Academy of Neurology. *Neurology.* 2013; 80(24): 2250–2257.

2. Ketcham CJ, Hall E, Bixby WR et al. A neuroscientific approach to the examination of concussions in student-athletes. *Journal of Visualized Experiments.* 2014(94).

3. Kelly KC, Jordan EM, Joyner AB, Burdette GT, Buckley TA. National Collegiate Athletic Association Division I athletic trainers' concussion-management practice patterns. *Journal of Athletic Training.* 2014; 49(5): 665–673.

4. Ellemberg D, Henry LC, Macciocchi SN, Guskiewicz KM, Broglio SP. Advances in sport concussion assessment: from behavioral to brain imaging measures. *Journal of Neurotrauma.* 2009; 26(12): 2365–2382.

5. Ruhe A, Fejer R, Gansslen A, Klein W. Assessing postural stability in the concussed athlete: what to do, what to expect, and when. *Sports Health.* 2014; 6(5): 427–433.

6. Peterson CL, Ferrara MS, Mrazik M, Piland S, Elliott R. Evaluation of neuropsychological domain scores and postural stability following cerebral concussion in sports. *Clinical Journal of Sport Medicine.* 2003; 13(4): 230–237.

7. Broglio SP, Puetz TW. The effect of sport concussion on neurocognitive function, self-report symptoms and postural control: a meta-analysis. *Sports Medicine.* 2008; 38(1): 53–67.

8. Makdissi M, Darby D, Maruff P, Ugoni A, Brukner P, McCrory PR. Natural history of concussion in sport: markers of severity and implications for management. *The American Journal of Sports Medicine.* 2010; 38(3): 464–471.

9. Karr JE, Areshenkoff CN, Garcia-Barrera MA. The neuropsychological outcomes of concussion: a systematic review of meta-analyses on the cognitive sequelae of mild traumatic brain injury. *Neuropsychology.* 2014; 28(3): 321–336.

10. Tsushima WT, Shirakawa N, Geling O. Neurocognitive functioning and symptom reporting of high school athletes following a single concussion. *Applied Neuropsychology Child.* 2013; 2(1): 13–16.

11. Henry LC, Elbin RJ, Collins MW, Marchetti G, Kontos AP. Examining recovery trajectories after sport-related concussion with a multimodal clinical assessment approach. *Neurosurgery*. 2015; 78(2): 232–241.

12. McCrea M, Guskiewicz KM, Marshall SW et al. Acute effects and recovery time following concussion in collegiate football players: the NCAA Concussion Study. *Journal of the American Medical Association*. 2003; 290(19): 2556–2563.

13. Fait P, Swaine B, Cantin JF, Leblond J, McFadyen BJ. Altered integrated locomotor and cognitive function in elite athletes 30 days postconcussion: a preliminary study. *The Journal of Head Trauma Rehabilitation*. 2013; 28(4): 293–301.

14. McCrea M, Barr WB, Guskiewicz K et al. Standard regression-based methods for measuring recovery after sport-related concussion. *Journal of the International Neuropsychological Society*. 2005; 11(1): 58–69.

15. Porcher NJ, Solecki TJ. A narrative review of sports-related concussion and return-to-play testing with asymptomatic athletes. *Journal of Chiropractic Medicine*. 2013; 12(4): 260–268.

16. Reynolds E, Collins MW, Mucha A, Troutman-Ensecki C. Establishing a clinical service for the management of sports-related concussions. *Neurosurgery*. 2014; 75 Suppl 4: S71–81.

17. Kelleher E, Taylor-Linzey E, Ferrigno L, Bryson J, Kaminski S. A community return-to-play mTBI clinic: results of a pilot program and survey of high school athletes. *Journal of Pediatric Surgery*. 2014; 49(2): 341–344.

18. Faltus J. Rehabilitation strategies addressing neurocognitive and balance deficits following a concussion in a female snowboard athlete: a case report. *International Journal of Sports Physical Therapy*. 2014; 9(2): 232–241.

19. McCrory P, Meeuwisse W, Aubry M et al. Consensus statement on Concussion in Sport – The 4th International Conference on Concussion in Sport held in Zurich, November 2012. *Physical Therapy in Sport*. 2013; 14(2): e1–e13.

20. Taylor AM. Neuropsychological evaluation and management of sport-related concussion. *Current Opinion in Pediatrics*. 2012; 24(6): 717–723.

21. Webbe FM, Zimmer A. History of neuropsychological study of sport-related concussion. *Brain Injury*. 2015; 29(2): 129–138.

22. Killam C, Cautin RL, Santucci AC. Assessing the enduring residual neuropsychological effects of head trauma in college athletes who participate in contact sports. *Archives of Clinical Neuropsychology*. 2005; 20(5): 599–611.

23. Belanger HG, Vanderploeg RD. The neuropsychological impact of sports-related concussion: a meta-analysis. *Journal of the International Neuropsychological Society*. 2005; 11(4): 345–357.

24. McCrea M, Iverson GL, Echemendia RJ, Makdissi M, Raftery M. Day of injury assessment of sport-related concussion. *British Journal of Sports Medicine*. 2013; 47(5): 272–284.

25. Bene ER, Sepulveda AM. Clinical test instrument development to identify and track recovery from concussion. *Seminars in Speech and Language*. 2014; 35(3): 173–185.

26. Moser RS, Iverson GL, Echemendia RJ et al. Neuropsychological evaluation in the diagnosis and management of sports–related concussion. *Archives of Clinical Neuropsychology*. 2007; 22(8): 909–916.

27. McCrory P, Makdissi M, Davis G, Collie A. Value of neuropsychological testing after head injuries in football. *British Journal of Sports Medicine*. 2005; 39 Suppl 1: i58–63.

28. Barr WB, McCrea M. Sensitivity and specificity of standardized neurocognitive testing immediately following sports concussion. *Journal of the International Neuropsychological Society*. 2001; 7(6): 693–702.

29. Barr WB. An evidence based approach to sports concussion: confronting the availability cascade. *Neuropsychology Review*. 2013; 23(4): 271–272.

30. Maroon JC, Lovell MR, Norwig J, Podell K, Powell JW, Hartl R. Cerebral concussion in athletes: evaluation and neuropsychological testing. *Neurosurgery*. 2000; 47(3): 659–669.

31. Scorza KA, Raleigh MF, O'Connor FG. Current concepts in concussion: evaluation and management. *American Family Physician*. 2012; 85(2): 123–132.

32. Rahman-Filipiak AA, Woodard JL. Administration and environment considerations in computer-based sports-concussion assessment. *Neuropsychology Review*. 2013; 23(4): 314–334.

33. Guise BJ, Thompson MD, Greve KW, Bianchini KJ, West L. Assessment of performance validity in the Stroop Color and Word Test in mild traumatic brain injury patients: a criterion-groups validation design. *Journal of Neuropsychology*. 2014; 8(1): 20–33.

34. Cernich A, Reeves D, Sun W, Bleiberg J. Automated Neuropsychological Assessment Metrics sports medicine battery. *Archives of Clinical Neuropsychology*. 2007; 22 Suppl 1: S101–114.

35. Segalowitz SJ, Mahaney P, Santesso DL, MacGregor L, Dywan J, Willer B. Retest reliability in adolescents of a computerized neuropsychological battery used to assess recovery from concussion. *NeuroRehabilitation*. 2007; 22(3): 243–251.

36. De Marco AP, Broshek DK. Computerized cognitive testing in the management of youth sports-related concussion. *Journal of Child Neurology*. 2014; 31(1): 68–75.

37. Resch JE, McCrea MA, Cullum CM. Computerized neurocognitive testing in the management of sport-related concussion: an update. *Neuropsychology Review*. 2013; 23(4): 335–349.

38. Bauer RM, Iverson GL, Cernich AN, Binder LM, Ruff RM, Naugle RI. Computerized neuropsychological assessment devices: joint position paper of the American Academy of Clinical Neuropsychology and the National Academy of Neuropsychology. *The Clinical Neuropsychologist*. 2012; 26(2): 177–196.

39. Meehan WP, 3rd, d'Hemecourt P, Collins CL, Taylor AM, Comstock RD. Computerized neurocognitive testing for the management of sport-related concussions. *Pediatrics*. 2012; 129(1): 38–44.

40. Choe MC, Giza CC. Diagnosis and management of acute concussion. *Seminars in Neurology*. 2015; 35(1): 29–41.

41. McKay CD, Brooks BL, Mrazik M, Jubinville AL, Emery CA. Psychometric properties and reference values for the ImPACT neurocognitive test battery in a sample of elite youth ice hockey players. *Archives of Clinical Neuropsychology*. 2014; 29(2): 141–151.

42. Schatz P, Pardini JE, Lovell MR, Collins MW, Podell K. Sensitivity and specificity of the ImPACT Test Battery for concussion in athletes. *Archives of Clinical Neuropsychology*. 2006; 21(1): 91–99.

43. Schatz P, Sandel N. Sensitivity and specificity of the online version of ImPACT in high school and collegiate athletes. *The American Journal of Sports Medicine*. 2013; 41(2): 321–326.

44. Iverson GL, Lovell MR, Collins MW. Validity of ImPACT for measuring processing speed following sports-related concussion. *Journal of Clinical and Experimental Neuropsychology*. 2005; 27(6): 683–689.

45. Schatz P, Maerlender A. A two-factor theory for concussion assessment using ImPACT: memory and speed. *Archives of Clinical Neuropsychology*. 2013; 28(8): 791–797.

46. Newman JB, Reesman JH, Vaughan CG, Gioia GA. Assessment of processing speed in children with mild TBI: a "first look" at the validity of pediatric ImPACT. *The Clinical Neuropsychologist*. 2013; 27(5): 779–793.

47. Bruce J, Echemendia R, Meeuwisse W, Comper P, Sisco A. 1 year test-retest reliability of ImPACT in professional ice hockey players. *The Clinical Neuropsychologist*. 2014; 28(1): 14–25.

48. Resch J, Driscoll A, McCaffrey N et al. ImPact test-retest reliability: reliably unreliable? *Journal of Athletic Training*. 2013; 48(4): 506–511.

49. Collie A, Maruff P, Makdissi M, McCrory P, McStephen M, Darby D. CogSport: reliability and correlation with conventional cognitive tests used in postconcussion medical evaluations. *Clinical Journal of Sport Medicine*. 2003; 13(1): 28–32.

50. Gioia GA. Multimodal evaluation and management of children with concussion: using our heads and available evidence. *Brain Injury*. 2015; 29(2): 195–206.

51. Haran FJ, Alphonso AL, Creason A et al. Reliable change estimates for assessing recovery from concussion using the ANAM4 TBI-MIL. *The Journal of Head Trauma Rehabilitation*. 2015; 31(5): 329–338.

52. Reeves D, Thorne R, Winter A, Hegge F. The united tri-service cognitive performance assessment battery *Report 89–1*. 1989; San Diego, California: US Naval Aerospace Medical Research Laboratory and Walter Reed Army Institute of Research.

53. Norris JN, Carr W, Herzig T, Labrie DW, Sams R. ANAM4 TBI reaction time-based tests have prognostic utility for acute concussion. *Military Medicine*. 2013; 178(7): 767–774.

54. Erlanger D, Kaushik T, Cantu R et al. Symptom-based assessment of the severity of a concussion. *Journal of Neurosurgery*. 2003; 98(3): 477–484.

55. Broglio SP, Sosnoff JJ, Ferrara MS. The relationship of athlete-reported concussion symptoms and objective measures of neurocognitive function and postural control. *Clinical Journal of Sport Medicine*. 2009; 19(5): 377–382.

56. Collins MW, Grindel SH, Lovell MR et al. Relationship between concussion and neuropsychological performance in college football players. *The Journal of the American Medical Association*. 1999; 282(10): 964–970.

57. McCauley SR, Wilde EA, Barnes A et al. Patterns of early emotional and neuropsychological sequelae after mild traumatic brain injury. *Journal of Neurotrauma*. 2014; 31(10): 914–925.

58. Okonkwo DO, Tempel ZJ, Maroon J. Sideline assessment tools for the evaluation of concussion in athletes: a review. *Neurosurgery*. 2014; 75 Suppl 4: S82–95.

59. Covassin T, Schatz P, Swanik CB. Sex differences in neuropsychological function and post-concussion symptoms of concussed collegiate athletes. *Neurosurgery*. 2007; 61(2): 345–350.

60. Pedersen HA, Ferraro FR, Himle M, Schultz C, Poolman M. Neuropsychological factors related to college ice hockey concussions. *American Journal of Alzheimer's Disease and Other Dementias*. 2014; 29(3): 201–204.

61. Van Kampen DA, Lovell MR, Pardini JE, Collins MW, Fu FH. The "value added" of neurocognitive testing after sports-related concussion. *The American Journal of Sports Medicine*. 2006; 34(10): 1630–1635.

62. Lau BC, Collins MW, Lovell MR. Sensitivity and specificity of subacute computerized neurocognitive testing and symptom evaluation in predicting outcomes after sports-related concussion. *The American Journal of Sports Medicine*. 2011; 39(6): 1209–1216.

63. Meehan WP, 3rd, d'Hemecourt P, Comstock RD. High school concussions in the 2008–2009 academic year: mechanism, symptoms, and management. *The American Journal of Sports Medicine.* 2010; 38(12): 2405–2409.

64. Lau BC, Collins MW, Lovell MR. Cutoff scores in neurocognitive testing and symptom clusters that predict protracted recovery from concussions in high school athletes. *Neurosurgery.* 2012; 70(2): 371–379.

65. Pleacher MD, Dexter WW. Concussion management by primary care providers. *British Journal of Sports Medicine.* 2006; 40(1): e2.

66. Meyer JE, Arnett PA. Changes in symptoms in concussed and non-concussed athletes following neuropsychological assessment. *Developmental Neuropsychology.* 2015; 40(1): 24–28.

67. Covassin T, Crutcher B, Wallace J. Does a 20 minute cognitive task increase concussion symptoms in concussed athletes? *Brain Injury.* 2013; 27(13–14): 1589–1594.

68. Putukian M. The acute symptoms of sport-related concussion: diagnosis and on-field management. *Clinics in Sports Medicine.* 2011; 30(1): 49–61, viii.

69. Broglio SP, Cantu RC, Gioia GA et al. National Athletic Trainers' Association position statement: management of sport concussion. *Journal of Athletic Training.* 2014; 49(2): 245–265.

70. Kirkwood MW, Yeates KO, Taylor HG, Randolph C, McCrea M, Anderson VA. Management of pediatric mild traumatic brain injury: a neuropsychological review from injury through recovery. *The Clinical Neuropsychologist.* 2008; 22(5): 769–800.

71. Makdissi M, Cantu RC, Johnston KM, McCrory P, Meeuwisse WH. The difficult concussion patient: what is the best approach to investigation and management of persistent (>10 days) postconcussive symptoms? *British Journal of Sports Medicine.* 2013; 47(5): 308–313.

72. Echemendia RJ, Iverson GL, McCrea M et al. Advances in neuropsychological assessment of sport-related concussion. *British Journal of Sports Medicine.* 2013; 47(5): 294–298.

73. Moser RS, Schatz P, Lichtenstein JD. The importance of proper administration and interpretation of neuropsychological baseline and postconcussion computerized testing. *Applied Neuropsychology Child.* 2015; 4(1): 41–48.

74. Echemendia RJ, Herring S, Bailes J. Who should conduct and interpret the neuropsychological assessment in sports-related concussion? *British Journal of Sports Medicine.* 2009; 43 Suppl 1: i32–35.

75. Iverson G. Predicting slow recovery from sport-related concussion: the new simple-complex distinction. *Clinical Journal of Sport Medicine.* 2007; 17(1): 31–37.

76. Lau BC, Kontos AP, Collins MW, Mucha A, Lovell MR. Which on-field signs/symptoms predict protracted recovery from sport-related concussion among high school football players? *The American Journal of Sports Medicine.* 2011; 39(11): 2311–2318.

77. Iverson GL, Gaetz M, Lovell MR, Collins MW. Relation between subjective fogginess and neuropsychological testing following concussion. *Journal of the International Neuropsychological Society.* 2004; 10(6): 904–906.

78. Collins MW, Iverson GL, Lovell MR, McKeag DB, Norwig J, Maroon J. On-field predictors of neuropsychological and symptom deficit following sports-related concussion. *Clinical Journal of Sport Medicine.* 2003; 13(4): 222–229.

79. Field M, Collins MW, Lovell MR, Maroon J. Does age play a role in recovery from sports-related concussion? A comparison of high school and collegiate athletes. *Journal of Pediatrics.* 2003; 142(5): 546–553.

80. Zuckerman SL, Lee YM, Odom MJ, Solomon GS, Forbes JA, Sills AK. Recovery from sports-related concussion: Days to return to neurocognitive baseline in adolescents

versus young adults. *Surgical Neurology International*. 2012; 3: 130.

81. Sim A, Terryberry-Spohr L, Wilson KR. Prolonged recovery of memory functioning after mild traumatic brain injury in adolescent athletes. *Journal of Neurosurgery*. 2008; 108(3): 511–516.

82. Register-Mihalik JK, Kontos DL, Guskiewicz KM, Mihalik JP, Conder R, Shields EW. Age-related differences and reliability on computerized and paper-and-pencil neurocognitive assessment batteries. *Journal of Athletic Training*. 2012; 47(3): 297–305.

83. Covassin T, Elbin RJ, Harris W, Parker T, Kontos A. The role of age and sex in symptoms, neurocognitive performance, and postural stability in athletes after concussion. *The American Journal of Sports Medicine*. 2012; 40(6): 1303–1312.

84. Covassin T, Elbin RJ, 3rd, Larson E, Kontos AP. Sex and age differences in depression and baseline sport-related concussion neurocognitive performance and symptoms. *Clinical Journal of Sport Medicine*. 2012; 22(2): 98–104.

85. Pellman EJ, Lovell MR, Viano DC, Casson IR. Concussion in professional football: recovery of NFL and high school athletes assessed by computerized neuropsychological testing—Part 12. *Neurosurgery*. 2006; 58(2): 263–274.

86. Pellman EJ, Lovell MR, Viano DC, Casson IR, Tucker AM. Concussion in professional football: neuropsychological testing—Part 6. *Neurosurgery*. 2004; 55(6): 1290–1303.

87. Iverson GL, Brooks BL, Collins MW, Lovell MR. Tracking neuropsychological recovery following concussion in sport. *Brain Injury*. 2006; 20(3): 245–252.

88. Dougan BK, Horswill MS, Geffen GM. Athletes' age, sex, and years of education moderate the acute neuropsychological impact of sports-related concussion: a meta-analysis. *Journal of the International Neuropsychological Society*. 2014; 20(1): 64–80.

89. Collins MW, Field M, Lovell MR et al. Relationship between postconcussion headache and neuropsychological test performance in high school athletes. *The American Journal of Sports Medicine*. 2003; 31(2): 168–173.

90. Grady MF. Concussion in the adolescent athlete. *Current Problems in Pediatric and Adolescent Health Care*. 2010; 40(7): 154–169.

91. Frommer LJ, Gurka KK, Cross KM, Ingersoll CD, Comstock RD, Saliba SA. Sex differences in concussion symptoms of high school athletes. *Journal of Athletic Training*. 2011; 46(1): 76–84.

92. Zuckerman SL, Apple RP, Odom MJ, Lee YM, Solomon GS, Sills AK. Effect of sex on symptoms and return to baseline in sport-related concussion. *Journal of Neurosurgery Pediatrics*. 2014; 13(1): 72–81.

93. Stulemeijer M, van der Werf S, Borm GF, Vos PE. Early prediction of favourable recovery 6 months after mild traumatic brain injury. *Journal of Neurology, Neurosurgery, and Psychiatry*. 2008; 79(8): 936–942.

94. Brown DA, Elsass JA, Miller AJ, Reed LE, Reneker JC. Differences in symptom reporting between males and females at baseline and after a sports-related concussion: a systematic review and meta-analysis. *Sports Medicine*. 2015; 45(7): 1027–1040.

95. Kerr HA. Concussion risk factors and strategies for prevention. *Pediatric Annals*. 2014; 43(12): e309–315.

96. Babikian T, McArthur D, Asarnow RF. Predictors of 1-month and 1-year neurocognitive functioning from the UCLA longitudinal mild, uncomplicated, pediatric traumatic brain injury study. *Journal of the International Neuropsychological Society*. 2013; 19(2): 145–154.

97. Hou R, Moss-Morris R, Peveler R, Mogg K, Bradley BP, Belli A. When a minor head injury results in enduring symptoms: a prospective investigation of risk factors for postconcussional syndrome after mild traumatic brain injury. *Journal of Neurology, Neurosurgery, and Psychiatry*. 2012; 83(2): 217–223.

98. Broshek DK, De Marco AP, Freeman JR. A review of post-concussion syndrome and psychological factors associated with concussion. *Brain Injury*. 2015; 29(2): 228–237.

99. Al-Ozairi A, McCullagh S, Feinstein A. Predicting posttraumatic stress symptoms following mild, moderate, and severe traumatic brain injury: the role of post-traumatic amnesia. *The Journal of Head Trauma Rehabilitation*. 2015; 30(4): 283–289.

100. Wood RL, O'Hagan G, Williams C, McCabe M, Chadwick N. Anxiety sensitivity and alexithymia as mediators of postconcussion syndrome following mild traumatic brain injury. *The Journal of Head Trauma Rehabilitation*. 2014; 29(1): E9–e17.

101. Waldron-Perrine B, Hennrick H, Spencer RJ, Pangilinan PH, Bieliauskas LA. Postconcussive symptom report in polytrauma: influence of mild traumatic brain injury and psychiatric distress. *Military Medicine*. 2014; 179(8): 856–864.

102. Yang J, Peek-Asa C, Covassin T, Torner JC. Post-concussion symptoms of depression and anxiety in division I collegiate athletes. *Developmental Neuropsychology*. 2015; 40(1): 18–23.

103. King NS, Kirwilliam S. Permanent postconcussion symptoms after mild head injury. *Brain Injury*. 2011; 25(5): 462–470.

104. Meares S, Shores EA, Taylor AJ et al. The prospective course of postconcussion syndrome: the role of mild traumatic brain injury. *Neuropsychology*. 2011; 25(4): 454–465.

105. Adeyemo BO, Biederman J, Zafonte R et al. Mild traumatic brain injury and ADHD: a systematic review of the literature and meta-analysis. *Journal of Attention Disorders*. 2014; 18(7): 576–584.

106. Bonfield CM, Lam S, Lin Y, Greene S. The impact of attention deficit hyperactivity disorder on recovery from mild traumatic brain injury. *Journal of Neurosurgery Pediatrics*. 2013; 12(2): 97–102.

107. McCauley SR, Boake C, Levin HS, Contant CF, Song JX. Postconcussional disorder following mild to moderate traumatic brain injury: anxiety, depression, and social support as risk factors and comorbidities. *Journal of Clinical and Experimental Neuropsychology*. 2001; 23(6): 792–808.

108. Tator CH, Davis H. The postconcussion syndrome in sports and recreation: clinical features and demography in 138 athletes. *Neurosurgery*. 2014; 75 Suppl 4: S106–112.

109. Pineau H, Marchand A, Guay S. Objective neuropsychological deficits in post-traumatic stress disorder and mild traumatic brain injury: what remains beyond symptom similarity? *Behavioral Sciences (Basel, Switzerland)*. 2014; 4(4): 471–486.

110. Shandera-Ochsner AL, Berry DT, Harp JP et al. Neuropsychological effects of self-reported deployment-related mild TBI and current PTSD in OIF/OEF veterans. *Clin Neuropsychology*. 2013; 27(6): 881–907.

111. Nelson LD, Guskiewicz KM, Marshall SW et al. Multiple self-reported concussions are more prevalent in athletes with ADHD and learning disability. *Clinical Journal of Sport Medicine*. 2015; 26(2): 120–127.

112. Mautner K, Sussman WI, Axtman M, Al-Farsi Y, Al-Adawi S. Relationship of attention deficit hyperactivity disorder and postconcussion recovery in youth athletes. *Clinical Journal of Sport Medicine*. 2015; 25(4): 355–360.

113. Mannix R, Iverson GL, Maxwell B, Atkins JE, Zafonte R, Berkner PD. Multiple prior concussions are associated with symptoms in high school athletes. *Annals of Clinical and Translational Neurology*. 2014; 1(6): 433–438.

114. Guskiewicz KM, McCrea M, Marshall SW et al. Cumulative effects associated with recurrent concussion in collegiate football players: the NCAA Concussion Study. *The Journal of the American Medical Association*. 2003; 290(19): 2549–2555.

115. Makdissi M, Davis G, Jordan B, Patricios J, Purcell L, Putukian M. Revisiting the modifiers: how should the evaluation and management of acute concussions differ in specific groups? *British Journal of Sports Medicine*. 2013; 47(5): 314–320.

116. Schatz P, Moser RS, Covassin T, Karpf R. Early indicators of enduring symptoms in high school athletes with multiple previous concussions. *Neurosurgery*. 2011; 68(6): 1562–1567.

117. Eisenberg MA, Andrea J, Meehan W, Mannix R. Time interval between concussions and symptom duration. *Pediatrics*. 2013; 132(1): 8–17.

118. Valovich McLeod TC, Bay RC, Lam KC, Chhabra A. Representative baseline values on the Sport Concussion Assessment Tool 2 (SCAT2) in adolescent athletes vary by gender, grade, and concussion history. *The American Journal of Sports Medicine*. 2012; 40(4): 927–933.

119. Covassin T, Moran R, Wilhelm K. Concussion symptoms and neurocognitive performance of high school and college athletes who incur multiple concussions. *The American Journal of Sports Medicine*. 2013; 41(12): 2885–2889.

120. Morgan CD, Zuckerman SL, Lee YM et al. Predictors of postconcussion syndrome after sports-related concussion in young athletes: a matched case-control study. *Journal of Neurosurgery Pediatrics*. 2015; 15(6): 589–598.

121. Abrahams S, Fie SM, Patricios J, Posthumus M, September AV. Risk factors for sports concussion: an evidence-based systematic review. *British Journal of Sports Medicine*. 2014; 48(2): 91–97.

122. Wasserman EB, Kerr ZY, Zuckerman SL, Covassin T. Epidemiology of sports-related concussions in National Collegiate Athletic Association Athletes from 2009–2010 to 2013–2014: symptom prevalence, symptom resolution time, and return-to-play time. *The American Journal of Sports Medicine*. 2015; 44(1): 226–233.

123. Corwin DJ, Zonfrillo MR, Master CL et al. Characteristics of prolonged concussion recovery in a pediatric subspecialty referral population. *Journal of Pediatrics*. 2014; 165(6): 1207–1215.

124. Delaney JS, Al-Kashmiri A, Correa JA. Mechanisms of injury for concussions in university football, ice hockey, and soccer. *Clinical Journal of Sport Medicine*. 2014; 24(3): 233–237.

125. Belanger HG, Curtiss G, Demery JA, Lebowitz BK, Vanderploeg RD. Factors moderating neuropsychological outcomes following mild traumatic brain injury: a meta-analysis. *Journal of the International Neuropsychological Society*. 2005; 11(3): 215–227.

126. Lees–Haley PR, Brown RS. Neuropsychological complaint base rates of 170 personal injury claimants. *Archives of Clinical Neuropsychology*. 1993; 8(3): 203–209.

127. Iverson GL, Schatz P. Advanced topics in neuropsychological assessment following sport-related concussion. *Brain Injury*. 2015; 29(2): 263–275.

128. Schatz P, Ferris CS. One-month test-retest reliability of the ImPACT test battery. *Archives of Clinical Neuropsychology*. 2013; 28(5): 499–504.

129. Broglio SP, Ferrara MS, Macciocchi SN, Baumgartner TA, Elliott R. Test-retest reliability of computerized concussion assessment programs. *Journal of Athletic Training*. 2007; 42(4): 509–514.

130. Randolph C. Baseline neuropsychological testing in managing sport-related concussion: does it modify risk? *Current Sports Medicine Reports*. 2011; 10(1): 21–26.

131. MacDonald J, Duerson D. Reliability of a computerized neurocognitive test in baseline concussion testing of high school athletes. *Clinical Journal of Sport Medicine*. 2015; 25(4): 367–372.

132. Echemendia RJ, Bruce JM, Bailey CM, Sanders JF, Arnett P, Vargas G. The utility of post-concussion neuropsychological data

in identifying cognitive change following sports-related MTBI in the absence of baseline data. *The Clinical Neuropsychologist.* 2012; 26(7): 1077–1091.

133. Elbin RJ, Kontos AP, Kegel N, Johnson E, Burkhart S, Schatz P. Individual and combined effects of LD and ADHD on computerized neurocognitive concussion test performance: evidence for separate norms. *Archives of Clinical Neuropsychology.* 2013; 28(5): 476–484.

134. Reed N, Murphy J, Dick T et al. A multimodal approach to assessing recovery in youth athletes following concussion. *Journal of Visualized Experiments.* 2014(91): 51892.

135. Shuttleworth-Edwards AB, Whitefield-Alexander VJ, Radloff SE, Taylor AM, Lovell MR. Computerized neuropsychological profiles of South African versus US athletes: a basis for commentary on cross-cultural norming issues in the sports concussion arena. *The Physician and Sportsmedicine.* 2009; 37(4): 45–52.

136. Lehman Blake M, Ott S, Villanyi E, Kazhuro K, Schatz P. Influence of language of administration on impact performance by bilingual spanish-english college students. *Archives of Clinical Neuropsychology.* 2015; 30(4): 302–309.

137. Ott S, Schatz P, Solomon G, Ryan JJ. Neurocognitive performance and symptom profiles of Spanish-speaking Hispanic athletes on the ImPACT test. *Archives of Clinical Neuropsychology.* 2014; 29(2): 152–163.

138. Jones NS, Walter KD, Caplinger R, Wright D, Raasch WG, Young C. Effect of education and language on baseline concussion screening tests in professional baseball players. *Clinical Journal of Sport Medicine.* 2014; 24(4): 284–288.

139. Moser RS, Schatz P, Neidzwski K, Ott SD. Group versus individual administration affects baseline neurocognitive test performance. *The American Journal of Sports Medicine.* 2011; 39(11): 2325–2330.

140. Covassin T, Weiss L, Powell J, Womack C. Effects of a maximal exercise test on neurocognitive function. *British Journal of Sports Medicine.* 2007; 41(6): 370–374.

141. Patel AV, Mihalik JP, Notebaert AJ, Guskiewicz KM, Prentice WE. Neuropsychological performance, postural stability, and symptoms after dehydration. *Journal of Athletic Training.* 2007; 42(1): 66–75.

142. Kit KA, Mateer CA, Tuokko HA, Spencer-Rodgers J. Influence of negative stereotypes and beliefs on neuropsychological test performance in a traumatic brain injury population. *Journal of the International Neuropsychological Society.* 2014; 20(2): 157–167.

143. Blaine H, Sullivan KA, Edmed SL. The effect of varied test instructions on neuropsychological performance following mild traumatic brain injury: an investigation of "diagnosis threat." *Journal of Neurotrauma.* 2013; 30(16): 1405–1414.

144. Rabinowitz AR, Merritt VC, Arnett PA. The return-to-play incentive and the effect of motivation on neuropsychological test-performance: implications for baseline concussion testing. *Developmental Neuropsychology.* 2015; 40(1): 29–33.

145. Schatz P, Glatts C. "Sandbagging" baseline test performance on ImPACT, without detection, is more difficult than it appears. *Archives of Clinical Neuropsychology.* 2013; 28(3): 236–244.

146. Kirkwood MW, Kirk JW, Blaha RZ, Wilson P. Noncredible effort during pediatric neuropsychological exam: a case series and literature review. *Child Neuropsychology.* 2010; 16(6): 604–618.

147. Provance AJ, Terhune EB, Cooley C et al. The relationship between initial physical examination findings and failure on objective validity testing during neuropsychological evaluation after pediatric mild traumatic brain injury. *Sports Health.* 2014; 6(5): 410–415.

148. Hunt TN, Ferrara MS, Miller LS, Macciocchi S. The effect of effort on baseline neuropsychological test scores in high school football athletes. *Archives of Clinical Neuropsychology*. 2007; 22(5): 615–621.

149. Szabo AJ, Alosco ML, Fedor A, Gunstad J. Invalid performance and the ImPACT in national collegiate athletic association division I football players. *Journal of Athletic Training*. 2013; 48(6): 851–855.

150. Kuhn AW, Solomon GS. Supervision and computerized neurocognitive baseline test performance in high school athletes: an initial investigation. *Journal of Athletic Training*. 2014; 49(6): 800–805.

151. Larrabee GJ. Detection of malingering using atypical performance patterns on standard neuropsychological tests. *The Clinical Neuropsychologist*. 2003; 17(3): 410–425.

152. Hinton-Bayre AD. Choice of reliable change model can alter decisions regarding neuropsychological impairment after sports-related concussion. *Clinical Journal of Sport Medicine*. 2012; 22(2): 105–108.

153. Erdal K. Neuropsychological testing for sports-related concussion: how athletes can sandbag their baseline testing without detection. *Archives of Clinical Neuropsychology*. 2012; 27(5): 473–479.

154. Lin LF, Liou TH, Hu CJ et al. Balance function and sensory integration after mild traumatic brain injury. *Brain Injury*. 2015; 29(1): 41–46.

155. Zhou G, Brodsky JR. Objective vestibular testing of children with dizziness and balance complaints following sports-related concussions. *Otolaryngology—Head and Neck Surgery*. 2015; 152(6): 1133–1139.

156. Alsalaheen BA, Whitney SL, Marchetti GF et al. Relationship between cognitive assessment and balance measures in adolescents referred for vestibular physical therapy after concussion. *Clinical Journal of Sport Medicine*. 2015; 26(1): 46–52.

157. Honaker JA, Lester HF, Patterson JN, Jones SM. Examining postconcussion symptoms of dizziness and imbalance on neurocognitive performance in collegiate football players. *Otology and Neurotology*. 2014; 35(6): 1111–1117.

158. Valovich McLeod TC, Hale TD. Vestibular and balance issues following sport-related concussion. *Brain Injury*. 2015; 29(2): 175–184.

159. Corwin DJ, Wiebe DJ, Zonfrillo MR et al. Vestibular deficits following youth concussion. *Journal of Pediatrics*. 2015; 166(5): 1221–1225.

160. Guskiewicz KM, Ross SE, Marshall SW. Postural stability and neuropsychological deficits after concussion in collegiate athletes. *Journal of Athletic Training*. 2001; 36(3): 263–273.

161. Cripps A, Livingston SC. The value of balance-assessment measurements in identifying and monitoring acute postural instability among concussed athletes. *Journal of Sport Rehabilitation*. 2013; 22(1): 67–71.

162. Howell DR, Osternig LR, Chou LS. Dual-task effect on gait balance control in adolescents with concussion. *Archives of Physical Medicine and Rehabilitation*. 2013; 94(8): 1513–1520.

163. Heitger MH, Jones RD, Macleod AD, Snell DL, Frampton CM, Anderson TJ. Impaired eye movements in post-concussion syndrome indicate suboptimal brain function beyond the influence of depression, malingering or intellectual ability. *Brain*. 2009; 132(Pt 10): 2850–2870.

164. Powers KC, Kalmar JM, Cinelli ME. Recovery of static stability following a concussion. *Gait and Posture*. 2014; 39(1): 611–614.

165. Greenwald BD, Cifu DX, Marwitz JH et al. Factors associated with balance deficits on admission to rehabilitation after traumatic brain injury: a multicenter analysis. *The Journal of Head Trauma Rehabilitation*. 2001; 16(3): 238–252.

166. Howell DR, Osternig LR, Chou LS. Return to activity after concussion affects dual-task gait balance control recovery. *Medicine and Science in Sports and Exercise*. 2015; 47(4): 673–680.

167. Guskiewicz KM. Balance assessment in the management of sport-related concussion. *Clinics in Sports Medicine*. 2011; 30(1): 89–102, ix.

168. Guskiewicz KM, Register-Mihalik J, McCrory P et al. Evidence-based approach to revising the SCAT2: introducing the SCAT3. *British Journal of Sports Medicine*. 2013; 47(5): 289–293.

169. Khanna NK, Baumgartner K, LaBella CR. Balance error scoring system performance in children and adolescents with no history of concussion. *Sports Health*. 2015; 7(4): 341–345.

170. Guskiewicz KM, Riemann BL, Perrin DH, Nashner LM. Alternative approaches to the assessment of mild head injury in athletes. *Medicine and Science in Sports and Exercise*. 1997; 29(7 Suppl): S213–221.

171. Murray N, Salvatore A, Powell D, Reed-Jones R. Reliability and validity evidence of multiple balance assessments in athletes with a concussion. *Journal of Athletic Training*. 2014; 49(4): 540–549.

172. King LA, Horak FB, Mancini M et al. Instrumenting the balance error scoring system for use with patients reporting persistent balance problems after mild traumatic brain injury. *Archives of Physical Medicine and Rehabilitation*. 2014; 95(2): 353–359.

173. Furman GR, Lin CC, Bellanca JL, Marchetti GF, Collins MW, Whitney SL. Comparison of the balance accelerometer measure and balance error scoring system in adolescent concussions in sports. *The American Journal of Sports Medicine*. 2013; 41(6): 1404–1410.

174. Quatman-Yates C, Hugentobler J, Ammon R, Mwase N, Kurowski B, Myer GD. The utility of the balance error scoring system for mild brain injury assessments in children and adolescents. *The Physician and Sportsmedicine*. 2014; 42(3): 32–38.

175. Valovich TC, Perrin DH, Gansneder BM. Repeat administration elicits a practice effect with the balance error scoring system but not with the standardized assessment of concussion in high school athletes. *Journal of Athletic Training*. 2003; 38(1): 51–56.

176. Mulligan IJ, Boland MA, McIlhenny CV. The balance error scoring system learned response among young adults. *Sports Health*. 2013; 5(1): 22–26.

177. Graves BS. University football players, postural stability, and concussions. *Journal of Strength and Conditioning Research*. 2015; 30(2): 579–583.

178. Cavanaugh JT, Guskiewicz KM, Giuliani C, Marshall S, Mercer V, Stergiou N. Detecting altered postural control after cerebral concussion in athletes with normal postural stability. *British Journal of Sports Medicine*. 2005; 39(11): 805–811.

179. Quatman-Yates CC, Bonnette S, Hugentobler JA et al. Postconcussion postural sway variability changes in youth: the benefit of structural variability analyses. *Pediatric Physical Therapy*. 2015; 27(4): 316–327.

180. Ustinova KI, Silkwood-Sherer DJ. Postural perturbations induced by a moving virtual environment are reduced in persons with brain injury when gripping a mobile object. *Journal of Neurologic Physical Therapy*. 2014; 38(2): 125–133.

181. Teel EF, Slobounov SM. Validation of a virtual reality balance module for use in clinical concussion assessment and management. *Clinical Journal of Sport Medicine*. 2015; 25(2): 144–148.

182. Slobounov S, Tutwiler R, Sebastianelli W, Slobounov E. Alteration of postural responses to visual field motion in mild traumatic brain injury. *Neurosurgery*. 2006; 59(1): 134–139.

183. Slobounov S, Slobounov E, Newell K. Application of virtual reality graphics in assessment of concussion. *Cyberpsychology and Behavior*. 2006; 9(2): 188–191.

184. Teel EF, Gay MR, Arnett PA, Slobounov SM. Differential sensitivity between a virtual reality balance module and clinically used concussion balance modalities. *Clinical Journal of Sport Medicine*. 2015; 26(2): 162–166.

185. Slobounov S, Cao C, Sebastianelli W, Slobounov E, Newell K. Residual deficits from concussion as revealed by virtual time-to-contact measures of postural stability. *Clinical Neurophysiology*. 2008; 119(2): 281–289.

186. Catena RD, van Donkelaar P, Chou LS. Different gait tasks distinguish immediate vs. long-term effects of concussion on balance control. *Journal of Neuroengineering and Rehabilitation*. 2009; 6: 25.

187. Catena RD, van Donkelaar P, Chou LS. The effects of attention capacity on dynamic balance control following concussion. *Journal of Neuroengineering and Rehabilitation*. 2011; 8: 8.

188. Maerlender A, Rieman W, Lichtenstein J, Condiracci C. Programmed physical exertion in recovery from sports-related concussion: a randomized pilot study. *Developmental Neuropsychology*. 2015; 40(5): 273–278.

189. Chiu SL, Osternig L, Chou LS. Concussion induces gait inter-joint coordination variability under conditions of divided attention and obstacle crossing. *Gait and Posture*. 2013; 38(4): 717–722.

190. Powers KC, Kalmar JM, Cinelli ME. Dynamic stability and steering control following a sport-induced concussion. *Gait and Posture*. 2014; 39(2): 728–732.

191. Baker CS, Cinelli ME. Visuomotor deficits during locomotion in previously concussed athletes 30 or more days following return to play. *Physiological Reports*. 2014; 2(12).

192. Buckley TA, Munkasy BA, Tapia-Lovler TG, Wikstrom EA. Altered gait termination strategies following a concussion. *Gait and Posture*. 2013; 38(3): 549–551.

193. Pearson BC, Armitage KR, Horner CW, Carpenter RH. Saccadometry: the possible application of latency distribution measurement for monitoring concussion. *British Journal of Sports Medicine*. 2007; 41(9): 610–612.

194. Kelty-Stephen DG, Qureshi Ahmad M, Stirling L. Use of a tracing task to assess visuomotor performance for evidence of concussion and recuperation. *Psychological Assessment*. 2015; 27(4) 1379–1387.

195. Maruta J, Ghajar J. Detecting eye movement abnormalities from concussion. *Progress in Neurological Surgery*. 2014; 28: 226–233.

196. Honaker JA, Criter RE, Patterson JN, Jones SM. Gaze stabilization test asymmetry score as an indicator of previous concussion in a cohort of collegiate football players. *Clinical Journal of Sport Medicine*. 2015; 25(4): 361–366.

197. Galetta KM, Morganroth J, Moehringer N et al. Adding vision to concussion testing: a prospective study of sideline testing in youth and collegiate athletes. *Journal of Neuro-Ophthalmology*. 2015; 35(3): 235–241.

198. Vernau BT, Grady MF, Goodman A et al. Oculomotor and neurocognitive assessment of youth ice hockey players: baseline associations and observations after concussion. *Developmental Neuropsychology*. 2015; 40(1): 7–11.

199. Leong DF, Balcer LJ, Galetta SL, Evans G, Gimre M, Watt D. The King-Devick test for sideline concussion screening in collegiate football. *Journal of Optometry*. 2015; 8(2): 131–139.

200. King D, Hume P, Gissane C, Clark T. Use of the King-Devick test for sideline concussion screening in junior rugby league. *Journal of the Neurological Sciences*. 2015; 357(1–2): 75–79.

201. Seidman DH, Burlingame J, Yousif LR et al. Evaluation of the King-Devick test as a concussion screening tool in high school football players. *Journal of the Neurological Sciences*. 2015; 356(1–2): 97–101.

202. Samadani U, Ritlop R, Reyes M et al. Eye tracking detects disconjugate eye movements associated with structural traumatic brain injury and concussion. *Journal of Neurotrauma*. 2015; 32(8): 548–556.

203. Ellis MJ, Cordingley D, Vis S, Reimer K, Leiter J, Russell K. Vestibulo-ocular dysfunction in pediatric sports-related concussion. *Journal of Neurosurgery Pediatrics*. 2015; 16(3): 248–255.

204. Maruta J, Suh M, Niogi SN, Mukherjee P, Ghajar J. Visual tracking synchronization as a metric for concussion screening. *The Journal of Head Trauma Rehabilitation*. 2010; 25(4): 293–305.

205. Alhilali LM, Yaeger K, Collins M, Fakhran S. Detection of central white matter injury underlying vestibulopathy after mild traumatic brain injury. *Radiology*. 2014; 272(1): 224–232.

206. King D, Gissane C, Hume PA, Flaws M. The King-Devick test was useful in management of concussion in amateur rugby union and rugby league in New Zealand. *Journal of the Neurological Sciences*. 2015; 351(1–2): 58–64.

207. Barnett BP, Singman EL. Vision concerns after mild traumatic brain injury. *Current Treatment Options in Neurology*. 2015; 17(2): 329.

208. Master CL, Scheiman M, Gallaway M et al. Vision diagnoses are common after concussion in adolescents. *Clinical Pediatrics*. 2015; 55(3): 260–267.

209. Soldatovic-Stajic B, Misic-Pavkov G, Bozic K, Novovic Z, Gajic Z. Neuropsychological and neurophysiological evaluation of cognitive deficits related to the severity of traumatic brain injury. *European Review for Medical and Pharmacological Sciences*. 2014; 18(11): 1632–1637.

210. Lavoie ME, Dupuis F, Johnston KM, Leclerc S, Lassonde M. Visual p300 effects beyond symptoms in concussed college athletes. *Journal of Clinical and Experimental Neuropsychology*. 2004; 26(1): 55–73.

211. Ozen LJ, Itier RJ, Preston FF, Fernandes MA. Long-term working memory deficits after concussion: electrophysiological evidence. *Brain Injury*. 2013; 27(11): 1244–1255.

212. Moore RD, Hillman CH, Broglio SP. The persistent influence of concussive injuries on cognitive control and neuroelectric function. *Journal of Athletic Training*. 2014; 49(1): 24–35.

213. Gay M, Ray W, Johnson B, Teel E, Geronimo A, Slobounov S. Feasibility of EEG measures in conjunction with light exercise for return-to-play evaluation after sports-related concussion. *Developmental Neuropsychology*. 2015; 40(4): 248–253.

214. Moore RD, Sauve W, Ellemberg D. Neurophysiological correlates of persistent psycho-affective alterations in athletes with a history of concussion. *Brain Imaging and Behavior*. 2015; 10(4): 1108–1116.

215. Prichep LS, McCrea M, Barr W, Powell M, Chabot RJ. Time course of clinical and electrophysiological recovery after sport-related concussion. *The Journal of Head Trauma Rehabilitation*. 2013; 28(4): 266–273.

216. Rogers JM, Fox AM, Donnelly J. Impaired practice effects following mild traumatic brain injury: an event-related potential investigation. *Brain Injury*. 2015; 29(3): 343–351.

217. De Beaumont L, Brisson B, Lassonde M, Jolicoeur P. Long-term electrophysiological changes in athletes with a history of multiple concussions. *Brain Injury*. 2007; 21(6): 631–644.

218. Dupuis F, Johnston KM, Lavoie M, Lepore F, Lassonde M. Concussions in athletes produce brain dysfunction as revealed by event-related potentials. *Neuroreport*. 2000; 11(18): 4087–4092.

219. Baillargeon A, Lassonde M, Leclerc S, Ellemberg D. Neuropsychological and neurophysiological assessment of sport concussion in children, adolescents and adults. *Brain Injury*. 2012; 26(3): 211–220.

220. Corradini PL, Persinger MA. Spectral power, source localization and microstates to quantify chronic deficits from 'mild' closed head injury: correlation with classic neuropsychological tests. *Brain Injury*. 2014; 28(10): 1317–1327.

221. Kutcher JS, McCrory P, Davis G, Ptito A, Meeuwisse WH, Broglio SP. What evidence exists for new strategies or technologies in the diagnosis of sports concussion and assessment of recovery? *British Journal of Sports Medicine*. 2013; 47(5): 299–303.

222. Gaetz M, Bernstein DM. The current status of electrophysiologic procedures for the assessment of mild traumatic brain injury. *The Journal of Head Trauma Rehabilitation*. 2001; 16(4): 386–405.

223. Rapp PE, Keyser DO, Albano A et al. Traumatic brain injury detection using electrophysiological methods. *Frontiers in Human Neuroscience*. 2015; 9: 11.

224. Diaz DS. Management of athletes with post-concussion syndrome. *Seminars in Speech and Language*. 2014; 35(3): 204–210.

225. Gurley JM, Hujsak BD, Kelly JL. Vestibular rehabilitation following mild traumatic brain injury. *NeuroRehabilitation*. 2013; 32(3): 519–528.

226. Gottshall K. Vestibular rehabilitation after mild traumatic brain injury with vestibular pathology. *NeuroRehabilitation*. 2011; 29(2): 167–171.

227. Gurr B, Moffat N. Psychological consequences of vertigo and the effectiveness of vestibular rehabilitation for brain injury patients. *Brain Injury*. 2001; 15(5): 387–400.

228. Broglio SP, Collins MW, Williams RM, Mucha A, Kontos AP. Current and emerging rehabilitation for concussion: a review of the evidence. *Clinics in Sports Medicine*. 2015; 34(2): 213–231.

229. Ustinova KI, Chernikova LA, Dull A, Perkins J. Physical therapy for correcting postural and coordination deficits in patients with mild-to-moderate traumatic brain injury. *Physiotherapy Theory and Practice*. 2015; 31(1): 1–7.

230. Ustinova KI, Perkins J, Leonard WA, Hausbeck CJ. Virtual reality game-based therapy for treatment of postural and co-ordination abnormalities secondary to TBI: a pilot study. *Brain Injury*. 2014; 28(4): 486–495.

231. Reneker JC, Cook CE. Dizziness after sports-related concussion: can physiotherapists offer better treatment than just 'physical and cognitive rest'? *British Journal of Sports Medicine*. 2015; 49(8): 491–492.

232. Ellis MJ, Leddy JJ, Willer B. Physiological, vestibulo-ocular and cervicogenic post-concussion disorders: an evidence-based classification system with directions for treatment. *Brain Injury*. 2015; 29(2): 238–248.

233. Schneider KJ, Meeuwisse WH, Nettel-Aguirre A et al. Cervicovestibular rehabilitation in sport-related concussion: a randomised controlled trial. *British Journal of Sports Medicine*. 2014; 48(17): 1294–1298.

234. Alsalaheen BA, Whitney SL, Mucha A, Morris LO, Furman JM, Sparto PJ. Exercise prescription patterns in patients treated with vestibular rehabilitation after concussion. *Physiotherapy Research International*. 2013; 18(2): 100–108.

235. Webb TS, Whitehead CR, Wells TS, Gore RK, Otte CN. Neurologically-related sequelae associated with mild traumatic brain injury. *Brain Injury*. 2015; 29(4): 430–437.

236. Alsalaheen BA, Mucha A, Morris LO et al. Vestibular rehabilitation for dizziness and balance disorders after concussion. *Journal of Neurologic Physical Therapy*. 2010; 34(2): 87–93.

237. Clark JF, Colosimo A, Ellis JK et al. Vision training methods for sports concussion mitigation and management. *Journal of Visualized Experiments*. 2015(99): e52648.

238. Yadav NK, Thiagarajan P, Ciuffreda KJ. Effect of oculomotor vision rehabilitation on the visual-evoked potential and visual attention in mild traumatic brain injury. *Brain Injury*. 2014; 28(7): 922–929.

239. Thiagarajan P, Ciuffreda KJ. Effect of oculomotor rehabilitation on vergence responsivity in mild traumatic brain injury. *Journal of Rehabilitation Research and Development*. 2013; 50(9): 1223–1240.

240. Thiagarajan P, Ciuffreda KJ, Capo-Aponte JE, Ludlam DP, Kapoor N. Oculomotor neuro-rehabilitation for reading in mild traumatic brain injury (mTBI): an integrative approach. *NeuroRehabilitation*. 2014; 34(1): 129–146.

241. Thiagarajan P, Ciuffreda KJ. Versional eye tracking in mild traumatic brain injury (mTBI): effects of oculomotor training (OMT). *Brain Injury*. 2014; 28(7): 930–943.

242. Thiagarajan P, Ciuffreda KJ. Effect of oculomotor rehabilitation on accommodative responsivity in mild traumatic brain injury. *Journal of Rehabilitation Research and Development*. 2014; 51(2): 175–191.

243. Cournoyer J, Tripp BL. Concussion knowledge in high school football players. *Journal of Athletic Training*. 2014; 49(5): 654–658.

244. Cusimano MD, Chipman M, Donnelly P, Hutchison MG. Effectiveness of an educational video on concussion knowledge in minor league hockey players: a cluster randomised controlled trial. *British Journal of Sports Medicine*. 2014; 48(2): 141–146.

245. Kroshus E, Daneshvar DH, Baugh CM, Nowinski CJ, Cantu RC. NCAA concussion education in ice hockey: an ineffective mandate. *British Journal of Sports Medicine*. 2014; 48(2): 135–140.

246. Mrazik M, Perra A, Brooks BL, Naidu D. Exploring minor hockey players' knowledge and attitudes toward concussion: implications for prevention. *The Journal of Head Trauma Rehabilitation*. 2015; 30(3): 219–227.

247. Ponsford J, Willmott C, Rothwell A et al. Impact of early intervention on outcome after mild traumatic brain injury in children. *Pediatrics*. 2001; 108(6): 1297–1303.

248. Register-Mihalik JK, Guskiewicz KM, McLeod TC, Linnan LA, Mueller FO, Marshall SW. Knowledge, attitude, and concussion-reporting behaviors among high school athletes: a preliminary study. *Journal of Athletic Training*. 2013; 48(5): 645–653.

249. Kay MC, Welch CE, Valovich McLeod TC. Positive and negative factors that influence concussion reporting among secondary-school athletes. *Journal of Sport Rehabilitation*. 2015; 24(2): 210–213.

250. Williamson IJ, Goodman D. Converging evidence for the under-reporting of concussions in youth ice hockey. *British Journal of Sports Medicine*. 2006; 40(2): 128–132.

251. Kurowski B, Pomerantz WJ, Schaiper C, Gittelman MA. Factors that influence concussion knowledge and self-reported attitudes in high school athletes. *The Journal of Trauma and Acute Care Surgery*. 2014; 77 (3 Suppl 1): S12–17.

252. Chrisman SP, Quitiquit C, Rivara FP. Qualitative study of barriers to concussive symptom reporting in high school athletics. *The Journal of Adolescent Health*. 2013; 52(3): 330–335.e333.

253. Kroshus E, Baugh CM, Hawrilenko M, Daneshvar DH. Pilot randomized evaluation of publically available concussion education materials: evidence of a possible negative effect. *Health Education and Behavior*. 2015; 42(2): 153–162.

254. Guskiewicz KM. When treating sport concussion, check the boxes, but also go the extra mile. *Journal of Athletic Training*. 2013; 48(4): 441.

255. Kroshus E, Baugh CM, Daneshvar DH, Nowinski CJ, Cantu RC. Concussion reporting intention: a valuable metric for predicting reporting behavior and evaluating concussion education. *Clinical Journal of Sport Medicine*. 2015; 25(3): 243–247.

256. Kroshus E, Baugh CM, Daneshvar DH, Viswanath K. Understanding concussion reporting using a model based on the theory of planned behavior. *The Journal of Adolescent Health*. 2014; 54(3): 269–274. e262.

257. Register-Mihalik JK, Linnan LA, Marshall SW, Valovich McLeod TC, Mueller FO, Guskiewicz KM. Using theory to understand high school aged athletes' intentions to report sport-related concussion: implications for concussion education initiatives. *Brain Injury*. 2013; 27(7–8): 878–886.

258. Mannings C, Kalynych C, Joseph MM, Smotherman C, Kraemer DF. Knowledge assessment of sports-related concussion among parents of children aged 5 years to 15 years enrolled in recreational tackle football. *The Journal of Trauma and Acute Care Surgery*. 2014; 77(3 Suppl 1): S18–22.

259. Babul S. Addressing the need for standardized concussion care in Canada: Concussion awareness training tool. *Canadian Family Physician Medecin de Famille Canadien*. 2015; 61(8): 660–662.

260. Stoller J, Carson JD, Garel A et al. Do family physicians, emergency department physicians, and pediatricians give consistent sport-related concussion management advice? *Canadian Family Physician Medecin de Famille Canadien*. 2014; 60(6): 548, 550–542.

261. Broshek DK, Samples H, Beard J, Goodkin HP. Current practices of the child neurologist in managing sports concussion. *Journal of Child Neurology*. 2014; 29(1): 17–22.

262. Lebrun CM, Mrazik M, Prasad AS et al. Sport concussion knowledge base, clinical practises and needs for continuing medical education: a survey of family physicians and cross-border comparison. *British Journal of Sports Medicine*. 2013; 47(1): 54–59.

263. Zemek R, Eady K, Moreau K et al. Knowledge of paediatric concussion among front-line primary care providers. *Paediatrics and Child Health*. 2014; 19(9): 475–480.

CHAPTER 7

Return to activity following concussion

Introduction

As reviewed in detail in Chapter 2, the initial insult of a concussion not only causes direct focal cerebral/neuronal injury, but it propagates a cascade of extracellular and intracellular reactions.[1–5] Numerous preclinical studies have characterized this process of secondary injury and the vulnerable state in which the brain is placed in following concussion. In tandem, increasing knowledge is growing in regard to a hypermetabolic/vascular response following a repeat head injury within this acute window period, causing the rare case of sudden death (termed second impact syndrome) and also the long-term effects of repeated subconcussion/concussion leading to Chronic Traumatic Encephalopathy (CTE) (refer to Chapters 7 and 9, respectively). Due to this growing body of literature and cases, there has been a paradigm shift within the past decade. Initially, there was a shift from returning a player back to the field the same day of concussion—or development of concussion-like symptoms—if they met specific criteria,[6–8] to a more cautious approach: "When in doubt, sit them out."[9] However, this has now evolved to the current recommendation by the International Consensus Conference on Concussion, the American Academy of Neurology, the National Athletic Trainers Association, and the Institute of Medicine to *not* return any player the same day of injury.[10–15]

Those charged with determining the appropriate return to learn, work, and play of an athlete following concussion reach toward these guidelines in order to obtain a consensus statement on the proper protocol to return a player to activity. These guidelines do clearly recommend for a "*gradual* return to activity," but do not provide a defined algorithm specifically for the pediatric population or the return to learning process.[16,17] It is the lack of clarity in defined guidelines that can lead to an ambiguous care of athletes and early return to activity.[18] A Canadian study retrospectively reviewed charts of pediatric patients that sustained a concussion, and found that 45% had a premature return to school or sport—this was classified as those that were observed to have an exacerbation in symptoms.[19] Our incomplete understanding of how the known pathophysiology relates to predictive measures (acute assessment scales, neuropsychology testing, advanced neuroimaging modalities, biomarkers, etc.) and return to activity is really the root of why there is limited guidance in return to activity.[20] A need exists for clearly defined guidelines to assist the medical personnel taking care of the concussed athlete, remove any conflict of interest between athlete-parent-coach-doctor,[21] and also litigation prevention through concise documentation. In 2013, a review of pediatric primary care providers showed that only 10 out of 91 medical records with a diagnosis of concussion had distinct cognitive rest recommendations.[22]

What is most difficult in attempting to determine succinct guidelines is that our preclinical and clinical conclusions are riddled with conflicting data. Previously, a pronounced emphasis was on prolonged rest following concussion but recent literature has shown that prolonged rest is detrimental on outcomes following concussion.[23] It has been postulated that lack of activity and social limitations only heightens anxiety and depression that are shown to exacerbate postconcussive symptoms.[2]

Hopefully, as research continues to understand the postconcussive period, a clearer and succinct return-to-activity protocol will be available. The goal of this chapter is to present preclinical and clinical studies (specific to return to learn or play) along with the most recent guidelines to provide the reader with an enriched understanding of how to return the pediatric and adult patient to the academic environment, the work place, driving, and finally physical activity (Figure 7.1). It is necessary to understand that though robust preclinical models have been established, the translatability to humans is always a concern. For example, most preclinical studies use rodent subjects, but it is apparent that their smooth, lissencephalic cortex is very different than the human brain and therefore may react differently to external forces. On the other hand, human retrospective and prospective studies also have limitations due to their inherent bias, which will be discussed in more detail.

Return to activity

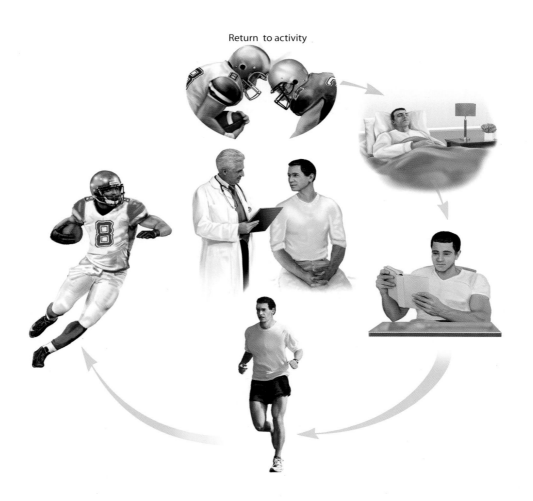

Figure 7.1 Schematic depiction of return to activity following a concussion. After a concussive injury, the athlete is to be removed from play and determination made if higher medical assessment is required. Following a short rest period (dictated by symptomatology), the athlete progresses through the return to learn followed by escalation in physical activity. Once asymptomatic with full exertion, the athlete is evaluated and potentially cleared for return to full contact activities. The advancement through each successive phase of the return to activity is under the guidance of a medical professional versed in caring for concussed athletes.

Return to learn

Preclinical and clinical research

As mentioned, the brain can be taxed during the metabolically disturbed postconcussive state. Creed et al. highlighted this postconcussive state in the rat TBI model displaying that, though rats had early recoverable behavior deficits in memory and spatial acquisition, progressive secondary injury seen as white matter degeneration occurred for up to 2 weeks following injury.[24] It was proposed that cognitive stress during this time period could potentiate further secondary injury that may ultimately lead to irreversible structural changes or prolonged postconcussive symptoms. The emphasis on postconcussive management has been focused on return to play, and it wasn't until more recently that return to learn has become a focus in preclinical literature. Initial studies by Giza et al. demonstrated a detrimental effect in long-term cognitive outcomes in rats exposed to a cognitively stimulating environment in the first two week period following concussive injury. Those that had initiation of the stimulating environment 2 weeks after injury showed marked cognitive improvements.[25] Then in 2013, Briones et al. disputed these findings in a controlled cortical impact rat model in which the animals were either exposed to an enriched environment or standard environment for 4 weeks directly following injury. Those exposed to an early enriched environment showed a significant reduction in specific proinflammatory markers within the brain, an increase in anti-inflammatory markers, and an improvement in cognitive behavior testing.[26] Due to differences in study designs and timing of introduction of the enriched environment, it is difficult to compare these two studies directly. But, it does begin to potentially describe a delicate time window that early (less than 2 weeks from injury) cognitive use is detrimental, but not as deleterious as prolonged cognitive rest (more than one month from injury).

Due to the questionable applicability of preclinical results, researchers turned to the use of observational, retrospective, and randomized studies to analyze outcomes in concussed patients that had no rest, a brief period of rest, or prolonged rest following injury. Moser et al. in 2012 took all high school and collegiate athletes who presented with a concussion and instructed them to have a strict one week rest period starting from the time of presentation to the outpatient clinic. This stratified each patient into cohorts of 1–7 days, 8–30 days, and more than 31 days rest. Based on their time from injury to evaluate in addition to the prescribe one week of rest. The conclusion was that the group that had the longest rest period (more than 31 days) had overall improved outcomes (postconcussive assessment and cognitive testing).[27] But, there is a conceivable bias to this study in that a patient with less severe symptoms would delay presentation to a medical professional, therefore being stratified into the prolonged rest cohort. Also response bias from the athletes may have occurred when asked about their lack of or participation in activities prior to clinical evaluation. Similarly, another prospective single center study in 335 youth to collegiate athletes found that increased cognitive activity following injury was predictive of having longer duration of symptoms.[28]

Alternatively, studies have found limited benefit and potential harmful effects to any period of rest, and specific if its prolonged.[29–31] In 2002, De Krujik et al. randomized 107 adult patients (mean age 39.9) to either no rest versus 6 days of rest. No significant difference in outcomes were appreciated at 2 weeks, 3 or 6 months between the two groups. Also, Gibson et al. found no benefit of cognitive rest following concussion in a retrospective review of 135 patients, aged 8 to 26 years, who presented to a concussion clinic.[30]

Moor et al. performed in 2015 an observational study where pediatric students who were less adherent to physician recommendations of physical and cognitive rest were found to recover quicker.[29] Without the ability to randomize, it is necessary to attempt to separate the varying degrees of concussion based on initial presentation. For this reason, it is difficult to formulate conclusions from this study because an athlete who suffered from a more minor concussion may be more likely to ignore rest recommendations and return to activity sooner because his/her symptoms have subsided. But this finding began to question if any rest could be actually harmful.

In 2015, Thomas et al. performed a randomized study in pediatric patients who presented following a concussion with a negative head CT scan. They were randomized to either a one, two, or five day strict rest period followed by a stepwise return to activity. The five day rest period group showed a significant increase in daily postconcussive symptoms and a slower time to recover.[32] For this reason, the authors proposed the importance in cognitive rest but not to be prolonged. Though not a sound clinical trial, this randomized study provides evidence that surpasses the previously mentioned retrospective studies filled with bias, therefore cognitive rest, but not prolonged, has become the standard to our return-to-learn guidelines.

Return to learn guidelines

Though it is challenging to compare each of these studies together (due to their inherent bias, pediatric/adult population, and variable study design of duration and timing of activity progression), it does appear that (*i*) cognitive stress negatively affects the perturbed postinjurious brain, (*ii*) an initial rest period is necessary, and (*iii*) the actual timing is essential with regard to the period of rest and subsequent progression of activities. For this reason, we agree with published recommendations to allow several days of complete rest after a concussion, followed by a graded return-to-learn process.[1,33–36] Focus does need to be placed on prevention of excessive prolonged cognitive rest due to its detrimental effects seen in preclinical studies.[37]

The initial phase of the return-to-learn sequence should consists of a complete rest period for several days.[38,39] Clear instructions should be given to the athlete and parent to guide them in deciding how many days of rest should occur prior to follow-up appointment with a medical professional. During this time frame, the focus of the athlete is towards rest and complete limitation of cognitive stimulation that specifically aggravates symptoms. For this reason, it is necessary that the athlete be off all medications at the time for decision of activity progression.[40] The duration is dependent on the individual's *symptoms*. The patient does not need to be completely asymptomatic, but the symptoms should be tolerable, not exacerbated by mild cognitive activity (tolerate at least 30 minutes), of minimal duration, and amenable to rest.[1,35,41,42] Adolescent athletes, on average,

return to academics roughly 3 to 4 days after injury and are symptom free by 2 weeks.[43]

Once these criteria are met, it is necessary for the athlete to be evaluated by a medical professional to supervise their return-to-learn route. The purpose of this appointment is to (*i*) educate about concussion and concussion recovery, (*ii*) evaluate current status of symptoms, (*iii*) validate if the athlete is ready to progress or if more cognitive rest is needed based on symptomatology, neurocognitive/neuropsychological testing and other diagnostic tools (balance, oculomotor, reaction time, etc.), and (*iv*) establish an initial, individualized, and incremental return-to-learn schedule.[44] A multidisciplinary approach built around strong communication between, not only, the physician, school nurse, and athletic trainer, but also the athlete, athlete's parents, teachers, and coach is essential to safely and efficiently return to academics.[43]

Gioia et al. published the "PACE" model in 2015: Progressive Activities of Controlled Exertion to guide medical personnel in the return-to-learn process.[42] This model is composed of 10 different elements that are summarized into four different stages. The four stages are: "set the positive foundation," "define parameters of activity-exertion schedule," "teach activity, monitoring, and management skills," and lastly "reinforce progress to recovery." The initial and subsequent follow-up clinic appointments should be structured in this manner (Table 7.1).[42]

The essential component to the return-to-learn process is that it should be individualized and tailored by the presence or absence of symptoms.[41,42,45] Once the patient is asymptomatic following a progression to a normal scholastic schedule, a repeat assessment scale should be performed (ex. SCAT) along with neuropsychological testing if available.[46]

When to consider referral to a concussion specialist

The majority of athletes, 80% to 90%, will have *complete* resolution of their symptoms within 7 to 10 days following a concussion.[13] As mentioned, the athlete should take several days of rest till their symptoms subside, followed by assessment by a medical professor. Due to this fluid approach, the athlete may recover in a matter of days, allowing

Table 7.1   Approach to Return-to Learn in the Outpatient Setting, Developed from the PACE Model[42]

1. Concussion education	A large focus of the clinic appointment should be devoted to education of the athlete and family. Recommended topics of education include:
	• Secondary injury and role for gradual return to learn
	• Short-term symptoms that may affect academic tasks
	  • Of concussed student athletes[42]:
	    • 49% with slowed performance on academic work
	    • 54% with fatigue
	    • 58% with attention difficulties
	    • 66% with headaches
	  • Long-term effects of repeated injury (mild cognitive impairment, chronic traumatic encephalopathy)
	  • Current research for return-to-learn guidelines and limitations

2. Establish positive outlook towards recovery	Explain the typical recovery process and duration with positive emphasis on full recovery • 80%–90% of concussions have symptomatic resolution within 7–10 days[13] Due to publicized cases in professional athletes, recognize and address fears of prolonged recovery and permanent neurological deficits[47]
3. Explain process of return-to-learn	1–2 week progression in cognitive activities Individualized progression of activities tailored by symptom aggravation or improvement[41,42,45] Refer to Table 7.2 for more detailed return-to-learn plan[48]
4. Educate symptom monitoring and management skills	Describe how physical, cognitive, and emotional exertion can all affect the recovery of the brain but conversely, prolonged rest is also detrimental Symptom monitoring • Use of a symptom checklist to make student aware of symptoms and specific exacerbating factors • Determine average time to symptom exacerbation once begin academic work • Refer to Figure 7.2 for an example of a symptom monitoring tool[48] Management skills • Use understanding of exacerbating factors and time till symptom onset to recommend modification of daily class schedule and course work. This may include shortened class periods, scheduled breaks, reduction or extension in coursework and tests[49–51] • Progressive increase in daily activities with goal to stay below symptom threshold[1,33,42] • Other modifications: anxiety/stress management, sleep hygiene, limits on cell phone/video game/computer/television use, based on symptoms, reduction in stimulating social situations
5. Monitoring for recovery	Weekly reassessment with adjustments to academic work, as needed, with goal of progression Use of an assessment scale to monitor recovery Fluid communication between physician and school provider including updates on student's progress and further accommodations
6. Reinforce recovery	Positive emphasis on recovery and avoidance of nocebo effect[52]

for an earlier initiation of a graded return to learn. Because our current knowledge of the detrimental effects of prolonged rest following concussion is limited, if the athlete is still having persistent, non-improving symptoms after one week of the rest period, they should be evaluated by a clinician. Therefore, no athlete should exceed one week of rest without being evaluated by a physician. At this point, a thorough history should be obtained focusing on the patient's symptoms (frequency, duration, severity, etc.) and also evaluate for possible apprehensions or personal desires to not return to school. Psychological and physical factors associated with prolonged rest (depression, anxiety, deconditioning, etc.) may also cause "concussion like symptoms," and therefore this should be considered in patients with prolonged symptoms.[53,54] There may exist other motivators prolonging

Table 7.2 Sequential Stages of the Return-to-Learn Process

Stage	Activity	Objective
No activity	Complete cognitive rest—no school, no homework, no reading, no texting, no video games, no computer work	Recovery
Gradual reintroduction of cognitive activity	Relax previous restrictions on activities and add back for short periods of time (5–15 minutes at a time)	Gradual controlled increase in subsymptom threshold cognitive activities
Homework at home before school work at school	Homework in longer increments (20–30 minutes at a time)	Increase cognitive stamina by repetition of short periods of self-paced cognitive activity
School re-entry	Part day of school after tolerating 1–2 cumulative hours of homework at home	Return to school with accommodations to permit controlled subsymptom threshold increase in cognitive load
Gradual reintegration into school	Increase to full day of school	Accommodations decrease as cognitive stamina improves
Resumption of full cognitive workload	Introduce testing, catch up with essential work	Full return to school; may commence return-to-play protocol (see Table 7.3)

Source: Master CL et al., *Pediatric Annals*, 41(9), 1–6, 2012. With permission.

Cognitive Activity Monitoring (CAM) Log

Name: ____________________ Parent/Teacher: ____________________

DATE TIME							
LOCATION (circle one)	Home School	Home School	Home School	Home School	Home School	Home School	Home School
COGNITIVE ACTIVITY:							
DURATION:							
SYMPTOM (PRE/POST)	Rate 0–10	Rate 0–10	Rate 0–10	Rate 0–10	Rate 0–10	Rate 0–10	Rate 0–10
HEADACHE	__/__	__/__	__/__	__/__	__/__	__/__	__/__
FATIGUE	__/__	__/__	__/__	__/__	__/__	__/__	__/__
CONCENTRATION PROBLEMS	__/__	__/__	__/__	__/__	__/__	__/__	__/__
IRRITABILITY	__/__	__/__	__/__	__/__	__/__	__/__	__/__
FOGGINESS	__/__	__/__	__/__	__/__	__/__	__/__	__/__
LIGHT/NOISE SENSITIVITY	__/__	__/__	__/__	__/__	__/__	__/__	__/__
Other: ______	__/__	__/__	__/__	__/__	__/__	__/__	__/__
PRE-POST DIFFERENCE	____	____	____	____	____	____	____

Figure 7.2 **Example of a symptom monitoring log used during the return-to-learn phase.** (From Master CL et al. *Pediatric Annals*, 41(9):1–6, 2012.)

recovery such as cultural, social, secondary gain, or a negative outlook.[55] For example, if the symptoms appear minor, in concert with an anxious parent or athlete, it may be reasonable to introduce the return-to-learn protocol along with emphasis on recovery and calming of fears. If the athlete does have persistent, unremitting symptoms, a referral to a specialized concussion specialist should be considered.

Even after the athlete has initiated the return-to-learn process, referral to a specialist may still be warranted at a later date. It has been noted that, following concussion, one-third of children had the presence of *exertional* symptoms at

2 weeks postinjury,[42] but the overall recovery pattern should be a gradual *reduction* in symptoms over 1 to 2 weeks. Therefore, for the athlete that has initiated the return-to-learn process, a medical provider should also consider referral if the patient has extreme worsening of symptoms even after scaling back on activities, or is requiring a prolonged return to learn (persistence of symptoms after 3 to 4 weeks).[41]

Return-to-work guidelines

There is a paucity of literature on return-to-work recommendations for the adult population. Though the pediatric population is at an increased risk of concussion and more pronounced postconcussive symptoms in comparison to adults,[10,11,13,56,57] we still do not recommend a truncated return-to-work process in comparison to the pediatric return to learn. In view of our limited evidence, it is appropriate to err towards caution than risk long-term cognitive effects.

Similar to the pediatric return-to-learn guidelines, we feel that the adult should also have several days of complete rest following a concussion. Again, the determination of the length of this rest period should be based upon the presence of symptoms. The adult should initiate a return-to-work process that mirrors the pediatric return to learn, once he or she is able to tolerate more than 30 minutes of cognitive activity with minimal exacerbation of symptoms. This should be under the guidance and direction of the patient's primary care provider. It will be necessary for the provider to gauge the personality and work habits of the individual. Based on this the primary care provider will either need to emphasize the importance of a gradual return to activity in the highly career-driven individual, and in contrast, may need to push for a return to the workplace in someone that is less driven and has less motivation.

Depending on the patient's profession and ability to perform light duty, he/she should first perform similar occupational tasks at home (for example reading from a computer screen), being cognizant of tasks that exacerbate symptoms, and the time they are able to comfortably perform the task until symptoms begin to present again. Awareness of what activities exacerbate symptoms while at home will help to direct the specific tasks the person will be able to perform while on light duty at the workplace. Again, the emphasis is to remain below the symptom threshold. A Finnish study noted that 47% of adults returned to work one week following injury and only 71% returned one month following injury. It is pertinent to recognize the different societal influences of return to work and therefore there may be extremely circumstances beyond injury recovery that prevents someone from returning to work.[58,59]

It is conceivable that the return-to-work process could take roughly 1 to 2 weeks or less if light duty is available. The adult should return to full occupational duties as symptoms allow. A prospective review of mild to more severe traumatic brain injury found a variability in the likelihood of return to work that depended on a patient's specific occupation: professional/managerial (56%), technical/skill (40%), and manual labor (32%).[60] Intuitively, an individual who performs a manual labor job may require an extended duration of return to work compared to someone with an office job due to the specific occupation requirement.

For the adult whose career is dependent on manual labor, a similar rest period followed by progressive increase in cognitive activity should be undertaken, as detailed above. Progression to light duty, if available, should be considered in a way to prevent extensive time off from work. Once the individual is able to tolerate more than 24 hours with minimal to no symptoms, a similar return-to-play progression, discussed in detail below, should be performed prior to returning to a vocation that requires physical exertion.

Return-to-drive guidelines

Similar to return to work, a lack of recommendations exists with regard to return to driving following a traumatic brain injury.[61] A study evaluated patients for 24 hours following mild traumatic brain injury and revealed a reduced performance on an occupational therapy drive maze test. Due to these findings, the study recommended complete cessation from driving for at least 24 hours after injury.[55] We feel that individuals should not drive during the initial rest period following a concussion. After this, consideration for driving should only be made once the symptoms are minimal (as to not interfere with one's driving ability, including concentration, alertness, etc.) and not exacerbated by the required cognitive tasks of operating an automobile.

Return to play

The preclinical data that influences the return-to-play guidelines is more convincing than the literature reviewed for return to learn. It has been widely accepted that repeat head injury in the acute phase following concussion is harmful to the athlete. The specifics about the exact timing of returning an athlete to activity is still contested and the long-term effects of repetitive concussion are even more passionately debated.[2,10,62] We will review the preclinical and clinical data that influences the return-to-play guidelines and present an approach to managing the return to play of an athlete. For a more formal discussion regarding subconcussion and the long-term effects (cognitive impairment and chronic traumatic encephalopathy), refer to Chapter 9.

Preclinical and clinical research

The initial driving force to formulate the return-to-play guidelines was the concern of a repeat concussion during the postinjury period of brain recovery. It has been established in preclinical models that a repeat concussion has detrimental effects: worsening diffuse axonal and parenchymal injury, greater blood–brain barrier breakdown, increased microglial activation and gliosis, reduced performance on behavioral tests, and even increased mortality.[63–71] First shown in vitro by Weber et al. the initial injury actually primes the neuron and reduces its injury threshold for subsequent trauma.[67] Intuitively, a second concussion is found to have worse outcomes, but only if it occurs within a specific time frame following the first concussion. Through assessing the various study designs of each preclinical trial, it is possible to obtain a partial understanding of when specifically the animal is most at risk of a synergistic effect from repeat trauma. In mice, rat, and swine mild TBI models, results indicate that poorer outcomes, as mentioned above, exist when the animal receives a second injury minutes,[72] one,[63–66] three,[65,68,73] five,[68] or seven[71] days following the initial event.[74] Similarly, repeat head injuries demonstrated a worse outcome when occurring within 24 hours and 7 days in clinical studies.[65,69,70,75,76] But, multiple investigations, that had varying time points for secondary injury, did not see a worsening effect if the subsequent injury occurred more than one week following the first mild TBI.[65,66,68,73]

Interestingly, a nonrandomized, human, prospective study in young athletes exhibited no difference in outcomes (neuropsychological and balance testing) between the ones who received no rest following injury versus the players that had, on average, a three day rest period. But, most importantly this study demonstrated that there was a small but significant risk of repeat concussion seen in 7% of the studied population. Eighty percent of those with repeat concussion had the second concussion within the first 10 days following injury![77] Therefore, limitation of contact activity within the first 1 to 2 weeks following injury would prevent a large portion of potential repeat concussions and possible neurological injury.

As continued experimental evidence developed, a complex dilemma of specific timing to activity, types of activity, and prolonged lack of activity began to surface, making the return-to-play question more complicated than expected. Griesbach et al. emphasized that exercise was beneficial in the acute time period, but only following a two-week rest period. Specifically, after a two-week rest period, rats exercised on days 14 to 20 following injury had an up regulation of BDNF (promotes neuroplasticity) that correlated with improved behavior testing.[78] Interestingly, this effect was not seen in the rats that were immediately exercised following injury. Contradictory to this preclinical study, a clinical trial of 107 patients randomized to either 6 days of complete bed rest versus progression of activity starting on day one after concussion, found no statistical difference in post-traumatic symptoms at 6 months.[79] What is important to note of this study is that similar to the return-to-learn data, there was no added benefit to prolonged rest. Comparable to return to learn, return to play also appears advantageous when a gradual progression is implemented, in contrast to lack of or excessive exercise performed immediately following injury. This was revealed by a retrospective review of concussed college-age student athletes. This review found that those engaging in moderate levels of activity at follow-up (defined as school activity plus some light home physical activity, i.e. slow jogging, mowing the lawn) fared better than those that refrained from any activity or those that were taking part in high levels of activity.[80]

Return-to-play guidelines

The utmost role of proper return-to-play guidelines is to prevent any further harm to the athlete, either through early physical exertion worsening secondary injury or receiving a repeat concussion during the healing process. Therefore, the current consensus opinion in return to play recommends instructing concussed athletes to refrain from any contact activities that would make an athlete prone to repeat concussion. Further, the progression of increasing exercise intensity, from mild to moderate levels, should be dictated by the presence of symptoms.[10,11,13,46,81]

The initiation of exercise progression should be guided by a medical professional, and in fact, many states require medical evaluation prior to activity clearance.[1,82,83] Following the initial period of strict rest, a progression of cognitively demanding activities should be undertaken, as described in the return-to-learn process. This progression may last a few days to a few weeks depending on symptom severity. As stated by the Zurich Guidelines: "A sensible approach involves the gradual return to school and social activities before contact sports in a manner that does not result in significant exacerbation of symptoms."[82] Once symptoms are more mild, tolerable, and short lived for more than 24 hours and also neuropsychological testing is within a standard deviation of the mean, it is reasonable to initiate the return-to-play process.[84–86] Similar to the return-to-learn advancement, athletes should not be under the influence of any pharmacotherapy during the evaluation to determine initiation of return-to-play steps.

The return to play is a stepwise process in which each step should take roughly 24 hours.[10,48,82,87,88] If symptoms begin to develop, the athlete should stop and rest for 24 hours till symptoms subside. The athlete should then return to the previous step in which he or she was asymptomatic. Refer to Table 7.3 for the stepwise progression of return-to-play guidelines.[48] For guidance, May et al. published sport-specific, graded physical activities to assist in returning the athlete to either football, gymnastics, cheerleading, wrestling, soccer, basketball, lacrosse, baseball, softball, and ice hockey.[89] Completion of the return-to-play process and consideration for return to contact sports is made once the athlete is asymptomatic (at rest and with exertion) along with normalizing of their neurocognitive test scores. Some have advocated for the use of provocative testing in the clinic setting to assist in clearance.[90,91] For example, a graded treadmill test (Buffalo concussion treadmill

Table 7.3 Sequential Stages of the Return-to-Play Process

Rehabilitation Stage	Functional Exercise at Each Stage of Rehabilitation	Objective of Each Stage
1. No activity	Symptom limited physical and cognitive rest	Recovery
2. Light aerobic exercise	Walking, swimming or stationary cycling keeping intensity <70% maximum permitted heart rate	Increase HR
	No resistance training	
3. Sport-specific exercise	Skating drills in ice hockey, running drills in soccer	Add movement
	No head impact activities	
4. Non-contact training drills	Progression to more complex training drills, e.g., passing drills in football and ice hockey	Exercise, coordination and cognitive load
	May start progressive resistance training	
5. Full-contact practice	Following medical clearance participate in normal training activities	Restore confidence and assess functional skills by coaching staff
6. Return to play	Normal game play	

Source: McCrory P et al., *Physical Therapy in Sport*, 14(2), e1–e13, 2013.

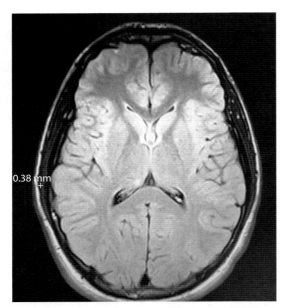

Brain MRI of a 14-year-old athlete with multiple, which was significant for a high-intensity lesion in the right pulvinar region.

References

1. Caskey RC, Nance ML. Management of pediatric mild traumatic brain injury. *Advances in Pediatrics*. 2014; 61(1): 271–286.

2. Choe MC, Giza CC. Diagnosis and management of acute concussion. *Seminars in Neurology*. 2015; 35(1): 29–41.

3. Giza CC, Hovda DA. The neurometabolic cascade of concussion. *Journal of Athletic Training*. 2001; 36(3): 228–235.

4. Giza CC, Hovda DA. The new neurometabolic cascade of concussion. *Neurosurgery*. 2014; 75 Suppl 4: S24–33.

5. Hovda DA. The neurophysiology of concussion. *Progress in Neurological Surgery*. 2014; 28: 28–37.

6. Cantu RC. Return to play guidelines after a head injury. *Clinics in Sports Medicine*. 1998; 17(1): 45–60.

7. Clacy A, Sharman R, Lovell G. Return-to-play confusion: considerations for sport-related concussion. *Journal of Bioethical Inquiry*. 2013; 10(1): 127–128.

8. Pellman EJ, Viano DC, Casson IR, Arfken C, Feuer H. Concussion in professional football: players returning to the same game—Part 7. *Neurosurgery*. 2005; 56(1): 79–90.

9. Miles CM. Concussion management: the current landscape. *Journal of the American Academy of Physician Assistants*. 2014; 27(2): 8–9.

10. Giza CC, Kutcher JS, Ashwal S et al. Summary of evidence-based guideline update: evaluation and management of concussion in sports: report of the Guideline Development Subcommittee of the American Academy of Neurology. *Neurology*. 2013; 80(24): 2250–2257.

11. Committee on Sports-Related Concussions in Y, Board on Children Y, Families, Institute of M, National Research C. The National Academies Collection: Reports funded by National Institutes of Health. In: Graham R, Rivara FP, Ford MA, Spicer CM, eds. *Sports-Related Concussions in Youth: Improving the Science, Changing the Culture*. Washington D.C.: National Academies Press.

12. Broglio SP, Cantu RC, Gioia GA et al. National Athletic Trainers' Association position statement: management of sport concussion. *Journal of Athletic Training*. 2014; 49(2): 245–265.

13. McCrory P, Meeuwisse WH, Aubry M et al. Consensus statement on concussion in sport: the 4th International Conference on Concussion in Sport, Zurich, November 2012. *Journal of Athletic Training*. 2013; 48(4): 554–575.

14. Harmon KG, Drezner J, Gammons M et al. American Medical Society for Sports Medicine position statement: concussion in sport. *Clinical Journal of Sport Medicine*. 2013; 23(1): 1–18.

15. Casa DJ, Guskiewicz KM, Anderson SA et al. National athletic trainers' association position statement: preventing sudden death in

sports. *Journal of Athletic Training*. 2012; 47(1): 96–118.

16. Craton N, Leslie O. Time to re-think the Zurich Guidelines?: a critique on the consensus statement on concussion in sport: the 4th International Conference on Concussion in Sport, held in Zurich, November 2012. *Clinical Journal of Sport Medicine*. 2014; 24(2): 93–95.

17. Davis GA, Purcell LK. The evaluation and management of acute concussion differs in young children. *British Journal of Sports Medicine*. 2014; 48(2): 98–101.

18. Heath CJ, Callahan JL. Self-reported concussion symptoms and training routines in mixed martial arts athletes. *Research in Sports Medicine (Print)*. 2013; 21(3): 195–203.

19. Carson JD, Lawrence DW, Kraft SA et al. Premature return to play and return to learn after a sport-related concussion: physician's chart review. *Canadian Family Physician Medecin de Famille Canadien*. 2014; 60(6): e310, e312–315.

20. Collins MW, Lovell MR, McKeag DB. Current issues in managing sports-related concussion. *The Journal of the American Medical Association*. 1999; 282(24): 2283–2285.

21. Partridge B. Dazed and confused: sports medicine, conflicts of interest, and concussion management. *Journal of Bioethical Inquiry*. 2014; 11(1): 65–74.

22. Arbogast KB, McGinley AD, Master CL, Grady MF, Robinson RL, Zonfrillo MR. Cognitive rest and school-based recommendations following pediatric concussion: the need for primary care support tools. *Clinical Pediatrics*. 2013; 52(5): 397–402.

23. Silverberg ND, Iverson GL. Is rest after concussion "the best medicine?": recommendations for activity resumption following concussion in athletes, civilians, and military service members. *The Journal of Head Trauma Rehabilitation*. 2013; 28(4): 250–259.

24. Creed JA, DiLeonardi AM, Fox DP, Tessler AR, Raghupathi R. Concussive brain trauma in the mouse results in acute cognitive deficits and sustained impairment of axonal function. *Journal of Neurotrauma*. 2011; 28(4): 547–563.

25. Giza CC, Griesbach GS, Hovda DA. Experience-dependent behavioral plasticity is disturbed following traumatic injury to the immature brain. *Behavioural Brain Research*. 2005; 157(1): 11–22.

26. Briones TL, Woods J, Rogozinska M. Decreased neuroinflammation and increased brain energy homeostasis following environmental enrichment after mild traumatic brain injury is associated with improvement in cognitive function. *Acta Neuropathologica Communications*. 2013; 1: 57.

27. Moser RS, Glatts C, Schatz P. Efficacy of immediate and delayed cognitive and physical rest for treatment of sports-related concussion. *Journal of Pediatrics*. 2012; 161(5): 922–926.

28. Brown NJ, Mannix RC, O'Brien MJ, Gostine D, Collins MW, Meehan WP, 3rd. Effect of cognitive activity level on duration of post-concussion symptoms. *Pediatrics*. 2014; 133(2): e299–304.

29. Moor HM, Eisenhauer RC, Killian KD et al. The relationship between adherence behaviors and recovery time in adolescents after a sports-related concussion: an observational study. *International Journal of Sports Physical Therapy*. 2015; 10(2): 225–233.

30. Gibson S, Nigrovic LE, O'Brien M, Meehan WP, 3rd. The effect of recommending cognitive rest on recovery from sport-related concussion. *Brain Injury*. 2013; 27(7–8): 839–842.

31. Buckley TA, Munkasy BA, Clouse BP. Acute cognitive and physical rest may not improve concussion recovery time. *The Journal of Head Trauma Rehabilitation*. 2015.

32. Thomas DG, Apps JN, Hoffmann RG, McCrea M, Hammeke T. Benefits of strict rest after acute concussion: a randomized controlled trial. *Pediatrics*. 2015; 135(2): 213–223.

33. Baker JG, Rieger BP, McAvoy K et al. Principles for return to learn after concussion. *International Journal of Clinical Practice*. 2014; 68(11): 1286–1288.

34. Eastman A, Chang DG. Return to Learn: a review of cognitive rest versus rehabilitation after sports concussion. *NeuroRehabilitation*. 2015; 37(2): 235–244.

35. Kutcher JS, Giza CC. Sports concussion diagnosis and management. *Continuum (Minneapolis, Minn)*. 2014; 20(6 Sports Neurology): 1552–1569.

36. DeMatteo C, Stazyk K, Giglia L et al. A balanced protocol for return to school for children and youth following concussive injury. *Clinical Pediatrics*. 2015; 54(8): 783–792.

37. Giza CC. Pediatric issues in sports concussions. *Continuum*. 2014; 20(6 Sports Neurology): 1570–1587.

38. Halstead ME, Walter KD. American Academy of Pediatrics. Clinical report—sport-related concussion in children and adolescents. *Pediatrics*. 2010; 126(3): 597–615.

39. Conder RL, Conder AA. Sports-related concussions. *North Carolina Medical Journal*. 2015; 76(2): 89–95.

40. Echemendia RJ, Giza CC, Kutcher JS. Developing guidelines for return to play: consensus and evidence-based approaches. *Brain Injury*. 2015; 29(2): 185–194.

41. Halstead ME, McAvoy K, Devore CD, Carl R, Lee M, Logan K. Returning to learning following a concussion. *Pediatrics*. 2013; 132(5): 948–957.

42. Gioia GA. Multimodal evaluation and management of children with concussion: using our heads and available evidence. *Brain Injury*. 2015; 29(2): 195–206.

43. Purcell L, Harvey J, Seabrook JA. Patterns of recovery following sport-related concussion in children and adolescents. *Clinical Pediatrics*. 2015.

44. Gardner A. The complex clinical issues involved in an athlete's decision to retire from collision sport due to multiple concussions: a case study of a professional athlete. *Frontiers in Neurology*. 2013; 4: 141.

45. Meehan WP, 3rd, Bachur RG. The recommendation for rest following acute concussion. *Pediatrics*. 2015; 135(2): 362–363.

46. Hall EE, Ketcham CJ, Crenshaw CR, Baker MH, McConnell JM, Patel K. Concussion management in collegiate student-athletes: return-to-academics recommendations. *Clinical Journal of Sport Medicine*. 2015; 25(3): 291–296.

47. Barr WB. An evidence based approach to sports concussion: confronting the availability cascade. *Neuropsychology Review*. 2013; 23(4): 271–272.

48. Master CL, Gioia GA, Leddy JJ, Grady MF. Importance of 'return-to-learn' in pediatric and adolescent concussion. *Pediatric Annals*. 2012; 41(9): 1–6.

49. McGrath N. Supporting the student-athlete's return to the classroom after a sport-related concussion. *Journal of Athletic Training*. 2010; 45(5): 492–498.

50. Olympia RP, Ritter JT, Brady J, Bramley H. Return to learning after a concussion and compliance with recommendations for cognitive rest. *Clinical Journal of Sport Medicine*. 2015.

51. Ransom DM, Vaughan CG, Pratson L, Sady MD, McGill CA, Gioia GA. Academic effects of concussion in children and adolescents. *Pediatrics*. 2015; 135(6): 1043–1050.

52. Colloca L, Finniss D. Nocebo effects, patient-clinician communication, and therapeutic outcomes. *The Journal of the American Medical Association*. 2012; 307(6): 567–568.

53. DiFazio M, Silverberg ND, Kirkwood MW, Bernier R, Iverson GL. Prolonged activity restriction after concussion: are we worsening outcomes? *Clinical Pediatrics*. 2015.

54. Karlin AM. Concussion in the pediatric and adolescent population: "different population, different concerns." *PM & R.* 2011; 3(10 Suppl 2): S369–379.

55. Bush SS, Ruff RM, Troster AI et al. Symptom validity assessment: practice issues and medical necessity NAN policy & planning committee. *Archives of Clinical Neuropsychology.* 2005; 20(4): 419–426.

56. Dessy A, Rasouli J, Gometz A, Choudhri T. A review of modifying factors affecting usage of diagnostic rating scales in concussion management. *Clinical Neurology and Neurosurgery.* 2014; 122: 59–63.

57. Foley C, Gregory A, Solomon G. Young age as a modifying factor in sports concussion management: what is the evidence? *Current Sports Medicine Reports.* 2014; 13(6): 390–394.

58. Waljas M, Iverson GL, Lange RT et al. Return to work following mild traumatic brain injury. *The Journal of Head Trauma Rehabilitation.* 2014; 29(5): 443–450.

59. Shames J, Treger I, Ring H, Giaquinto S. Return to work following traumatic brain injury: trends and challenges. *Disability and Rehabilitation.* 2007; 29(17): 1387–1395.

60. Walker WC, Marwitz JH, Kreutzer JS, Hart T, Novack TA. Occupational categories and return to work after traumatic brain injury: a multicenter study. *Archives of Physical Medicine and Rehabilitation.* 2006; 87(12): 1576–1582.

61. Baker A, Unswo CA, Lannin NA. Fitness-to-drive after mild traumatic brain injury: mapping the time trajectory of recovery in the acute stages post injury. *Accident; Analysis and Prevention.* 2015; 79: 50–55.

62. Reynolds E, Collins MW, Mucha A, Troutman-Ensecki C. Establishing a clinical service for the management of sports-related concussions. *Neurosurgery.* 2014; 75 Suppl 4: S71–81.

63. Laurer HL, Bareyre FM, Lee VM et al. Mild head injury increasing the brain's vulnerability to a second concussive impact. *Journal of Neurosurgery.* 2001; 95(5): 859–870.

64. Bolton AN, Saatman KE. Regional neurodegeneration and gliosis are amplified by mild traumatic brain injury repeated at 24-hour intervals. *Journal of Neuropathology and Experimental Neurology.* 2014; 73(10): 933–947.

65. Huang L, Coats JS, Mohd-Yusof A et al. Tissue vulnerability is increased following repetitive mild traumatic brain injury in the rat. *Brain Research.* 2013; 1499: 109–120.

66. Friess SH, Ichord RN, Ralston J et al. Repeated traumatic brain injury affects composite cognitive function in piglets. *Journal of Neurotrauma.* 2009; 26(7): 1111–1121.

67. Weber JT. Experimental models of repetitive brain injuries. *Progress in Brain Research.* 2007; 161: 253–261.

68. Longhi L, Saatman KE, Fujimoto S et al. Temporal window of vulnerability to repetitive experimental concussive brain injury. *Neurosurgery.* 2005; 56(2): 364–374.

69. Goddeyne C, Nichols J, Wu C, Anderson T. Repetitive mild traumatic brain injury induces ventriculomegaly and cortical thinning in juvenile rats. *Journal of Neurophysiology.* 2015; 113(9): 3268–3280.

70. Raghupathi R, Mehr MF, Helfaer MA, Margulies SS. Traumatic axonal injury is exacerbated following repetitive closed head injury in the neonatal pig. *Journal of Neurotrauma.* 2004; 21(3): 307–316.

71. Donovan V, Kim C, Anugerah AK et al. Repeated mild traumatic brain injury results in long-term white-matter disruption. *Journal of Cerebral Blood Flow and Metabolism.* 2014; 34(4): 715–723.

72. Dapul HR, Park J, Zhang J et al. Concussive injury before or after controlled cortical impact exacerbates histopathology and

Return to activity

functional outcome in a mixed traumatic brain injury model in mice. *Journal of Neurotrauma.* 2013; 30(5): 382–391.

73. Weil ZM, Gaier KR, Karelina K. Injury timing alters metabolic, inflammatory and functional outcomes following repeated mild traumatic brain injury. *Neurobiology of Disease.* 2014; 70: 108–116.

74. Schneider KJ, Iverson GL, Emery CA, McCrory P, Herring SA, Meeuwisse WH. The effects of rest and treatment following sport-related concussion: a systematic review of the literature. *British Journal of Sports Medicine.* 2013; 47(5): 304–307.

75. Terwilliger V, Pratson L, Vaughan C, Gioia G. Additional post-concussion impact exposure may affect recovery in adolescent athletes. *Journal of Neurotrauma.* 2015.

76. Collins MW, Lovell MR, Iverson GL, Cantu RC, Maroon JC, Field M. Cumulative effects of concussion in high school athletes. *Neurosurgery.* 2002; 51(5): 1175–1179.

77. McCrea M, Guskiewicz K, Randolph C et al. Effects of a symptom-free waiting period on clinical outcome and risk of reinjury after sport-related concussion. *Neurosurgery.* 2009; 65(5): 876–882.

78. Griesbach GS, Hovda DA, Molteni R, Wu A, Gomez-Pinilla F. Voluntary exercise following traumatic brain injury: brain-derived neurotrophic factor upregulation and recovery of function. *Neuroscience.* 2004; 125(1): 129–139.

79. Kruijk JR, Leffers P, Meerhoff S, Rutten J, Twijnstra A. Effectiveness of bed rest after mild traumatic brain injury: a randomised trial of no versus six days of bed rest. *Journal of Neurology, Neurosurgery, and Psychiatry.* 2002; 73(2): 167–172.

80. Majerske C, Mihalik J, Ren D, Collins M, Reddy C, Lovell M, Wagner AK. Concussion in sports: postconcussive activity levels, symptoms, and neurocognitive performance. *Journal of Athletic Training.* 2008; 43(3): 265–274.

81. Wells EM, Goodkin HP, Griesbach GS. Challenges in determining the role of rest and exercise in the management of mild traumatic brain injury. *Journal of Child Neurology.* 2015.

82. McCrory P, Meeuwisse W, Aubry M et al. Consensus statement on concussion in sport - the 4th international conference on concussion in sport held in Zurich, November 2012. *Physical Therapy in Sport.* 2013; 14(2): e1–e13.

83. Herring SA, Kibler WB, Putukian M. Team Physician Consensus Statement: 2013 update. *Medicine and Science in Sports and Exercise.* 2013; 45(8): 1618–1622.

84. Chermann JF, Klouche S, Savigny A, Lefevre N, Herman S, Bohu Y. Return to rugby after brain concussion: a prospective study in 35 high level rugby players. *Asian Journal of Sports Medicine.* 2014; 5(4): e24042.

85. Terrell TR, Cox CB, Bielak K, Casmus R, Laskowitz D, Nichols G. Sports concussion management: part II. *Southern Medical Journal.* 2014; 107(2): 126–135.

86. Terrell TR, Nobles T, Rader B et al. Sports concussion management: part I. *Southern Medical Journal.* 2014; 107(2): 115–125.

87. McClain R. Concussion and trauma in young athletes: prevention, treatment, and return-to-play. *Primary Care.* 2015; 42(1): 77–83.

88. McCrory P, Meeuwisse W, Johnston K et al. Consensus statement on concussion in sport - The 3rd international conference on concussion in sport held in Zurich, November 2008. *PM & R.* 2009; 1(5): 406–420.

89. May KH, Marshall DL, Burns TG, Popoli DM, Polikandriotis JA. Pediatric sports specific return to play guidelines following concussion. *International Journal of Sports Physical Therapy.* 2014; 9(2): 242–255.

90. Dematteo C, Volterman KA, Breithaupt PG, Claridge EA, Adamich J, Timmons BW.

Exertion testing in youth with mild traumatic brain injury/concussion. *Medicine and Science in Sports and Exercise.* 2015; 47(11): 2283–2290.

91. Leddy JJ, Baker JG, Kozlowski K, Bisson L, Willer B. Reliability of a graded exercise test for assessing recovery from concussion. *Clinical Journal of Sport Medicine.* 2011; 21(2): 89–94.

92. Darling SR, Leddy JJ, Baker JG et al. Evaluation of the Zurich Guidelines and exercise testing for return to play in adolescents following concussion. *Clinical Journal of Sport Medicine.* 2014; 24(2): 128–133.

93. Leddy JJ, Cox JL, Baker JG et al. Exercise treatment for postconcussion syndrome: a pilot study of changes in functional magnetic resonance imaging activation, physiology, and symptoms. *The Journal of Head Trauma Rehabilitation.* 2013; 28(4): 241–249.

94. Leddy JJ, Willer B. Use of graded exercise testing in concussion and return-to-activity management. *Current Sports Medicine Reports.* 2013; 12(6): 370–376.

95. Makdissi M, Darby D, Maruff P, Ugoni A, Brukner P, McCrory PR. Natural history of concussion in sport: markers of severity and implications for management. *The American Journal of Sports Medicine.* 2010; 38(3): 464–471.

96. Makdissi M, Davis G, Jordan B, Patricios J, Purcell L, Putukian M. Revisiting the modifiers: how should the evaluation and management of acute concussions differ in specific groups? *British Journal of Sports Medicine.* 2013; 47(5): 314–320.

97. Kerr HA. Concussion risk factors and strategies for prevention. *Pediatric Annals.* 2014; 43(12): e309–315.

98. Ponsford J, Willmott C, Rothwell A et al. Factors influencing outcome following mild traumatic brain injury in adults. *Journal of the International Neuropsychological Society.* 2000; 6(5): 568–579.

99. Kontos AP, Braithwaite R, Dakan S, Elbin RJ. Computerized neurocognitive testing within 1 week of sport-related concussion: meta-analytic review and analysis of moderating factors. *Journal of the International Neuropsychological Society.* 2014; 20(3): 324–332.

100. Babcock L, Byczkowski T, Wade SL, Ho M, Mookerjee S, Bazarian JJ. Predicting postconcussion syndrome after mild traumatic brain injury in children and adolescents who present to the emergency department. *The Journal of the American Medical Association Pedriatics.* 2013; 167(2): 156–161.

101. Pellman EJ, Lovell MR, Viano DC, Casson IR. Concussion in professional football: recovery of NFL and high school athletes assessed by computerized neuropsychological testing—Part 12. *Neurosurgery.* 2006; 58(2): 263–274.

102. Pellman EJ, Lovell MR, Viano DC, Casson IR, Tucker AM. Concussion in professional football: neuropsychological testing—Part 6. *Neurosurgery.* 2004; 55(6): 1290–1303.

103. Iverson GL, Brooks BL, Collins MW, Lovell MR. Tracking neuropsychological recovery following concussion in sport. *Brain Injury.* 2006; 20(3): 245–252.

104. Dougan BK, Horswill MS, Geffen GM. Athletes' age, sex, and years of education moderate the acute neuropsychological impact of sports-related concussion: a meta-analysis. *Journal of the International Neuropsychological Society.* 2014; 20(1): 64–80.

105. Collins MW, Field M, Lovell MR et al. Relationship between postconcussion headache and neuropsychological test performance in high school athletes. *The American Journal of Sports Medicine.* 2003; 31(2): 168–173.

106. Gessel LM, Fields SK, Collins CL, Dick RW, Comstock RD. Concussions among United States high school and collegiate athletes. *Journal of Athletic Training.* 2007; 42(4): 495–503.

107. Field M, Collins MW, Lovell MR, Maroon J. Does age play a role in recovery from

144. Henry LC, Tremblay S, Boulanger Y, Ellemberg D, Lassonde M. Neurometabolic changes in the acute phase after sports concussions correlate with symptom severity. *Journal of Neurotrauma*. 2010; 27(1): 65–76.

145. Chamard E, Lassonde M, Henry L et al. Neurometabolic and microstructural alterations following a sports-related concussion in female athletes. *Brain Injury*. 2013; 27(9): 1038–1046.

146. Mondello S, Schmid K, Berger RP et al. The challenge of mild traumatic brain injury: role of biochemical markers in diagnosis of brain damage. *Medicinal Research Reviews*. 2014; 34(3): 503–531.

CHAPTER 8

Neuroimaging in concussion

With Matthew T. Walker, M.D. and Monther Qandeel, M.D.

Introduction

The pathology associated with concussion can range from functional and microstructural alterations of the neurons, to macroscopic injury, like intracranial hemorrhage. Typically, macroscopic findings are better detected by standard conventional imaging and are seen only in a minute subset of those diagnosed with concussion, while the more characteristic microstructural and biochemical alterations require the use of more advanced neuroimaging techniques that are not commonly used in the typical acute clinical setting.

In this chapter we will review the standard imaging modalities (CT and MRI) used in the acute and chronic setting of a concussed athlete to rule out intracranial pathology or determine structural injury in those with persistent postconcussive symptoms. Further, we will review the more advanced neuroimaging techniques that have demonstrated their ability to evaluate in vivo injury at a microscale regarding structural integrity and even biochemical processes.

Clinical imaging modalities

Computed tomography (CT)

Though macrostructural pathology (subdural hemorrhage, epidural hemorrhage, traumatic subarachnoid hemorrhage, and diffuse cerebral edema) is uncommon in concussion, it still can occur and therefore must be ruled out in a subset of patients. As discussed in Chapter 4, the best imaging choice to assess for intracranial blood products in the acute setting is CT imaging. Borg et al. have estimated that CT brain abnormalities,

such as cerebral contusions, edema, and epidural/subdural hematomas (EDH/SDH), and skull fractures are present in only 5% of mTBI cases if GCS is 15, 20% with a GCS of 14, and 30% with a GCS of 13, while further studies have reported an even smaller percentage between 0.1% and 1%.[1–3] Therefore, the main role of CT imaging in concussion in the acute setting is to identify the clinically relevant intracranial lesions that may require neurosurgical intervention, hospitalization, or rigorous follow-up, but only a small subset of patients will be identified.[4]

Given the low positive yield of CT in an athlete following concussion, there has been significant disagreement on when to obtain cranial imaging depending on the medical subspecialty involved in making the decision.[5] As reviewed in Chapter 3, there are several decision-making guidelines, in both the pediatric and adult populations, elaborated in an attempt to increase the yield and to minimize the cost and risk of unnecessary ionizing radiation.

CT image findings

As discussed previously, acute CT abnormalities are estimated to occur in less than 5% of patients with concussion. Among these, cerebral contusions and subdural hematomas (SDHs) are the most common.[6–8]

Cerebral contusion

While the solid nature of the skull protects the brain against direct injury, it can also result in cerebral contusions, or brain "bruises," when there is friction between the two causing injury to the brain parenchyma and shearing of small blood vessels. Unlike the direct brain injury caused by depressed skull fractures, contusions in the setting of mTBI are indirectly caused by the acceleration/deceleration forces that induce movement of the brain, or massive brain slosh, relative to the fixed skull (Figure 2.2). These contusions tend to involve the cortex along the top of the gyri and are most prevalent along the inferior, lateral, and anterior surfaces of the frontal and temporal lobes where the inner skull surface is prominent.

Given the rich blood supply to the cerebral cortex, these contusions are frequently hemorrhagic and the blood can extend superficially into the subarachnoid and subdural spaces as well as deep into the white matter. This hemorrhage may be very subtle, and therefore difficult to detect by imaging. Hemorrhagic contusions can also occasionally be associated with intraventricular hemorrhage depending on the site of injury.

Subsequently, edema develops over hours and days after the injury, making the lesions more conspicuous on both CT and MRI imaging (Figure 4.4). These can be subtle initially, appearing as relatively small cortical/subcortical foci of hypoattenuation or hyperattenuation, depending on the absence or presence of associated hemorrhage. Over hours to days, they mature with more prominent hemorrhage and edema. Ultimately, they leave areas of gliosis; and chronically, necrosis resulting in cerebral volume loss, termed post-traumatic encephalomalacia.

Subdural hemorrhage

Subdural hemorrhage is blood localized to the potential space between the leptomeninges and the dura as a result of shearing of bridging veins between the cortex and dura, (Figures 4.5 and 4.9). These bridging veins are relatively fixed at the adjacent sinus or dura and cannot move to the same extent as the brain does, especially during a rotational movement. These veins are ensheathed with arachnoid trabeculae as they traverse the subarachnoid space but not in the subdural space and that is why the hemorrhage preferentially localizes to this space.[9] Other CT findings associated with mTBI include epidural

hematomas as well as skull fractures, which is further discussed in Chapter 4.

Conventional MRI (cMRI)

Unlike CT, cMRI is usually performed in the subacute and chronic settings when postconcussive symptoms persist for weeks or months after the injury. Compared to CT imaging, MRI provides increased sensitivity for detecting structural abnormalities but remains insensitive, even in symptomatic patients. Indeed, 43% to 68% of mild TBI patients show no abnormality by cMRI.[10,11] A conventional MRI study for head injury typically includes T1-weighted and T2-weighted fast spin echo sequences, fluid attenuated inversion recovery (FLAIR), and a heme-sensitive sequence such as T2*-weighted gradient echo sequence/gradient recovery echo (GRE). Susceptibility weighted imaging (SWI) is another heme-sensitive sequence, which is even more sensitive to blood products compared to GRE sequences, especially in smaller lesions.[12]

cMRI image findings

Cerebral contusion

In a relatively small sample of 21 consecutive mTBI patients, Hofman et al. showed MRI abnormalities acutely in 12 patients (57%), mainly on FLAIR and T2*-weighted imaging. The acute traumatic abnormalities detected were cortical contusions as areas of edema that appeared hyperintense. Such lesions were larger and more numerous on FLAIR compared to T2* when nonhemorrhagic. On the other hand, deoxyhemoglobin within the hemorrhagic lesions made them most conspicuous on T2*. The contusions were predominantly frontal and temporal in distribution. Follow-up MRI at 6 months did not show new lesions but showed more atrophy reflecting posttraumatic encephalomalacia and reactive gliosis in all patients with MRI abnormalities on the initial scan.[10]

Diffuse axonal injury

In addition to the superficially located contusions, the acceleration/deceleration forces in mTBI/concussion can also cause deep injuries by partially or completely shearing the fragile axons through inducing differential movement between tissues of dissimilar density or rigidity, therefore commonly occurring at the gray and white matter junction, or at locations with long projecting white matter tracts like the corpus callosum, brainstem, superior cerebellar peduncle, and internal capsule. This axonal injury is termed diffuse axonal injury (DAI) and though it varies in severity and manifestation, it is the most frequent explanation for coma and poor outcome associated with significant closed head injury when involvement occurs within the brainstem.[13–17]

In mTBI, as opposed to moderate and severe TBI, DAI lesions tend to be fewer in number and subcortical in distribution, as opposed to the larger number of lesions and more central distribution involving the brainstem and corpus callosum. Just like contusions, DAI lesions can be nonhemorrhagic or hemorrhagic and their MRI appearance differs accordingly. The hemorrhage originates from the DAI-associated capillary injury and is therefore a specific but not necessarily sensitive, indirect sign of DAI. Hemorrhage is best detected by the heme-sensitive sequences. In a study of 20 consecutive patients with mTBI and normal head CT scans, Mittl et al. have shown MRI evidence of DAI in six patients (30%) defined as a white matter abnormality on either T2 or T2* imaging.[18]

As discussed in Chapter 2, axonal ultrastructural analysis has shown that shearing leads to immediate and delayed mechanical disruption and buckling of the microtubules, which subsequently triggers progressive microtubular disassembly leading to failure of axonal transport and axonal swelling (Figure 2.11).[19–25] Over the following months, secondary disconnection and ultimately Wallerian degeneration occurs. Given that DAI is largely a microscopic injury and therefore a subtler lesion, the extent of the damage is significantly underestimated by both CT and conventional cMRI, but multiple newer imaging techniques can better visualize this type of tissue damage.

Diffusion weighted imaging (DWI)

While cMRI sequences are estimated to show evidence of hemorrhagic and nonhemorrhagic DAI in an additional 30% of CT negative mTBI patients,[18] both modalities remain insensitive for detection of abnormalities in patients in the acute setting,[26] even when symptoms are present. They are also inconsistent in predicting the functional outcome of mTBI. Huisman et al. showed in 2003 that DWI, when obtained in the acute setting of closed head injury, can show more lesions than T2/FLAIR and GRE sequences, though it was more likely to miss hemorrhagic lesions. Additionally, DWI is less sensitive to patient motion than the other sequences and yields higher contrast-to-noise ratios and therefore increased lesion conspicuity.[26]

The apparent diffusion coefficient (ADC) value of these DWI positive lesions can vary: decreased, unchanged, or increased. While the detailed cellular basis for this variability of ADC is beyond the scope of this chapter, reduced ADC may reflect more severe tissue damage because it usually represents cytotoxic edema. Trauma-induced axotomy and the formation of retraction balls with concomitant cytoskeletal collapse along the severed axons probably also contribute to reduced ADC.[27] On the other hand, increased ADCs most likely reflect vasogenic edema and less severe injury. Therefore, DWI can provide additional, unique information about the physiologic state of brain tissue and severity of tissue damage, independently of other imaging findings and clinical assessments that may better predict the long-term prognosis.

Diffusion tensor imaging (DTI)

While DWI studies the water diffusion characteristics in tissues without representation of directionality, DTI utilizes the same basic principles but also takes into account directionality of the diffusion, allowing the calculation of several measures, like fractional anisotropy and mean diffusivity, that more precisely represent the diffusion characteristics of the tissue. The tissue characteristics measured by DTI are represented through mathematical values and color-coded maps. Because water normally diffuses more readily along the long axis of axons than it does in the other directions, DTI can study the microstructure of the neural tissue, not only mapping the white matter tracts but also assessing microstructural integrity. Damage to the cytoskeleton and failure of axonal transport mechanisms from DAI can therefore affect the tissue characteristics measured by DTI.

Multiple studies have analyzed these alterations in the diffusivity parameters in the setting of mTBI. However, the alterations were not very consistent among different studies. Niogi et al., in a review of DTI and adult mTBI,[28] showed DTI results can vary depending on the time of imaging and the part of the brain imaged. This variability in diffusivity alterations probably also reflects differing underlying pathophysiological processes and also varying stages of evolution of the axonal pathology.[29] Among these values, Niogi et al. reviewed fractional anisotropy (FA), which is the directionality of molecular displacement by diffusion. FA has been shown in multiple studies to decrease in the acute post-traumatic setting both within lesions and in the normally appearing tissue, reflecting the widespread extent of DAI. On the other hand, few studies confirmed increased FA, along with decreased ADC, in the first 72 hours postinjury. This probably reflects swelling of the still intact axons that would restrict the interstitial space, making it more anisotropic with a net increase in FA. Chronically, Wallerian degeneration ensues with axonal degeneration followed by myelin degeneration and astrocytic infiltration. Wallerian degeneration is associated with decreased ADC and FA, as expected. The mean diffusivity—another diffusion value measure—was also not very consistent. It was felt that axial and radial diffusivity may offer more specific insight into the neuropathology of mTBI, but more longitudinal studies are necessary to better understand the pathological process from acute to chronic injury states.

Using the results from studies that have performed Region of Interest (ROI) analysis to examine several regions throughout the brain, Niogi et al. found that the frontal and temporal white matter structures demonstrated the most abnormal FA profiles, in both the acute and chronic phases. Specifically, the anterior corona radiata, uncinate fasciculus, superior longitudinal fasciculus, and the anterior corpus callosum were the most commonly injured tracts.[30–32] A few of the more recent studies have shown correlations between abnormal FA in specific white matter tracts and impairment in certain cognitive domains. For example, loss of the integrity of frontal and temporal white matter pathways correlated with deficits in executive attention and memory, while FA of the uncinate fasciculus bilaterally correlated with verbal memory. With large-scale multicenter studies, quantitative DTI may serve a predictive role in mTBI/concussion in the future.[33,34]

Experimental imaging modalities

As mentioned, the largely microstructural and biochemical nature of a concussion causes this injury to be frequently invisible or significantly underestimated by conventional imaging tools.[4] Through the advancement of neuroimaging for concussion, researchers have been able to better understand the pathophysiological response of a neuron following injury, and therefore more appropriately study concussed athletes.

Functional MRI (fMRI)

Functional MRI (fMRI) is a noninvasive study that can assess regional brain activity while performing or not performing a specific task (resting state fMRI or task-based fMRI), which is achieved indirectly by imaging the regional differences in cerebral blood flow using blood oxygenation level dependent (BOLD) imaging. Under normal physiologic conditions, regional blood flow in the brain is tightly linked to oxygen and carbon dioxide. When a specific part of the brain cortex is activated, the increased metabolic need leads to increased extraction of oxygen from the local capillaries with an initial drop in oxyhemoglobin levels. After a short lag of 26 seconds, the regional blood flow increases providing a surplus of oxyhemoglobin and leading to deoxyhemoglobin washout. This physiologic response of decreased levels of deoxyhemoglobin is what is imaged in fMRI. Because deoxygenated hemoglobin is paramagnetic whereas oxygenated hemoglobin is not, the relative decrease in the deoxyhemoglobin in the activated cortex leads to proton dephasing by inducing local magnetic field inhomogeneities and a net minimal but measurable decrease in signal on a heavily T2* weighted sequence such as BOLD imaging.

While it may seem reasonable that functional connectivity abnormalities, as assessed by fMRI, should parallel structural connectivity abnormalities, as assessed by DTI, the relationship is more complex. This reflects that not every alteration in structural connectivity translates into changes in functional activity, and vice versa. Zhang et al. have failed to show consistent findings between the functional deficits and the white matter structural alterations in concussed individuals, using task-focused fMRI and DTI.[35] On the other hand, Sharp et al. studied functional and structural connectivity after traumatic brain injury and have shown lower default mode network functional connectivity in patients with more evidence of diffuse axonal injury within the adjacent corpus callosum, therefore providing evidence of a direct relationship.[36] These inconsistent findings may be attributable to the varying time windows of dynamic versus static changes in functional and structural connectivity following injury.

Task-based fMRI

The most widely used task-based fMRI design in clinical practice is the block design that uses repeated blocks of activity (paradigm) separated by blocks of inactivity or alternative activity. Multiple different paradigms can be used, depending on the intended purpose of the study, such as visual, motor, speech, and memory paradigms.

Multiple studies have shown the value of fMRI in studying concussion-associated brain dysfunction. Chen et al. evaluated the regional brain activations associated with a working memory task in a small group of concussed athletes (15 symptomatic, 1 asymptomatic) and eight matched control subjects.[37] The task-related responses and activation patterns were different in the symptomatic athletes with concussions compared to the asymptomatic and control subjects. Chen et al. later showed that abnormal prefrontal cortex activation patterns on fMRI, in symptomatic concussed athletes, did actually normalize once the symptoms improved while the fMRI abnormalities persisted in the athletes who remained symptomatic.[38] fMRI also provided increased sensitivity by being able to detect abnormalities in a group of athletes with mild PCS symptoms when neuropsychological evaluation did not.[39] In a small prospective study, Jantzen et al. compared fMRI and behavioral performance as tools to detect differences caused by concussion in neural functioning.[40] Preseason baseline fMRI and neuropsychological

evaluation values were obtained for eight collegiate football players. Four developed concussions during the season and were re-evaluated within one week of the injury. The other four uninjured control players were retested at the end of the season. Compared to baseline, the concussed players showed marked within-subject increases in the amplitude and extent of BOLD activity during a finger-sequencing task despite the absence of observed deficits in behavioral performance. These findings led the researchers to propose that prospective neuroimaging may have great potential for understanding concussion recovery and specific symptom development. It may even have a role in return-to-play decisions. Despite the great potential, the clinical utility of fMRI in the evaluation of concussed patients will likely remain limited given the time, complexity, and cost factors associated with the testing.

While the specifics of which tracts are most frequently or most severely affected and the correlations with functional deficits were not very consistent across the different studies, a general theme was that concussed patients showed larger cortical networks along with additional increases in activity outside of the shared region of interest (ROI) during encoding. In one study, the significantly larger cluster size during encoding was most prominent in the parietal cortex, right dorsolateral prefrontal cortex, and right hippocampus.[41] Additionally, there was a significantly larger BOLD signal percent change at the right hippocampus. On the other hand, there was no significant change in the cluster size or BOLD signal percent change at the shared ROIs during retrieval. It is hypothesized that such alterations reflect a compensatory response by the brain to maintain its function despite structural/functional disruption from mild TBI.

Resting-state fMRI (RsfMRI)

Even during resting conditions, when the subject is not performing any explicit task, the brain remains active both functionally and metabolically. This resting-state brain activity translates into spontaneous regional fluctuations in BOLD signal over time given regional alterations in deoxyhemoglobin to oxyhemoglobin ratio, as discussed previously. This resting brain activity is not random, given the underlying connectivity within the brain. Functionally connected but spatially distinct areas within the brain are expected to show synchronous coactivation resulting in temporally-synchronous hemodynamic and BOLD signal alterations. Repeated history of coactivation patterns within these regions identifies resting-state networks. Identification of the correlation patterns in these spontaneous fluctuations requires a series of extensive postprocessing steps. Unlike structural connectivity, functional connectivity is dynamic and often changes on the order of seconds, therefore making analysis quite challenging.

Widespread rsfMRI abnormalities, including both deficits and enhancements, in functional connectivity have been described and compared between mTBI patients and normal subjects. Stevens et al. demonstrated two forms of increased connectivity[42]; one where there is increased strength of integration in brain regions that are typically part of a network, and a second in "new" connectivity that was recruited between non network brain regions. Such connectivity enhancements probably reflect compensatory neural processes though the underlying etiology is more difficult to determine and is multifactorial; it may be directly related to neuronal injury or secondary to increased effort, psychological distress, pain, or similar recovery related factors.

MR spectroscopy (MRS)

MRS is a noninvasive MR imaging modality that can provide qualitative and quantitative assessment of the chemical composition of tissue. By measuring changes in specific metabolites, MRS can detect tissue injury at an earlier stage than conventional imaging. It has been shown to be more sensitive than the cMRI tool for imaging DAI, better reflecting the widespread nature of DAI when cMRI shows only focal abnormalities, such as punctate lesions. Choline (Cho) is one of the breakdown products of cellular membrane disruption and is expected to increase in areas affected by DAI. This has been reproduced across studies in both the abnormal and the normal appearing white matter. N-acetylaspartate (NAA) is another major metabolite detected by MRS and is considered a marker of neuronal and axonal health. In

clinical practice, these metabolites are commonly represented in a semiquantitative ratio relative to creatine (Cr) in order to correct for variable cellular density in different parts of the brain. Therefore, it is not surprising that DAI results in an initial increase in Cho and decrease in NAA (signifying cellular breakdown and neuronal injury), represented as a decrease in NAA/Cr and increase in Cho/Cr. Another metabolite measured by MRS in TBI is lactate, a marker of hypoxia and ischemia. Studies have documented the presence of lactate in the pericontusional edema surrounding a focal injury, and in some cases in the contralateral normal appearing white matter in mTBI. This evidence of widespread hypoxia and metabolic stress has been suggested as an explanation for the vulnerability of neurons to repeated concussion/subconcussive blows and even Second Impact Syndrome.[43–45]

The trend of these metabolic alterations posttrauma has varied among studies but a general tendency is gradual reversal of the decreased white matter NAA towards normal levels in 2 months for mTBI.[43] Other studies have shown recovery of the Cho values to control levels 6–12 months after injury,[46] even in patients with poor outcomes, whereas NAA remained low.[47] Additionally, the correlation between the degree of these alterations and long-term outcomes has varied according to the study. In one of the earlier studies, researchers have found elevated Cho values in all TBI patients, regardless of the severity, and concluded that the initial increase in Cho does not reflect the severity of the injury or correlates with outcome.[48] On the other hand, Holshouser et al. looked specifically at the value of MRS in predicting outcome in children with TBI, ranging from mild to severe, and showed that lower NAA/Cr ratios within the first 16 days postinjury correlated with worse neurologic outcomes at 6–12 months, compared to the children with good outcomes and the control group.[49] Interestingly, the authors also indicated that metabolite ratios in the normal appearing tissue was a stronger predictor of outcome than the spectra in the hemorrhagic/injured tissue.

Multiple complicating factors limit the value of these results, including the heterogeneity of the acquisition technique and the exact location from which the spectra were acquired, as different parts of the brain exhibit different baseline NAA/Cr ratios and are also affected to variable degrees by DAI. Additionally, most of these studies were semi-quantitative utilizing ratios assuming that Cr remains stable, however there is some evidence that Cr is affected by the metabolic state of tissue.[50] Despite the lack of consistency in the findings across studies, MRS seems to offer an advantage of sensitivity, compared to structural cMRI; but at this time, the exact clinical significance of these biochemical alterations months after injury is unknown and therefore application to return-to-play recommendations is not possible.

MR perfusion weighted imaging (PWI)

While BOLD signal in functional MRI is an indirect reflection of brain tissue perfusion, there are other noninvasive imaging techniques that are specifically designed to assess cerebral perfusion, such as dynamic contrast-enhanced (DCE) MR and CT, dynamic susceptibility contrast (DSC) MR, arterial spin labeling (ASL) MR, and single photon emission computed tomography (SPECT) imaging. While the technical differences between these techniques are beyond the scope of this chapter, most of them provide clinical value by providing a relative measurement of cerebral perfusion by comparing the region of interest to another, presumably healthy part of the brain. This technique then provides relative perfusion values, such as relative cerebral blood volume (rCBV) and relative cerebral blood flow (rCBF) of the specific region. While trauma-induced abnormalities of perfusion are well-described, and believed to reflect structural and functional brain alterations, such a relative approach to the perfusion assessment may not be the most sensitive method when studying a diffuse process like DAI.

By performing a group analysis on a military mTBI cohort, Liu et al. demonstrated the presence of perfusion deficits using DSC MR in the mTBI group relative to the controls.[51] The perfusion deficits consisted of multiple clusters of decreased rCBF in the cerebellum, cuneus, cingulate, and temporal gyrus. Additionally, the perfusion deficits in the cerebellum and anterior cingulate significantly correlated with neurocognitive results, such as measures of verbal memory, speed of reaction time, and self-report of stress symptoms.

In another study using true fast imaging with steady-state precession arterial spin labeling (True FISP ASL), Ge et al. have shown persistent hypoperfusion in chronically symptomatic mTBI patients (on average 26.5 months after injury) that was more severe in the thalami, compared to the white matter and basal ganglia.[52] The decreased CBF in the thalamus correlated significantly with several neuropsychological measures, including processing and response speed, memory, verbal fluency, and executive function.

Meier et al. designed a prospective study to longitudinally assess the recovery of perfusion deficits in the setting of mTBI and to compare the time course of CBF recovery with that of cognitive and behavioral symptoms.[53] From a cohort of collegiate football athletes, 17 subjects underwent serial ASL perfusion imaging along with neuropsychological testing at approximately one day, one week, and one month postconcussion. It was noted that over the course of the study there were initial changes in CBF that improved over time in the right insular and superior temporal cortex longitudinally of the concussed athletes in comparison to the control subjects. The authors also suggested that CBF might represent a potential prognostic biomarker as it was decreased in the dorsal midinsular cortex at one month postconcussion in athletes slower to recover and was also inversely related to the magnitude of initial symptoms.

Positron emission tomography (PET)

PET with the use of [18F]fluorodeoxy-glucose ([18F]-FDG) assesses the levels of glucose utilization in tissues and has been applied for use in experimental evaluation post TBI. One of the earliest studies by Humayun et al. in 1989 reported regional metabolic differences, both decreases and increases, in mTBI patients despite the lack of anatomical abnormalities.[54] Multiple subsequent studies similarly reported regional abnormalities on FDG PET caused by mTBI.[55–62] The FDG PET abnormalities were larger and more widespread compared to the anatomic abnormalities in the conventional studies.[63] Hypometabolism has been attributed to hypoxia, which is a significant contributing factor in the TBI-associated pathology. Bergsneider et al. have studied the global cerebral metabolic rate of glucose (CMRglc), using quantitative FDG

PET, and showed that TBI results in an intermediate metabolic reduction phase that is dynamic and begins to resolve about one month following injury.[64] FDG PET has also shown a positive correlation with neuropsychological testing, though this has not been studied as vigorously as with SPECT.[65]

Utilizing other radiotracers, such as ^{15}O-labelled gas PET and [11C]flumazenil PET, Shiga et al. were also able to demonstrate evidence of metabolic abnormalities despite the lack of relevant MRI findings in symptomatic TBI patients.[66]

Because of limited availability, cost, and radiation exposure, PET never gained popularity in clinical TBI assessment. However, this may change with the introduction of specialized ligands that can specifically bind to receptors that are unique to mTBI.[65]

Single photon emission computed tomography (SPECT)

SPECT has been utilized as a cheaper alternative to PET imaging. By injecting a radiotracer, such as 95mTc-hexamethylpropyleneamineoxime (HMPAO) or cobalt-57, SPECT can grossly measure regional CBF. With the assumption that flow parallels metabolic activity, SPECT abnormalities are indirectly considered alterations in metabolism. However, there is some evidence that this may not always be the case following TBI.[57]

In the acute post-traumatic setting, Audenaert et al. demonstrated frontal and temporal abnormalities on cobalt-57-SPECT despite the lack of CT or MR abnormalities in a subset of mTBI patients.[67] The authors were able to qualitatively correlate these abnormalities with neuropsychological testing in seven out of eight patients. On the other hand, despite the similar patient demographics, Hofman et al. were able to show only a weak correlation between the imaging findings and neurocognitive outcome, but did demonstrate that patients who had hypoperfusion on SPECT scans within the first five postinjury days subsequently developed atrophy at a six month follow-up, suggesting hypoxia as an underlying etiology for this atrophy.[10]

Ichise et al. evaluated chronic TBI patients, both "minor" and "major," comparing HMPAO SPECT to standard imaging techniques and neuropsychological performance.[68] SPECT detected more abnormalities than CT and MRI in both minor and major TBI subgroups, but was relatively more valuable in the minor TBI subgroup as this subgroup largely lacked abnormalities on initial CT and MRI. The authors also reported correlations between specific abnormal perfusion patterns, like anterior-posterior ratio (APR) and neuropsychological performance. Years after this, Bonne et al. sought to examine the correlation between neuropsychological deficits and rCBV by recruiting 28 chronically symptomatic male mTBI patients and comparing them with 20 matched controls.[69] While the mTBI patients showed regional hypoperfusion in frontal/prefrontal/temporal cortices and subcortical structures, hypoperfusion in the frontal, left posterior, and to a lesser extent, subcortical subgroups correlated with predictions in lesion location based on clinical neuropsychological deficits. In another study, hypoperfusion in the basal ganglia significantly correlated with the presence of postconcussive headaches.[70] Therefore, the use of SPECT imaging may have future potential to predict those athletes that may demonstrate specific clinical signs and symptoms warranting earlier rehabilitative and/or therapeutic interventions.

However, it should be kept in mind that SPECT imaging inherently suffers from significant limitations. For example, detecting SPECT abnormalities requires comparing the area of interest to other regions of the brain—presumably free of injury—but we know that mTBI is more frequently a diffuse brain process. Also, SPECT values are based on the assumption that blood flow parallels metabolic activity, which is not consistent, as previously mentioned.

Magnetoencephalography (MEG)

Though not widely used in clinical practice, MEG provides noninvasive functional mapping of the brain, with high spatial and temporal resolution, by recording the weak magnetic forces associated with the brain's electrical activity. Unlike EEG, the magnetic fields detected by MEG are not distorted by the skull and other tissues, allowing for greater accuracy of the signal. MEG is commonly performed with simultaneous EEG recording. MEG can be fused with structural imaging, such as CT and MRI, which produces functional/anatomic images of the brain, referred to as magnetic source imaging (MSI).

In a retrospective study of 30 adult patients with mTBI and persistent (over one year) post-concussive symptoms, abnormalities on MEG were found to be more sensitive than cMRI and SPECT.[70] Objective evidence of brain injury through positive image findings was present in only 4 patients by cMRI and 12 patients through the use of SPECT, while 19 patients showed abnormal activity (dipolar slow wave activity) by MEG. The researchers also documented significant correlations between regional MEG abnormal activity and certain cognitive deficits, such as temporal lobe activity and memory problems, parietal lobe and attention problems, and frontal lobe and executive function.

Conclusion

The advancement in neuroimaging techniques have provided researchers with in vivo evidence that the presumed neuronal response following injury seen in animal models parallels what occurs in the athlete following concussion. The previously held notion that concussion was only a functional and not structural injury has been debunked by these methods. Though standard neuroimaging is still needed to rule out the minute cohort of athletes that develop macrostructural injury, like hemorrhage, advancements in the understanding of concussive injury will only be furthered as we use more sophisticated imaging techniques to understand the microstructural and neurometabolic/chemical alterations of the neuron following injury. This exciting technology has the potential to improve concussion diagnosis, return-to-play standards, and possibibly even prognostication.

References

1. Borg J, Holm L, Cassidy JD et al. Diagnostic procedures in mild traumatic brain injury: results of the WHO Collaborating Centre Task Force on Mild Traumatic Brain Injury. *Journal of Rehabilitation Medicine.* 2004(43 Suppl): 61–75.

2. Dacey RG, Jr., Alves WM, Rimel RW, Winn HR, Jane JA. Neurosurgical complications after apparently minor head injury. Assessment of risk in a series of 610 patients. *Journal of Neurosurgery.* 1986; 65(2): 203–210.

3. Kuppermann N. Pediatric head trauma: the evidence regarding indications for emergent neuroimaging. *Pediatric Radiology.* 2008; 38 Suppl 4: S670–674.

4. Gonzalez PG, Walker MT. Imaging modalities in mild traumatic brain injury and sports concussion. *PM & R: The Journal of Injury, Function, and Rehabilitation.* 2011; 3(10 Suppl 2): S413–424.

5. Stiell IG, Wells GA, Vandemheen K et al. The Canadian CT Head Rule for patients with minor head injury. *Lancet.* 2001; 357(9266): 1391–1396.

6. Haydel MJ, Preston CA, Mills TJ, Luber S, Blaudeau E, DeBlieux PM. Indications for computed tomography in patients with minor head injury. *The New England Journal of Medicine.* 2000; 343(2): 100–106.

7. Borczuk P. Predictors of intracranial injury in patients with mild head trauma. *Annals of Emergency Medicine.* 1995; 25(6): 731–736.

8. Miller EC, Holmes JF, Derlet RW. Utilizing clinical factors to reduce head CT scan ordering for minor head trauma patients. *The Journal of Emergency Medicine.* 1997; 15(4): 453–457.

9. Yousem D, Grossman R. *Neuroradiology.* 3rd ed: Elsevier Health Sciences; 2010.

10. Hofman PA, Stapert SZ, van Kroonenburgh MJ, Jolles J, de Kruijk J, Wilmink JT. MR imaging, single-photon emission CT, and neurocognitive performance after mild traumatic brain injury. *AJNR American Journal of Neuroradiology.* 2001; 22(3): 441–449.

11. Hughes DG, Jackson A, Mason DL, Berry E, Hollis S, Yates DW. Abnormalities on magnetic resonance imaging seen acutely following mild traumatic brain injury: correlation with neuropsychological tests and delayed recovery. *Neuroradiology.* 2004; 46(7): 550–558.

12. Tong KA, Ashwal S, Holshouser BA et al. Hemorrhagic shearing lesions in children and adolescents with posttraumatic diffuse axonal injury: improved detection and initial results. *Radiology*. 2003; 227(2): 332–339.

13. Johnson VE, Stewart W, Smith DH. Axonal pathology in traumatic brain injury. *Experimental Neurology*. 2013; 246: 35–43.

14. Stone JL, Patel V, Bailes JE. The history of neurosurgical treatment of sports concussion. *Neurosurgery*. 2014; 75 Suppl 4: S3–s23.

15. Browne KD, Chen XH, Meaney DF, Smith DH. Mild traumatic brain injury and diffuse axonal injury in swine. *Journal of Neurotrauma*. 2011; 28(9): 1747–1755.

16. Gennarelli TA, Thibault LE, Adams JH, Graham DI, Thompson CJ, Marcincin RP. Diffuse axonal injury and traumatic coma in the primate. *Annals of Neurology*. 1982; 12(6): 564–574.

17. Kerr ZY, Collins CL, Mihalik JP, Marshall SW, Guskiewicz KM, Comstock RD. Impact locations and concussion outcomes in high school football player-to-player collisions. *Pediatrics*. 2014; 134(3): 489–496.

18. Mittl RL, Grossman RI, Hiehle JF et al. Prevalence of MR evidence of diffuse axonal injury in patients with mild head injury and normal head CT findings. *AJNR American Journal of Neuroradiology*. 1994; 15(8): 1583–1589.

19. Barkhoudarian G, Hovda DA, Giza CC. The molecular pathophysiology of concussive brain injury. *Clinics in Sports Medicine*. 2011; 30(1): 33–48, vii–iii.

20. Povlishock JT, Becker DP, Cheng CL, Vaughan GW. Axonal change in minor head injury. *Journal of Neuropathology and Experimental Neurology*. 1983; 42(3): 225–242.

21. Saatman KE, Abai B, Grosvenor A, Vorwerk CK, Smith DH, Meaney DF. Traumatic axonal injury results in biphasic calpain activation and retrograde transport impairment in mice. *Journal of Cerebral Blood Flow and Metabolism*. 2003; 23(1): 34–42.

22. Smith DH, Stewart W. Tackling concussion, beyond Hollywood. *The Lancet Neurology*. 2016; 15(7): 662–663.

23. Tang-Schomer MD, Patel AR, Baas PW, Smith DH. Mechanical breaking of microtubules in axons during dynamic stretch injury underlies delayed elasticity, microtubule disassembly, and axon degeneration. *Federation of American Societies for Experimental Biology Journal*. 2010; 24(5): 1401–1410.

24. Nakamura Y, Takeda M, Angelides KJ, Tanaka T, Tada K, Nishimura T. Effect of phosphorylation on 68 KDa neurofilament subunit protein assembly by the cyclic AMP dependent protein kinase in vitro. *Biochemical and Biophysical Research Communications*. 1990; 169(2): 744–750.

25. Zetterberg H, Smith DH, Blennow K. Biomarkers of mild traumatic brain injury in cerebrospinal fluid and blood. *Nature Reviews Neurology*. 2013; 9(4): 201–210.

26. Huisman TA, Sorensen AG, Hergan K, Gonzalez RG, Schaefer PW. Diffusion-weighted imaging for the evaluation of diffuse axonal injury in closed head injury. *Journal of Computer Assisted Tomography*. 2003; 27(1): 5–11.

27. Povlishock JT, Christman CW. The pathobiology of traumatically induced axonal injury in animals and humans: a review of current thoughts. *Journal of Neurotrauma*. 1995; 12(4): 555–564.

28. Niogi SN, Mukherjee P. Diffusion tensor imaging of mild traumatic brain injury. *The Journal of Head Trauma Rehabilitation*. 2010; 25(4): 241–255.

29. Salmond CH, Menon DK, Chatfield DA et al. Diffusion tensor imaging in chronic head injury survivors: correlations with learning and memory indices. *NeuroImage*. 2006; 29(1): 117–124.

30. Niogi SN, Mukherjee P, Ghajar J et al. Extent of microstructural white matter injury in postconcussive syndrome correlates with impaired cognitive reaction time: a 3T

diffusion tensor imaging study of mild traumatic brain injury. *AJNR American Journal of Neuroradiology*. 2008; 29(5): 967–973.

31. Little DM, Kraus MF, Joseph J et al. Thalamic integrity underlies executive dysfunction in traumatic brain injury. *Neurology*. 2010; 74(7): 558–564.

32. Kraus MF, Susmaras T, Caughlin BP, Walker CJ, Sweeney JA, Little DM. White matter integrity and cognition in chronic traumatic brain injury: a diffusion tensor imaging study. *Brain*. 2007; 130(Pt 10): 2508–2519.

33. Levin HS, Wilde E, Troyanskaya M et al. Diffusion tensor imaging of mild to moderate blast-related traumatic brain injury and its sequelae. *Journal of Neurotrauma*. 2010; 27(4): 683–694.

34. Niogi SN, Mukherjee P, Ghajar J et al. Structural dissociation of attentional control and memory in adults with and without mild traumatic brain injury. *Brain*. 2008; 131 (Pt 12): 3209–3221.

35. Zhang K, Johnson B, Pennell D, Ray W, Sebastianelli W, Slobounov S. Are functional deficits in concussed individuals consistent with white matter structural alterations: combined FMRI & DTI study. *Experimental Brain Research*. 2010; 204(1): 57–70.

36. Sharp DJ, Beckmann CF, Greenwood R et al. Default mode network functional and structural connectivity after traumatic brain injury. *Brain*. 2011; 134(Pt 8): 2233–2247.

37. Chen JK, Johnston KM, Frey S, Petrides M, Worsley K, Ptito A. Functional abnormalities in symptomatic concussed athletes: an fMRI study. *NeuroImage*. 2004; 22(1): 68–82.

38. Chen JK, Johnston KM, Petrides M, Ptito A. Recovery from mild head injury in sports: evidence from serial functional magnetic resonance imaging studies in male athletes. *Clinical Journal of Sport Medicine*. 2008; 18(3): 241–247.

39. Chen JK, Johnston KM, Collie A, McCrory P, Ptito A. A validation of the post concussion symptom scale in the assessment of complex concussion using cognitive testing

and functional MRI. *Journal of Neurology, Neurosurgery, and Psychiatry*. 2007; 78(11): 1231–1238.

40. Jantzen KJ, Anderson B, Steinberg FL, Kelso JA. A prospective functional MR imaging study of mild traumatic brain injury in college football players. *AJNR American Journal of Neuroradiology*. 2004; 25(5): 738–745.

41. Slobounov SM, Zhang K, Pennell D, Ray W, Johnson B, Sebastianelli W. Functional abnormalities in normally appearing athletes following mild traumatic brain injury: a functional MRI study. *Experimental Brain Research*. 2010; 202(2): 341–354.

42. Stevens MC, Lovejoy D, Kim J, Oakes H, Kureshi I, Witt ST. Multiple resting state network functional connectivity abnormalities in mild traumatic brain injury. *Brain Imaging and Behavior*. 2012; 6(2): 293–318.

43. Son BC, Park CK, Choi BG et al. Metabolic changes in pericontusional oedematous areas in mild head injury evaluated by 1H MRS. *Acta Neurochirurgica Supplement*. 2000; 76: 13–16.

44. Longhi L, Saatman KE, Fujimoto S et al. Temporal window of vulnerability to repetitive experimental concussive brain injury. *Neurosurgery*. 2005; 56(2): 364–374; discussion 364–374.

45. Vagnozzi R, Signoretti S, Cristofori L et al. Assessment of metabolic brain damage and recovery following mild traumatic brain injury: a multicentre, proton magnetic resonance spectroscopic study in concussed patients. *Brain*. 2010; 133(11): 3232–3242.

46. Cecil KM, Hills EC, Sandel ME et al. Proton magnetic resonance spectroscopy for detection of axonal injury in the splenium of the corpus callosum of brain-injured patients. *Journal of Neurosurgery*. 1998; 88(5): 795–801.

47. Belanger HG, Vanderploeg RD, Curtiss G, Warden DL. Recent neuroimaging techniques in mild traumatic brain injury. *The Journal of Neuropsychiatry and Clinical Neurosciences*. 2007; 19(1): 5–20.

48. Garnett MR, Blamire AM, Corkill RG, Cadoux-Hudson TA, Rajagopalan B, Styles P. Early proton magnetic resonance spectroscopy in normal-appearing brain correlates with outcome in patients following traumatic brain injury. *Brain*. 2000; 123 (Pt 10): 2046–2054.

49. Holshouser BA, Tong KA, Ashwal S. Proton MR spectroscopic imaging depicts diffuse axonal injury in children with traumatic brain injury. *AJNR American Journal of Neuroradiology*. 2005; 26(5): 1276–1285.

50. Castillo M, Kwock L, Mukherji SK. Clinical applications of proton MR spectroscopy. *AJNR American Journal of Neuroradiology*. 1996; 17(1): 1–15.

51. Liu W, Wang B, Wolfowitz R et al. Perfusion deficits in patients with mild traumatic brain injury characterized by dynamic susceptibility contrast MRI. *NMR in Biomedicine*. 2013; 26(6): 651–663.

52. Ge Y, Patel MB, Chen Q et al. Assessment of thalamic perfusion in patients with mild traumatic brain injury by true FISP arterial spin labelling MR imaging at 3T. *Brain Injury*. 2009; 23(7): 666–674.

53. Meier TB, Bellgowan PS, Singh R, Kuplicki R, Polanski DW, Mayer AR. Recovery of cerebral blood flow following sports-related concussion. *The Journal of the American Medical Association Neurology*. 2015; 72(5): 530–538.

54. Humayun MS, Presty SK, Lafrance ND et al. Local cerebral glucose abnormalities in mild closed head injured patients with cognitive impairments. *Nuclear Medicine Communications*. 1989; 10(5): 335–344.

55. Roberts MA, Manshadi FF, Bushnell DL, Hines ME. Neurobehavioural dysfunction following mild traumatic brain injury in childhood: a case report with positive findings on positron emission tomography (PET). *Brain Injury*. 1995; 9(5): 427–436.

56. Gross H, Kling A, Henry G, Herndon C, Lavretsky H. Local cerebral glucose metabolism in patients with long-term behavioral and cognitive deficits following mild traumatic brain injury. *The Journal of Neuropsychiatry and Clinical Neurosciences*. 1996; 8(3): 324–334.

57. Abu-Judeh HH, Singh M, Masdeu JC, Abdel-Dayem HM. Discordance between FDG uptake and technetium-99m-HMPAO brain perfusion in acute traumatic brain injury. *Journal of Nuclear Medicine: Official publication, Society of Nuclear Medicine*. 1998; 39(8): 1357–1359.

58. Umile EM, Sandel ME, Alavi A, Terry CM, Plotkin RC. Dynamic imaging in mild traumatic brain injury: support for the theory of medial temporal vulnerability. *Archives of Physical Medicine and Rehabilitation*. 2002; 83(11): 1506–1513.

59. Chen SH, Kareken DA, Fastenau PS, Trexler LE, Hutchins GD. A study of persistent post-concussion symptoms in mild head trauma using positron emission tomography. *Journal of Neurology, Neurosurgery, and Psychiatry*. 2003; 74(3): 326–332.

60. Ruff RM, Crouch JA, Troster AI et al. Selected cases of poor outcome following a minor brain trauma: comparing neuropsychological and positron emission tomography assessment. *Brain Injury*. 1994; 8(4): 297–308.

61. Provenzano FA, Jordan B, Tikofsky RS, Saxena C, Van Heertum RL, Ichise M. F-18 FDG PET imaging of chronic traumatic brain injury in boxers: a statistical parametric analysis. *Nuclear Medicine Communications*. 2010; 31(11): 952–957.

62. Peskind ER, Petrie EC, Cross DJ et al. Cerebrocerebellar hypometabolism associated with repetitive blast exposure mild traumatic brain injury in 12 Iraq war Veterans with persistent post-concussive symptoms. *NeuroImage*. 2011; 54 Suppl 1: S76–82.

63. Dubroff JG, Newberg A. Neuroimaging of traumatic brain injury. *Seminars in Neurology*. 2008; 28(4): 548–557.

64. Bergsneider M, Hovda DA, McArthur DL et al. Metabolic recovery following human traumatic brain injury based on FDG-PET:

time course and relationship to neurological disability. *The Journal of Head Trauma Rehabilitation*. 2001; 16(2): 135–148.

65. Lin AP, Liao HJ, Merugumala SK, Prabhu SP, Meehan WP, 3rd, Ross BD. Metabolic imaging of mild traumatic brain injury. *Brain Imaging and Behavior*. 2012; 6(2): 208–223.

66. Shiga T, Ikoma K, Katoh C et al. Loss of neuronal integrity: a cause of hypometabolism in patients with traumatic brain injury without MRI abnormality in the chronic stage. *European Journal of Nuclear Medicine and Molecular Imaging*. 2006; 33(7): 817–822.

67. Audenaert K, Jansen HM, Otte A et al. Imaging of mild traumatic brain injury using 57Co and 99mTc HMPAO SPECT as compared to other diagnostic procedures. *Medical Science Monitor*. 2003; 9(10): Mt112–117.

68. Ichise M, Chung DG, Wang P, Wortzman G, Gray BG, Franks W. Technetium-99m-HMPAO SPECT, CT and MRI in the evaluation of patients with chronic traumatic brain injury: a correlation with neuropsychological performance. *Journal of Nuclear Medicine*. 1994; 35(2): 217–226.

69. Bonne O, Gilboa A, Louzoun Y et al. Cerebral blood flow in chronic symptomatic mild traumatic brain injury. *Psychiatry Research*. 2003; 124(3): 141–152.

70. Lewine JD, Davis JT, Bigler ED et al. Objective documentation of traumatic brain injury subsequent to mild head trauma: multimodal brain imaging with MEG, SPECT, and MRI. *The Journal of Head Trauma Rehabilitation*. 2007; 22(3): 141–155.

The advent of subconcussion and chronic traumatic encephalopathy

With John Lee, M.D. Ph.D.

Introduction

In 2005, Omalu et al. published a seminal paper describing the pathological evidence of what was termed "Chronic Traumatic Encephalopathy" (CTE). This was described in a former NFL player who displayed a progressive mental decline with a myriad of cognitive, behavioral, and mood symptoms.[1] Over the past decade, an eruption of inquiry and scrutiny has surrounded the entity of CTE including the diagnosis, cause, and potential link with those sports at high risk of repetitive head trauma. Though scientific literature has exposed a relationship between repetitive head trauma and CTE for over a decade, the National Football League publically acknowledged its existence in March of 2016, after many years of contesting the presented data.[2] Unfortunately, our knowledge of this medical diagnosis remains incomplete, as there is limited prospective evidence to better evaluate its epidemiology. Due to the relatively small number of studied cases and conflicting results, the relationship between clinical symptoms and pathological disease burden continues to be highly debated.

In this chapter, we will describe the current understanding of CTE and its relation to repetitive concussive and even subconcussive injuries. We hope that through the presented literature, the reader will develop an enriched awareness of the preclinical and clinical research that describes CTE and subconcussion, while recognizing its limitations and the need for further study.

Subconcussion

A subconcussion results from sustained impact to the head or body that leads to an acceleration–deceleration event of the brain within the skull.[3] Similar to the diagnosis of concussion, a subconcussion does not need to involve a direct cranial impact. What distinguishes subconcussion from concussion is that with this mild insult the athlete does not have clinical signs, like they would in a concussion. As a single event, these mild injuries are clinically silent, but potentially accumulate over the course of years of athletic play to cause deleterious effects.[4] As seen in Figure 9.1,[3,5] these subconcussive events can have an astounding cumulative effect, potentially contributing to the development of CTE. This is important because the average high school and college player sustains a mean of 650–950 subconcussive impacts during a season.[6,7] To date, the only consistent risk factor for CTE, a progressive neurodegenerative syndrome, has been exposure to repeated mild traumatic brain injuries through years of athletic participation.[8–11]

As one can imagine, there are many challenges to effectively investigating subconcussion. Since subconcussion is a clinically silent head trauma, it is impossible for the athlete to quantify these events for a career, let alone a specific game.[12] Researchers have attempted to incorporate the use of helmet accelerometers in efforts to characterize specific angular acceleration and G forces experienced, during a practice or game, that do not lead to a symptomatic, concussive injury.

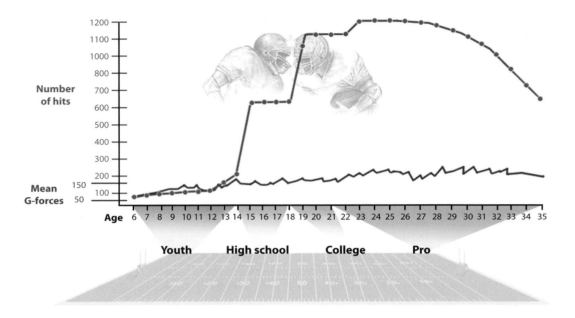

Figure 9.1 Graphical depiction of cumulative head impacts over a player's career. (From Bailes JE et al. *J Neurosurg.* Nov;119(5):1235–45 2013.)

However, without prospective data, it is difficult to determine the specific threshold of force required for a clinically silent phenomenon, and to determine what quantity and total force may lead to long-term deleterious clinical outcomes. Even the use of helmet accelerometers to determine the concussion threshold, a clinical diagnosis, has shown limitations and has been found to have a large range between individuals.[13–20]

Preclinical evidence of subconcussion

Due to the challenges in studying a clinically silent events in humans, researchers have turned to the use of low impact and repetitive TBI animal models in order to better characterize subconcussion. Animal models have been developed that use a single mild injury without acute behavioral changes (a subconcussive event). In these models, it has been observed that these subconcussive injuries still initiate a neuroinflammatory response within the brain similar to that described in more severe TBI.[21]

As the case reports of CTE began to appear, investigators increased experimental time points in order to evaluate the long-term effects of repetitive injury. What was concerning with these results was that in comparison to a single TBI, the repetitive mild TBI injury was remarkable for *progressive*

worsening neurological deficits at chronic time points. These studies demonstrated a gradation in clinical and pathological outcomes only occurring in those animals receiving repeated injury. These observations were made by measuring the following outcomes: and noted to be worse neuroinflammatory response, blood–brain barrier breakdown, diffuse axonal injury, gliosis, neuronal loss, cortical atrophy, mortality, and progressive behavioral deficits similar to human concussion/CTE symptomatology (impaired memory, balance/vestibular function, anxiety, depression).[22–35] In another study, Donovan et al. subjected a group of mice to a single and repetitive (2 total injuries, 1 week apart) mild TBI. The mice that received repetitive injury were found to have progressive white matter changes in the corpus callosum that were still persistent even at chronic time points (60 days from injury).[36] Mouzon et al. also saw a similar progression, histologically and with cognitive behavioral deficits, in a mouse repetitive mild TBI model. Both single and repetitive injury showed initial behavioral changes and cognitive deficits, but only in the repetitively injured animals (5 total injuries every 48 hours), in which those changes persisted even at 12 to 18 months from the injury.[37] The absence of findings in the single mildly injured animal, when compared to the findings in those with repetitive injuries, mirrors the results of an in vitro study performed by Weber et al. in 2007. This study emphasized the cumulative effect of injury following successive neuronal insults.[35] As mentioned in Chapter 4, many of these preclinical studies influenced recommendations for return to play because they mutually concluded that repetitive injuries, even subconcussive insults, caused long-term behavioral deficits and pathological changes.

Clinical evidence of subconcussion

Strong evidence has demonstrated, in preclinical animal models, that a repeat concussion has *acute* detrimental effects on a microscopic level (axonal, inflammatory, and vascular), along with consequences on global functioning of the animal.[28–33,36,38,39] What is more concerning is that though the vast majority of patients demonstrate symptomatic recovery following a concussive injury,[40–42] it appears that exposure to repetitive concussions has *chronic* deleterious consequences. Studies in football, hockey, soccer, rugby, and professional fighters have validated that exposure to repetitive head trauma and concussive injuries corresponds with a proinflammatory cerebral state,[43] cortical (cingulate, frontal lobe, precentral gyrus, thalamus, caudate, etc.) and hippocampal atrophy,[12,43–49] along with altered neural connectivity/functionality.[50–52] These complex insults to the brain are likely the culprit to the clinically demonstrated reduction in cognitive and memory abilities[50,53–56] and the increased incidence of long-term cognitive, behavioral, and motor impairment.[47,49,57–60]

Though all of these studies present data that single and repeat concussions are acutely and chronically detrimental with a cumulative effect, they do not address if specifically, subconcussion, without a significant enough injury to cause symptoms, also has this same cumulative influence leading to pathological changes in humans. To assess this, various groups analyzed a cohort of athletes during a season of play during which they did not experience a concussion, and therefore, were exposed only to the repetitive subconcussive blows associated with their contact sport. All groups found that players, though documented not to have sustained a concussion, had significant white matter changes (corpus callosum, amygdala) on diffusion tensor imaging (DTI) at the end of their regular season in comparison to preseason baseline testing. When retesting these players at 6 months after a rest period, these white matter changes were still present and had not yet improved.[61–64] In more detail, Lipton et al. showed abnormal white matter changes on DTI in a cohort of 37 soccer players, which were also correlated with a decline in neurocognitive performance. In this cohort, the average player headed the ball 432 times over one season, a potential subconcussion contributor.[65] Through DTI, it is evident that mild, asymptomatic, but repetitive subconcussive blows caused pathological (white matter alterations) and cognitive impairment. Likewise, Bazarian et al. obtained DTI on nine high school athletes participating in a contact sport (hockey or football) pre- and postseason, where only one of those athletes had experienced a concussion. Though a limited study due to sample size, this study found that in comparing the controls, those with subconcussive impacts, and the one athlete who suffered a concussion, exhibited a stepwise increase in white matter injury (changes in fractional anisotropy and medial diffusivity),[66] indicating that even those athletes exposed to *asymptomatic* subconcussions are still subject to injury.

Along with axonal injury seen on DTI, further imaging modalities have been used to assess changes in neurochemical and neuronal connectivity in players with profound concussive and subconcussive histories. Lin et al. performed magnetic resonance spectrometry (MRS) imaging on five former professional football, wrestling, and baseball players. During their 11 to 22 years of contact sports history, all athletes reported having a symptomatic concussion, in addition to definite recurring subconcussive impact exposure. These athletes demonstrated neurochemical alterations in comparison to the healthy controls, specifically in elevations of glutamate, glutamine, and choline.[67] Similarly, Koerte et al. found analogous alterations of neurochemicals consistent with markers of neuroinflammation in a cohort of retired soccer players (mean age 46.9 years old) who reported a history of repetitive subconcussive impacts.[68]

Using other MRI imaging modalities, Abbas et al. performed functional MRI (fMRI) on 22 collision sport athletes aged 14 to 22 years old, and compared them with 10 noncollision athletes. fMRI is an imaging modality that is able to indirectly assess brain connectivity through changes in blood flow. It is postulated that the brain has multiple pathways to perform a specific function. If one of these pathways becomes injured, following a mild TBI, the brain compensates by recruiting other tracts (hyperconnectivity) to assist in performing an activity/cognitive task. It was found that during the preseason testing of collision sport athletes, they were found to have increased connectivity, alluding to the fact that these players already had chronic injuries from subconcussive impacts. As postulated, there was an even greater increase in connectivity following the studied season of play, even though there were no self-reported concussive events.[69] Talavage et al. also performed fMRI on a cohort of high school football players. This cohort subdivided players without a diagnosis of concussion but with neurocognitive deficits (four players) and those without a concussion or neurocognitive deficits (four players).[70] Interestingly, the four players without a documented concussive injury but with neurocognitive deficits were found to be exposed to a greater total number and magnitude of collisions, when compared to those with normal neurocognitive testing. They were also found to have significant alterations on fMRI in the regions of the prefrontal cortex and cerebellum. Though these advanced neuroimaging techniques are in their infancy of development and many questions circulate as to what the exact meaning of these functional and neurochemical alterations are, this still provides striking evidence that subconcussive injuries without exposure to concussion causes cerebral physiological alterations and has potential harmful clinical consequences.

Though there are numerous limitations in the growing body of evidence about subconcussion in laboratory and clinical literature, the acute physiological changes seen by dynamic neuroimaging as well as the chronic effects seen in neuropsychological and epidemiological studies make it difficult to ignore the notion that subconcussive injuries, though mild and asymptomatic, but when repetitive in nature can lead to cumulative neurological injury. It is imperative for the medical community to disseminate this information to the athlete and athletic associations in order to influence policies for safe return-to-activity recommendations, alterations to hazardous rules of play, and also improvements in protective equipment.

Chronic traumatic encephalopathy

History

Dr. Harrison Martland, a forensic pathologist from New Jersey, termed in 1928 "punch drunk" a condition of cognitive delay and impaired gait seen only in professional boxers, which was later termed "dementia pugilistica" in 1937 by J.A. Millspaugh.[71–74] Through years of pathological study, dementia pugilistica was found to be characterized by postmortem studies in boxers as a deposition of protein aggregates of amyloid and neurofibrillary tangles.[75] Then in 1957, MacDonald Critchley, a British neurologist, coined the term "Chronic Traumatic Encephalopathy" or CTE when studying a cohort of boxers displaying Parkinsonian symptoms.[76] Since then, many other historical terms have been used to describe a similar clinical presentation in those subjected to repeated blows to the head: traumatic encephalitis, cumulative encephalopathy of the boxer, psychopathic deterioration of pugilists, chronic boxer's encephalopathy, and traumatic boxer's encephalopathy.[73,77]

In 2005, Dr. Bennet Omalu described similar histological features following the death of a prominent former NFL player, who developed severe, progressive cognitive and behavioral symptoms. The athlete portrayed similar pathological findings, however, the brain appeared grossly normal without any cavum septum pellucidum, cerebellar scarring, or other changes as typically seen in boxers characterized with dementia pugilistica.[1,78] In the following years, many prominent professional athletes were found to display similar clinical symptomatology, tragically ending their lives, and upon pathological evaluation of their brains, they were all noted to have a similar histological pattern.[73,79]

After a decade of research, led by Dr. Bennet Omalu and Dr. Ann McKee, there has been over 160 pathologically diagnosed cases of CTE, and over 85% of those were found among athletes in either boxing or American football.[9] A retrospective review of these cases determined that the only consistent link among these athletes, in developing this progressive neurodegenerative syndrome, was an exposure to years of repetitive head injuries, with the mean length of exposure to contact sports of 15.4 years.[80,81] CTE has been found in a wide variety of people exposed to repetitive head injury:[10] American football players, boxers, wrestlers, mixed martial artists, ice hockey players, soccer players, rugby players, military personnel, seizure patients, mentally disabled persons with a history of head banging, and physical abuse victims.[1,5,78,79,82–90] Though a small sample, Gavett et al. estimated that 3.7% of NFL players could be affected by CTE.[91,92] The lack of prospective data, the presence of asymptomatic players with possible CTE, and selection bias—influenced by who donates their brain for evaluation—combine to create limitations to obtaining a true incidence of CTE.

Pathological diagnosis of CTE

Currently, the definitive diagnosis of CTE can only be done postmortem.[93] It is characterized by a multifocal cortical and subcortical tauopathy in the form of neurofibrillary tangles and neuropil threads seen more prominently in sulcal depths, superficial cortical layers II and III, and, most specifically, surrounding blood vessels (perivascular)[1,5,8,10,11,78,94–98] (Figure 9.2). Interestingly, the perivascular location of tauopathy corresponds with the areas of axonal injury and inflammation seen in autopsy specimens following a head injury.[81,99,100]

A tauopathy is a group of neurodegenerative diseases that are characterized by intracellular or extracellular aggregations of tau within the brain—Alzheimer's being the most common tauopathy.[101] The tau protein is normally found associated with microtubules, a cell structural protein that assists in axonal transport, within the axon of a neuron but is also found in glial cells.[102,103] In nonpathological states, tau is phosphorylated (by kinases) and dephosphorylated (by phosphatases) at sites along the length of the protein in order to aid in normal CNS development, but this homeostasis is altered after injury exposure (Figure 9.3).[104] Following a pathological insult, the tau protein (soluble form)

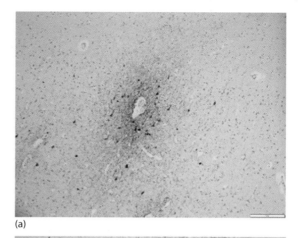

(a)

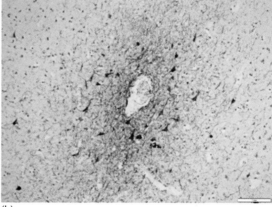

(b)

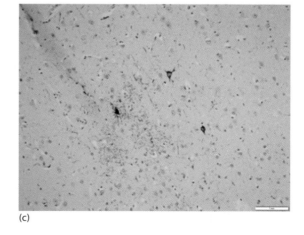

(c)

Figure 9.2 Pathological *perivascular* aggregation of phosphorylated tau protein at 10× (a) and 20× (b) and abnormal neuritic and neuronal hyperphosphorylated tau at 20× (c) in the cortices of a 23-year-old male with probable CTE.

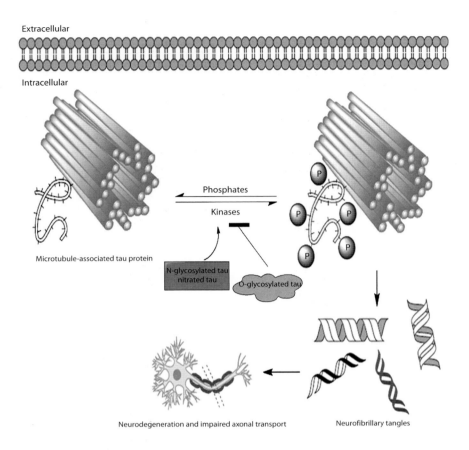

Extracellular

Intracellular

Phosphates

Kinases

Microtubule-associated tau protein

N-glycosylated tau nitrated tau

O-glycosylated tau

Neurodegeneration and impaired axonal transport

Neurofibrillary tangles

Figure 9.3 Neurofibrillary tangle formation involves an imbalance between tau kinase and tau phosphatase activity. If tau kinase activity is increased, and the phosphatase activity is decreased, hyperphosphorylation persists and can result in the formation of neurofibrillary tangles. Neurofibrillary tangles contribute to poor outcome by disrupting axonal transport and eventually causing the hierarchical spread of neurodegeneration. Neurodegeneration ultimately causes the classic symptoms seen in patients suspected of having chronic traumatic encephalopathy. (From Lucke-Wold BP et al. *J Neurotrauma.* Jul 1;31(13):1129–38, 2014.)

becomes preferentially hyperphosphorylated at specific sites (associated with development of neurodegenerative disease, see Figure 9.4[104]), leading to destabilization of the microtubule, and release of the insoluble form of hyperphosphorylated tau. These tau proteins clump together and are moved from the neuron's axon to the cytoplasm of the neuronal soma, seen histologically as neurofibrillary tangles or neuropil threads[104,105] (Figure 9.5). In other neurodegenerative diseases, tau aggregations also occur in oligodendrocytes (affecting maintenance of myelin), astrocytes (potentially altering the blood–brain barrier integrity), and microglial cells (Figure 9.6).[103] The specifics regarding tau accumulation based on location and even isoform

type, and how this translates to clinical disease in CTE, is still under active investigation.[103] Areas of active and future investigation regarding location should include delineation of both anatomic and microscopic locations of abnormal tau. For isoform subtypes, these investigations should determine whether the tau inclusions are 3R and/or 4R tau as well as if there are differences between the neuronal and glial tau inclusions in isoform expression in CTE.

In an attempt to characterize pathological findings of CTE, Omalu et al. in 2014 described four different phenotypes based on histomorphological findings.[34,97,106] The following year, McKee et al. developed a CTE staging system based specifically

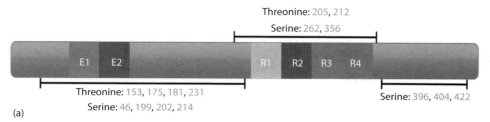

Threonine: 205, 212
Serine: 262, 356

E1 E2 R1 R2 R3 R4

Threonine: 153, 175, 181, 231
Serine: 46, 199, 202, 214

Serine: 396, 404, 422

(a)

Antibody		Phosphorylation site recognized	Tau form/location recognized
AT8		Serine **199** and **202**; Threonine **205**	Intra- and extracellular
AT100		Threonine **212** and Serine **214**	Intra- and extracellular
AT270		Threonine **181**	Intra- and extracellular
PHF1		Serine **396** and **404**	Intra- and extracellular
pS262		Serine **262**	Pretangle
TG3		Threonine **231**	Pretangle
pT153		Threonine **153**	Pretangle
12E8		Serine **262** and **356**	Intracellular
pS214		Serine **214**	Intracellular
pT175/181		Threonine **175** and **181**	Intracellular
pS422		Serine **422**	Intracellular
pS46		Serine **46**	Intracellular
CP13		Serine **202**	Unknown

(b)

Figure 9.4 (a) Potential phosphorylation sites along the tau protein that are associated with development of neuro-degenerative diseases. (b) Binding of specific antibodies, like PHF-1, have been found to be affected when phosphorylation occurs along one of these specific sites (for example serine 396 and 404). (From Lucke-Wold BP et al. *J Neurotrauma*. Jul 1;31(13):1129–38, 2014.)

on overall tau deposition severity.[5,11,107,108] There were a total of four different stages and each was determined by extent of gross macroscopic and microscopic findings. A fascinating observation is that the severity of pathology correlates with the number of years played in contact sports (Table 9.1).[11] It was proposed that earlier stages of the disease with low tau burden could possibly be reversible and not lead to chronic neurological symptoms, but this notion assumes that CTE occurs sequentially through these stages. But, without the ability for in vivo prospective characterization, there is no evidence to support this argument.

Co-existing proteinopathies/ neurodegerative diseases in CTE

Besides tau accumulation, the occurrence of supplementary cellular deposits such as β-amyloid, TDP-43, and α-synuclein in confirmed CTE cases is becoming better understood as more diagnosed CTE cases are examined. Since the diagnosis of CTE is dependent on the distribution of tau, these proteinopathies are not a primary distinguishing feature for diagnosis of CTE, but do appear to coexist as a secondary feature in a large percentage of cases. Regarding this overlap of specific protein deposition with other

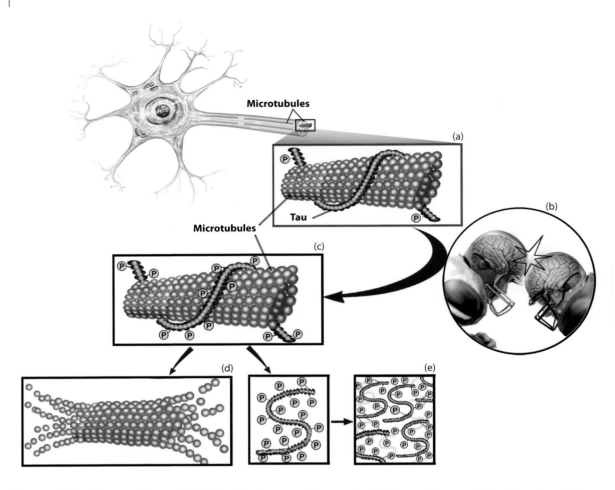

Figure 9.5 **Cartoon schematic depicting development of tauopathy.** (a) Tau protein associated with and providing stability to the microtubule fiber within an axon of a neuron. (b) A concussive or subconcussive injury occurs leading to primary and secondary neuronal injury. (c) The stressed state of the neuron leads to a preference of hyperphosphorylated tau. (d) Hyperphosphorylation destabilizes the microtubule fiber with dissociation of the tau. (e) Non soluble hyperphosphorylated tau fragments then aggregate to form neurofibrillary tangles and neuropil threads.

neurodegenerative diseases like Alzheimer's, Parkinson's, and amyotrophic lateral sclerosis, the assessment of confirmed CTE diagnoses and retrospective review of these patients' clinical course has led to an appreciation of these similar diseases co-occurring with CTE. Stein et al. noted that only 63% of their diagnosed CTE cases were considered "pure CTE," without another neurodegenerative co-diagnosis.[5,10]

Next, we will review these secondary characteristics of CTE histology, specifically amyloid, TDP-43, and α-synuclein and their relation to the likely noncoincidental overlap with co-occurring neurodegenerative diseases and CTE (Table 9.2[109]).

β-Amyloid and Alzheimer's disease

The β-Amyloid precursor protein (APP) is a cell adhesion protein found in the membrane of normal neurons that aids in the movement of molecules (axonal transport).[102] Following cellular stress/injury, β-APP becomes cleaved forming β amyloid, which aggregates to form plaques.[101] Amyloid plaques are a common pathological feature of normal aging, but are the histological finding in Alzheimer's disease (AD). AD is a neurodegenerative dementia associated with an accumulation of tau and amyloid, in the form of neurofibrillary tangles and neuritic β-amyloid plaques.[101,110–112] Though

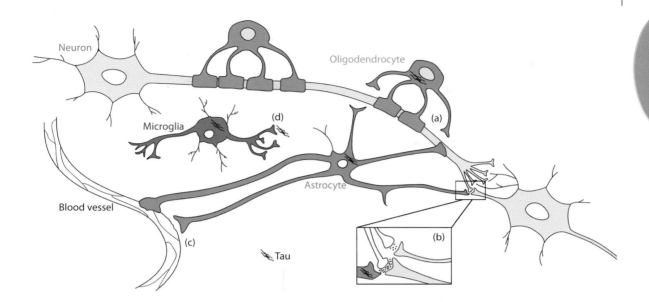

Figure 9.6 Schematic of functional consequences associated with tau pathology in glial cells. Tau overexpression disrupts oligodendrocyte (blue) and astrocyte (green) physiology and has been shown to lead to deficits in (a) myelin sheath integrity, (b) glutamate buffering at the synapse, and (c) maintenance of the BBB. These consequences are associated with neuronal degenerative changes and neuronal death. (d) Microglial cells (purple) have been shown to contribute to the spread of tau pathology across brain regions. (From Kahlson MA, Colodner KJ. *J Exp Neurosci*. Feb 10;9(Suppl 2):43–50, 2016.)

perivascular and sulcal depth tau accumulations are pathognomonic for CTE, a high prevalence of β-amyloid deposits has also been seen in CTE. McKee et al. noted the presence of β-amyloid in 44% of her CTE cases, which was more frequently seen in older CTE patients (over 65 years old) or with more advanced disease.[8,10,113] Therefore, what distinguishes AD from CTE is not the protein accumulation, but its specific location of aggregation seen in the brain. Unlike CTE, AD does not have the typical random perivascular or sulcal depth tau predominance, but rather, is found diffusely in a more orderly laminar distribution throughout the brain.[10,107,114] Also, though CTE is shown to have amyloid deposition, AD has more prominent neuritic amyloid plaques in comparison.[101,110]

It has been postulated that the inflammatory cascade that initiates the stereotypical tauopathy of CTE could also initiate the characteristic amyloid and tauopathy deposition in AD in the same patient.[115,116] It is currently unknown if this trigger leads to the development of AD in someone who would not have developed this disease without a history of head injury, or if the insult causes earlier onset in someone already susceptible to developing AD-like changes. A fascinating study by Tajiri et al., in 2013, used genetically engineered mice that were susceptible to developing AD. Following mild TBI, the susceptible mice were found to have an earlier onset of β-amyloid deposits leading to earlier cognitive symptoms in comparison to the mice that also received mild TBI, but were not genetically susceptible.[117]

Though the above argument appears pathophysiologically plausible, epidemiological studies have provided mixed results regarding the correlation between AD and TBI.[118] A review of 811,622 Swedish military cadets found no association between the clinical diagnosis of AD and a history of both mild and severe TBI.[119] In contrast, a meta-analysis of AD patients[120] and a retrospective review of NFL football players[121] did find a correlation between TBI and AD. Other studies found a similar association but only when the TBI occurred after 65 years old,[122] the TBI was associated with loss of consciousness,[75,102,116,123–130] or the TBI was of more moderate to severe nature.[111,124,128,130] A great limitation to most of these studies is that

Table 9.1 Description of McKee et al.'s Four Stages of CTE

Stage	Macroscopic Abnormalities (ventricular enlargement, cerebral and mammillary body atrophy, pallor of substantia nigra)	Septal Defects (cavum septum pellucidum, septal fenestrations)	Presence of β–Amyloid	Location of Neurofibrillary Tangles and Neuropil Threads	Schematic of Tau Distribution
1	Minimal	None	None	Focal areas, predominately perivascular and sulcal depths	
2	50%	50%	None	Multiple foci, with superficial extension	
3	Most cases, mild	50%	13%	Diffuse spread, involving the mesial temporal structures and 33% with cerebellar involvement. Spares rolandic and cingulate gyrus.	
4	Majority of cases, severe	66%	Not mentioned directly but states that 12% of cases had comorbid Alzheimer's Disease	Dense, widespread deposition	

Source: Table inserts from Stein TD et al. *Alzheimer's Research & Therapy.* 6:4. Copyright © 2014 BioMed Central Ltd.

Table 9.2 Classic Protein Aggregates Associated with Specific Neurodegenerative Diseases

Neurodegenerative Disease	Primary Histological Proteinopathy
Chronic Traumatic Encephalopathy	Primary: neurofibrillary tangles, hyperphosphorylated tau, and neuropil threads in sulcal depths and around *perivascular spaces* in a *patchy* distribution pattern Secondary: • Amyloid (52% of CTE patients, associated with older age)[113] • TDP-43 • α−synuclein
Alzheimer's disease	Neuritic β-amyloid plaques, neurofibrillary tangles, neuropil threads in a laminar and *orderly* distribution, and/or TDP-43
Parkinson's disease	α-synuclein
Amyotrophic lateral sclerosis	TDP-43

the diagnosis of AD was based solely on clinical criteria and not neuropathological specimens.[81]

Another proposed correlation between AD and CTE is the APOE4 allele. The presence of the APOE4 allele is a known risk factor for AD. It has been seen previously that a greater presence of this allele exists in individuals exposed to chronic head trauma and this also correlated with a reduction in cognitive test scores following injury[131] and an increased severity in chronic neurological deficits.[132] However, extensive investigations by McKee et al. (68 total CTE cases) and Maroon et al. (80 total CTE cases), did not show any statistical difference in presence of the APOE4 gene in the cohort of confirmed CTE cases compared to the general population.[9,11] Therefore, further research is needed to determine if there is an association between the presence of the APOE4 allele and CTE.

TDP-43 and amyotrophic lateral sclerosis

Similar to β−amyloid, TDP-43 is also seen in CTE but not required for a diagnosis of CTE. TDP-43 resides within the nucleus and is believed to regulate gene expression. In disease states, phosphorylated TDP-43 is found as cytoplasmic aggregates.[133] It is the main proteinopathy associated with amyotrophic lateral sclerosis (ALS) and in some cases of frontotemporal lobar degeneration (FTLD), as well as a secondary feature in Alzheimer's, Parkinson's, and Huntington's disease.[134,135]

Similar to amyloid, TDP-43 appears to be more prevalent in advanced cases of CTE, where over 50% of stage 1 and virtually all stage 4 cases of CTE displayed TDP-43 accumulations.[5,10] McKee et al. described three cases (10% of cohort) of patients diagnosed with CTE who had extensive

TDP-43 deposition; interestingly, they also had the classic upper and lower motor neuron clinical symptoms of ALS (muscle weakness and atrophy along with spasticity).[107,135] Multiple epidemiological studies have shown as much as a three to four fold increased risk to development of ALS in the setting of repeat head injuries, but this has not been a consistent finding.[121,136–138] Similar to AD, the causation between TBI and ALS may be linked through the progressive inflammatory state, following repetitive head injuries, that leads to protein aggregation (either tau, amyloid, or TDP-43).

α−Synuclein and Parkinson's disease

Last, α-synuclein has also been found in 22% of CTE cases.[11] α−Synuclein is a protein that exists normally in postsynaptic neuronal terminals. Parkinson's disease is the most common disease associated with aggregates of α−synuclein, occurring in the substantia nigra as lewy bodies.[139] A review by Gardner et al. of 52,393 patients over the age of 55 who presented to the ED, following either a mild or moderate/severe TBI, were found to be at a 24% and 50% increased risk of developing PD, respectively.[139] One could argue possible bias and challenges with determining causation because, for example, say a patient was not yet diagnosed with PD but had early cardinal signs of bradykinesia and postural instability making them more susceptible to TBI. Further, a case control study of 196 PD patients by Bower et al. also demonstrated an increased frequency of head trauma in comparison to the general public.[140] Further studies need to be performed to understand the relationship between TBI and PD.

Laboratory evidence and proposed molecular mechanism of CTE

As stated above, the manifestation of tau protein aggregates in the perivascular space and sulcal depths, occasionally with coexistent amyloid, TDP-43, and α–synuclein, was established as the pathological identification of CTE following neuropathological exploration.[98] It is believed that concussive/subconcussive blows produce an acceleration-deceleration force upon the movable brain within the skull.[8] This slosh effect leads to primary stretching and tearing of axons and white matter tracts, along with an insinuating secondary injury of cerebral/neuronal edema, metabolic derangements, and an inflammatory cascade as discussed in Chapter 2. When this adverse state is placed into perpetual motion through repeated injury, ensuing injury occurs and is believed to be the cause of CTE.[73,96,107,141,142] Through our knowledge of other neurodegenerative diseases (AD and PD), clinical scientists assumed that a neuronal insult could signal protein aggregation. However, it was unknown if concussion/subconcussions could be the specific initiator for the pathology that has been observed epidemiologically.

Research labs have validated that only through repetitive, and not single, mild TBI, could tau become phosphorylated and aggregate.[34,113,143] It was shown that repetitive acceleration-deceleration injury also caused β–amyloid accumulation in the mouse,[144] swine,[145] and rabbit.[146] Through different euthanasia time points, it appeared that β–amyloid plaques developed more acutely following TBI

while neurofibrillary tangles were a more chronic finding.[101] This may explain why neurofibrillary tangles, hyperphosphorylated tau, and neuropil threads have emerged as the diagnostic criteria for CTE. Lastly, Yang et al. was able to demonstrate in the rat cortical impact model that TDP-43 cleavage occurred after TBI, producing neurotoxicity.[133] In clinical studies, patients with severe TBI and following mild concussion had significant histological staining for APP and β–amyloid deposition.[99,147] Therefore, these preclinical and clinical studies scientifically validate that even mild head injuries can initiate the cascade leading to tau, amyloid, and TDP-43 accumulation.

What was most interesting among these outcomes was that the instigator to develop a neurodegenerative disease appeared to be a more severe or repetitive injury, not occurring following a single mild injury. This established a theory of clinical threshold, in which there exists a certain critical threshold of protein aggregation that causes symptomatology.[148] It assumes that all healthy individuals accumulate protein plaques with aging, but never reach the critical threshold level to display symptomatology. If the person is exposed to a single severe TBI or repetitive mild TBIs, this pushes them closer, if not past, the critical threshold and symptoms become present (Figure 9.7[148]).

In the normal physiological state, tau becomes phosphorylated and unphosphorylated by kinases. The functioning of these kinases is hampered by the release of excitatory neurotransmitters, like

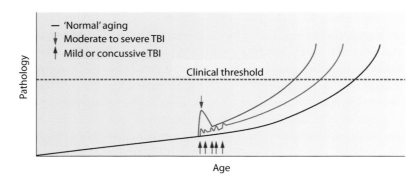

Figure 9.7 Neurodegenerative progression in a (a) normal aging individual, (b) following repetitive mild TBIs or (c) severe TBI. Once the threshold is reached, clinical symptoms appear. (Reprinted by permission from Macmillan Publishers Ltd: *Nat Rev Neurol*, Smith DH et al. Chronic neuropathologies of single and repetitive TBI: substrates of dementia? Apr;9(4):211–21, copyright 2013.)

glutamate, and the presence of reactive oxygen species due to focal microhemorrhage.[149] This leads to the preference of tau to remain hyperphosphorylated, detach from the microtubule, microtubule/neuronal destabilization, and accumulation of the non-soluble tau products.[104,142]

In recent studies, microglia have been found to have a role in phagocytosis of these tau accumulations, but the chronic inflammatory state following injury affects this mechanism for aggregate clearance.[34,43,150–152] It has been suggested that repetitive TBI and this perpetual chronic inflammatory state obstructs the microglial's ability to clear protein accumulations.[101,102] As the neuroinflammatory state effects aggregate clearance, increasing tau deposition and depleting the brain reserve, the threshold for clinical symptomatology is reached, and CTE becomes apparent.[3,153–155] Interestingly, in a preclinical study, through the use of monoclonal antibodies that reduce inflammatory cells, there was a reduction in APP accumulation and neuronal loss following TBI.[156]

But, what happens in those individuals that receive a head injury that does not push them past the critical threshold—can they still develop the disease? More recently, preclinical studies have begun to challenge this theory of disease evolution, specifically looking at the rate of protein aggregation following injury. With local injection of non-soluble tau or amyloid, researchers have found diffuse protein aggregation and deposition concerning for a "prion-like" effect, leading to exponential accumulation.[101,157–162] This indicates that the pathological protein aggregate can then influence the soluble, nonpathological protein and transform into the non-soluble state. If tau deposition has a prion-like effect, the inciting injury will induce immediate alterations in tau. Even after the removal/prevention of further injuries, the tau aggregates will influence conversion of the normal tau, propagating neuronal destabilization and neurotoxicity.

McKee et al. stated that, in their cohort, the total number of years playing football was actually more significant for development of CTE than total reported concussions;[11] other studies have demonstrated that up to 16% of confirmed CTE were not known to have a history of concussion.[81] It is unknown to what extent this can be attributed to recall bias, but this evidence potentially alludes to the fact that accumulation of subconcussions is actually more detrimental than concussions itself. This may be due to the fact that the clinical symptoms of concussion cause the player to remove him/herself from activity allowing this neuroinflammatory state to subside prior to repeat injury. With subconcussive blows, the player continues to participate in their sport propagating secondary injury, and producing a chronic neuroinflammatory state that can lead to perpetual tau accumulation and progressive neurodegeneration.[88,91,163,164]

Symptomatology of CTE

Due to the neurodegenerative nature of CTE, an initial injury and resultant secondary injury causes tau deposition and pathological changes. At a certain threshold of disease burden, symptoms become clinically evident. For this reason, there is a latent period between injury and clinical presentation.[95] Interestingly, Stern, McKee, and Omalu et al. all found that about 10% of histologically diagnosed cases of CTE were asymptomatic on retrospective review, potentially dying prior to symptom onset.[3,11,165]

The average age of symptom appearance occurs around 40 to 45 years of age, roughly 14.5 years after retiring from sport.[11,81] Maroon et al. evaluated the 153 known CTE cases and found that the average age of death occurred between 60 and 69 years (range 17–98), which is for below the national average of 78.8.[9,166] Through reviewing all cases of CTE, it became evident that CTE had a different clinical presentation in comparison to previously documented cases of dementia pugilistica. Multiple groups began to distinguish "classic" versus "modern" CTE: classic CTE had more pronounced motor/Parkinsonian-type symptoms as seen in boxers, versus modern CTE presented with neuropsychiatric and behavioral symptoms—with progression to dementia—seen more in contact sports (specifically football).[97,167]

The symptomatology of "modern" CTE was found, mostly through retrospective reviews of autopsy-confirmed CTE cases, to be dominated by three cardinal features: cognitive, behavioral, and mood impairments (Table 9.3).[12,92,109,118,165,168]

◆ Cognitive symptoms: memory difficulties, dementia, decreased attention and concentration
◆ Behavioral: personality changes, violence, erratic/impulsive behavior, suicidality
◆ Mood: depression, hopelessness, disinhibition, anger, irritability, labile mood

Stern et al. further classified two distinct phenotypes based on which symptoms were more prominent at onset within their cohort (n = 36).[165] It was seen that patients that developed first behavior or mood symptoms typically had an earlier onset of presentation (average age of death, 51 years). These patients would eventually develop cognitive symptoms with later progression of the disease state. The second phenotype typically was dominated by cognitive symptoms. This group was noted to have a later presentation (average age of death, 69 years), and typically did not develop behavior or mood symptoms.

As previously discussed, there may be a correlation between Alzheimer's disease and CTE, but this is still debated.[169,170] What appears to be more convincing from an epidemiological standpoint is increased risk of the younger onset of cognitive

impairment and dementia with CTE, specifically a non-Alzheimer's type.[58,119,148,155] It was found in one large military cohort study of 188,700 soldiers, there existed a 60% increased risk in dementia over 9 years following a TBI.[171] Other groups have found similar results but only with specific features. An increased risk of dementia occurred under the following circumstances: only following a moderate to severe TBI,[172] in retired NFL players who experienced more than three concussions,[58] if the concussion resulted in persistent neurological deficits,[173] or if the TBI occurred only at a young or older age,[122,174] however, this finding of age at first exposure has not been consistent.[175] Following a meta-analysis of 78,000 mild TBI patients, Godbolt et al. determined that there was still limited evidence to support for or against the association of TBI and dementia.[174]

Originally acknowledged in case reports by Omalu et al., it was noted that there appeared to be a correlation between suicide and CTE.[85] Bryan et al. analyzed a military cohort and found that there existed an increased risk of suicide as TBI exposure increased.[176] Maroon et al. looked specifically at all confirmed CTE cases and noted the prevalence of suicide to be 11.7%, an increase from the

Table 9.3 Detailed Cognitive, Behavioral, Mood, and Motor Symptoms Associated with CTE

Cognitive Features	Behavioral Features	Mood Features	Motor Features
Memory impairment[a]	Physical violence[a]	Depression[a]	Ataxia[b]
Executive dysfunction[a]	Verbal violence[a]	Hopelessness[a]	Dysarthria[b]
Impaired attention[a]	Explosivity[a]	Suicidality[b]	Parkinsonism[b]
Dysgraphia[b]	Loss of control[a]	Anxiety[b]	Gait[b]
Lack of insight	Short fuse[a]	Fearfulness[b]	Tremor[b]
Perseveration	Impulsivity[b]	Irritability[b]	Masked facies[b]
Language difficulties	Paranoid delusions[b]	Apathy[b]	Rigidity[b]
Dementia	Aggression	Loss of interest[b]	Weakness
Alogia	Rage	Labile emotions	Spasticity
Visuospatial difficulties	Inappropriate speech	Fatigue	Clonus
Cognitive impairment	Boastfulness	Flat affect	
Reduced intelligence	Childish behavior	Insomnia	
	Socially inappropriate	Mania	
	Disinhibited behavior	Euphoria	
	Personality changes	Mood swings	
	Psychosis	Prolix	
	Social isolation		

Source: Reproduced with permission from Montenegro PH et al. *Brain Pathology Brain Pathol.* 2015 May;25(3):304–17.
[a] Core diagnostic clinical feature, defined as any feature that appeared in 70% or more of the neuropathologically confirmed chronic traumatic encephalopathy (CTE) cases without comorbid disease.
[b] Supportive diagnostic feature, defined as any feature that appeared in neuropathologically confirmed CTE cases without comorbid disease.

national average of 1.5% to 4.8%, but likely due to the small cohort of CTE cases, no significance was found.[9] Until prospective CTE data is obtained, it will be difficult to determine the true statistical effect of CTE on suicidality.[177]

Other epidemiological studies have reviewed the connection between CTE and depressive symptoms.[59,178,179] In a review of retired football players, roughly 10% have been found to have the diagnosis of depression, which associates with the number of previous concussions.[59,178] Further, Strain et al. obtained MRI imaging on 26 ex-NFL players of which 5 had depressive symptoms, 21 were without, and compared them to 22 normal controls without depression.[180] Interestingly, white matter injury within the forceps minor (tract connecting the frontal lobes) on DTI was 100% sensitive and 95% specific for identifying those athletes with depression. The culmination of these results enforce the notion that repetitive head injuries and resultant white matter injury can potentially increase the risk of future clinically diagnosed depression. In combination with the fact that repetitive head trauma increases the risk of CTE, it is very easy to suggest that CTE and depression coexist.[59,178]

Clinical diagnosis of CTE

Currently, is only a neuropathological diagnosis, and therefore can only be diagnosed on postmortem analysis. But a groups have developed clinical criteria to assist in premortem diagnosis, but the criteria have not been prospectively contested. Jordan et al. proposed conditions such that they stratify a patient into "definite, probable, possible, and improbable CTE" based on clinical presentation and lack of any alternative diagnosis. "Definite" CTE does require a pathological diagnosis consistent with our current diagnostic criteria.[181] Victoroff et al. also proposed a set of clinical signs and symptoms for CTE diagnosis, but without the requirement of postmortem tissue.[182]

Due to the limitations of Victoroff and Jordan's diagnostic clinical criteria for CTE, Montenigro et al. took an intriguing stance in that they proposed a scheme to diagnose what they termed "traumatic encephalopathy syndrome, (TES)" (Table 9.4).[168] The emphasis was to strictly describe the clinical progression that has been typically seen

in patients diagnosed with CTE. They chose not to use the term CTE because CTE is considered a histological entity. Therefore, use of "syndrome" was chosen to denote this as a description of a clinical, not neuropathological, diagnosis. Also, they felt that CTE was not appropriate because the use of the word "chronic" with a connotation of stability, does not correctly describe the progressive clinical course that is seen in patients ultimately diagnosed with CTE. The diagnosis of TES requires five specific criteria (Table 9.4). Based on the dominant presenting symptom, the patient is subgrouped into either: TES behavioral/mood variant, TES cognitive variant, TES mixed variant, or TES dementia. The variants then can have an additional modifier if motor features are present. The group does caution that TES has unknown specificity for pathological diagnosis of CTE and recommends this classification scheme to only be used for research purposes.

Currently, there are no guidelines, due to lack of prospective evidence, to assist a clinician in the diagnosis of CTE premortem. If CTE is suspected, it is necessary to obtain a thorough history, specifically detailing occurrence of repetitive head trauma, and neurological exam with focus on the clinical hallmarks noted above, and also to rule out other possible neurological and psychiatric disorders. Laboratory (B12, folate, TSH, RPR/syphilis, HIV testing) and imaging studies (MRI) should be obtained in order to rule out other conditions associated with dementia or behavioral symptoms. Imaging may also give clues of repetitive trauma such as cerebral atrophy, cavum septum pellucidum, thinning of the corpus

Table 9.4 Clinical Criteria Developed by Montenigro et al. for the Diagnosis of Traumatic Encephalopathy Syndrome (TES)

Patient Must Exhibit these 5 Criteria:	• History of Repetitive Head Trauma • >12 months of symptoms • 1 core clinical feature (cognitive, behavioral, or mood symptom) • >1 supportive feature (impulsivity, anxiety, apathy, paranoia, suicidality, headache, motor signs, decline • Rule out all other neurological disorders delayed onset

callosum (classic findings of dementia pugilistica) (see Figure 9.8), but these findings are not specific.[183–185] Another commonly confused term with CTE is post-traumatic encephalopathy (PTE). PTE is secondary to a traumatic insult to the brain that leads to brain tissue loss, which can be visualized on cranial imaging. Unlike CTE, this is not a

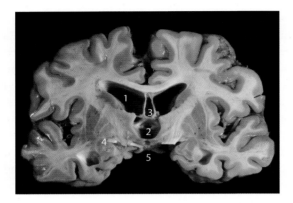

Figure 9.8 Cavum septum pellucidum: (3) a cystic cavity that exists within the septum pellucidum of the brain (2). This has been seen most commonly in dementia pugilistica, advanced stages of CTE, but also is a normal variant in humans. Cavum septum pellucidum: a cystic cavity.

progressive neurodegenerative disease associated with protein accumulations. Further advanced neuroimaging modalities (PET and fMRI), are purely investigational and currently not recommended for routine clinical use.[42]

Future directions in CTE

There are numerous obstacles that arise due to the challenges of prospective design in a disease that is only diagnosed postmortem. As mentioned above, clinical criteria has been developed in efforts to stratify which patients, based on symptoms, are more or less likely to be diagnosed with CTE. This will not be established as a valid clinical tool until more patients who have been evaluated and assigned to a "definite, probable, possible, and improbable CTE" subgroup or "TES" diagnosis is compared in concert with neuropathology. For this reason, there has been a push to develop premortem modalities to diagnosis CTE.[186] An exciting field of study is through the use of biomarkers for prognosis and outcome predictions following TBI. This will be discussed in more detail in Chapter 10, but some works have specifically shown potential for CTE prognostications. Ho et al. found in 2012 that there was an increase in serum

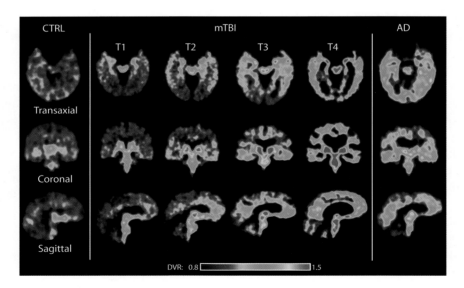

Figure 9.9 Distribution of signal intensity through the use of a tau and amyloid PET radionuclide. Recognize the low signal intensity within the healthy controls (CTRL) versus the graded progression of tau/amyloid signal within the cortical, subcortical, midbrain, and mesial temporal structures in the mild TBI patient (mTBI). The distribution of signal is also different in comparison between the mTBI and AD patient. (From Barrio JR et al. *Proc Natl Acad Sci U S A.* Apr 21;112(16):E2039–47, 2015.)

monocyte chemotactic protein-1 (MCP) following TBI, and this correlated with those more likely to be diagnosed with AD on postmortem studies.[187] Another group found that following severe TBI (n = 21) versus control group (n = 15), CSF samples in the severe TBI group were found to have a significant increase in TDP-43.[133] Further work and postmortem studies would need to be performed to determine if this has a potential predictive value for development of CTE, but it is interesting to note the overlap with known associations with AD and even TDP-43 accumulations in CTE. Biomarkers in TBI are in their infancy; similar literature regarding their predictive value for development of CTE is sparse.

With the development of radionuclide tracers for tau and amyloid, the possibility of premortem diagnosis of CTE through positron emission tomography (PET imaging) is becoming a realistic possibility. Starting in 2013, use of this technology was originally applied in very small cohorts of NFL players[188,189] and also has more recently shown to be able to predict between a patient with and without dementia who suffered from a TBI, based on amyloid signal.[190] In 2015, Barrio et al. published a landmark paper regarding this technology. A total of 14 mild TBI patients and 28 healthy controls received PET imaging with the use of a tau and amyloid marker. They found a significant difference in the mild TBI patients in the areas of the frontal cortex, subcortical structures, amygdala, and dorsal midbrain in comparison to the healthy controls. Also, the signal distribution varied distinctly from the AD patients (n = 24) mirroring what has been seen histologically (Figure 9.9[191]). Another interesting feature was that there appeared to be four distinct phenotypes of progressive increasing signal in the brainstem, amygdala, and also in an anterior to posterior cortical direction which intuitively resembles the biomechanics of an anterior/posterior acceleration-deceleration injury with the brainstem acting as a fulcrum (Figure 9.10[191]).

Conclusion

Stated in 2013 by the Zurich Guidelines: "Clinicians need to be mindful of the potential for long-term problems in the management of all athletes. However, it was agreed that chronic traumatic encephalopathy (CTE) represents a distinct tauopathy with an unknown incidence in athletic populations. It was further agreed that an exact cause-and-effect relationship has not been fully demonstrated between CTE and concussions or exposure to contact sports. At present, the interpretation of causation in the modern CTE case studies should proceed cautiously."[42,192] Since the release of this statement, there has been more evidence in regard to the histological diagnosis of CTE, retrospective review of these players developing a typical history of symptomatology and comorbid diseases, and even a proposed pathophysiological mechanism for the development of this progressive proteinopathy.

Though a large percentage of NFL players that have died and donated their brains for pathological examination have been diagnosed with CTE,

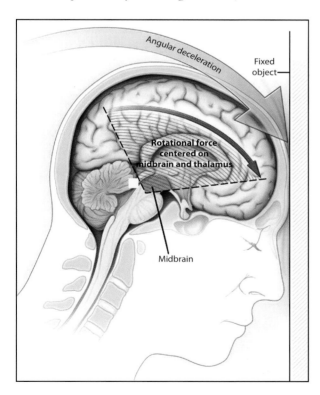

Figure 9.10 Proposed hypothesis of increased PET signal in the dorsal midbrain. Following an acceleration-deceleration force, the brainstem acts as a fulcrum as the movable brain sloshes forward and back within the fixed skull.

not all players with exposure to repetitive head trauma have autopsy-confirmed CTE.[5,8,11,193] McKee, Omalu, and Hazrati's reported from their earlier CTE cohorts that 35% (n = 6), 20% (17), and 50% (3) were negative for CTE even though they had a history of multiple TBIs.[8,11,193] This current literature has contradictions and obvious limitations possibly due to its retrospective nature, inherent selection bias (players with symptoms are more likely to donate their brain for analysis),[97] recall/reporting bias (unable to recount number of concussions), and also inability to truly quantify total subconcussive exposures;[194,195] this can only be resolved by further prospective trials.[186,196,197] Nevertheless, the growing body of evidence continues to reflect a correlation between subconcussive injuries and the increased incidence of CTE endorsed by not only animal, but also human data. Only through recognition of this disease and continued research can we begin to tackle questions such as:

◆ What is the threshold of injury (severity and frequency) required to develop tauopathy? What are the other genetic or environmental factors that influence this?
◆ What is the safest return-to-activity measures to reduce the risk of CTE and how should this be influenced by development of post-concussive syndrome?
◆ What is the relationship between burden of protein aggregates seen neuropathologically and correlation with symptoms?
◆ Is there a pure form of CTE and how does this relate to other neurodegenerative diseases?

Many have agreed that caution should always be taken when analyzing results of retrospective data and call towards prospective studies, however, as the Zurich Guidelines state, the present findings should not be ignored or negated.[9,42,198–200] It is a disservice to the athlete and their health to ignore the growing body of CTE literature. It is the responsibility of the medical provider to educate all athletes on the potential risks of chronic head injuries and adopt into their practice teachings of injury prevention and proper return to activity based on our current understanding. Hopefully through stronger studies and development of clinical diagnostic tests, will we be able to definitively care for the concussed athlete through sound evidence-based medicine.

References

1. Omalu BI, DeKosky ST, Minster RL, Kamboh MI, Hamilton RL, Wecht CH. Chronic traumatic encephalopathy in a National Football League player. *Neurosurgery*. 2005; 57(1): 128–134.

2. Martin J. NFL acknowledges CTE link with football. Now what? 2016; http://www.cnn.com/2016/03/15/health/nfl-cte-link/. Accessed September 17, 2016, 2016.

3. Bailes JE, Petraglia AL, Omalu BI, Nauman E, Talavage T. Role of subconcussion in repetitive mild traumatic brain injury. *Journal of Neurosurgery*. 2013; 119(5): 1235–1245.

4. Bailes JE, Dashnaw ML, Petraglia AL, Turner RC. Cumulative effects of repetitive mild traumatic brain injury. *Progress in Neurological Surgery*. 2014; 28: 50–62.

5. Stein TD, Alvarez VE, McKee AC. Chronic traumatic encephalopathy: a spectrum of neuropathological changes following repetitive brain trauma in athletes and military personnel. *Alzheimer's Research & Therapy*. 2014; 6(1): 4.

6. Broglio SP, Eckner JT, Martini D, Sosnoff JJ, Kutcher JS, Randolph C. Cumulative head impact burden in high school football. *Journal of Neurotrauma*. 2011; 28(10): 2069–2078.

7. Guskiewicz KM, Mihalik JP. Biomechanics of sport concussion: quest for the elusive injury threshold. *Exercise and Sport Sciences Reviews*. 2011; 39(1): 4–11.

8. Omalu B, Bailes J, Hamilton RL et al. Emerging histomorphologic phenotypes of chronic traumatic encephalopathy in American athletes. *Neurosurgery*. 2011; 69(1): 173–183.

9. Maroon JC, Winkelman R, Bost J, Amos A, Mathyssek C, Miele V. Chronic traumatic encephalopathy in contact sports: a systematic review of all reported pathological cases. *PLoS One*. 2015; 10(2): e0117338.

10. McKee AC, Stein TD, Kiernan PT, Alvarez VE. The neuropathology of chronic traumatic encephalopathy. *Brain Pathology (Zurich, Switzerland)*. 2015; 25(3): 350–364.

11. McKee AC, Stern RA, Nowinski CJ et al. The spectrum of disease in chronic traumatic encephalopathy. *Brain*. 2013; 136(Pt 1): 43–64.

12. Bernick C, Banks S. What boxing tells us about repetitive head trauma and the brain. *Alzheimer's Research & Therapy*. 2013; 5(3): 23.

13. Zhang L, Yang KH, King AI. A proposed injury threshold for mild traumatic brain injury. *Journal of Biochemical Engineering*. 2004; 126(2): 226–236.

14. Broglio SP, Schnebel B, Sosnoff JJ et al. Biomechanical properties of concussions in high school football. *Medicine and Science in Sports and Exercise*. 2010; 42(11): 2064–2071.

15. Beckwith JG, Greenwald RM, Chu JJ et al. Head impact exposure sustained by football players on days of diagnosed concussion. *Medicine and Science in Sports and Exercise*. 2013; 45(4): 737–746.

16. Funk JR, Duma SM, Manoogian SJ, Rowson S. Biomechanical risk estimates for mild traumatic brain injury. *Annual Proceedings/Association for the Advancement of Automotive Medicine Association for the Advancement of Automotive Medicine*. 2007; 51: 343–361.

17. Guskiewicz KM, Mihalik JP, Shankar V et al. Measurement of head impacts in collegiate football players: relationship between head impact biomechanics and acute clinical outcome after concussion. *Neurosurgery*. 2007; 61(6): 1244–1252.

18. Greenwald RM, Gwin JT, Chu JJ, Crisco JJ. Head impact severity measures for evaluating mild traumatic brain injury risk exposure. *Neurosurgery*. 2008; 62(4): 789–798.

19. Crisco JJ, Wilcox BJ, Machan JT et al. Magnitude of head impact exposures in individual collegiate football players. *Journal of Applied Biomechanics*. 2012; 28(2): 174–183.

20. Pellman EJ, Viano DC, Tucker AM, Casson IR, Waeckerle JF. Concussion in professional football: reconstruction of game impacts and injuries. *Neurosurgery*. 2003; 53(4): 799–812.

21. Shultz SR, MacFabe DF, Foley KA, Taylor R, Cain DP. Sub-concussive brain injury in the Long-Evans rat induces acute neuroinflammation in the absence of behavioral impairments. *Behavioural Brain Research*. 2012; 229(1): 145–152.

22. Creeley CE, Wozniak DF, Bayly PV, Olney JW, Lewis LM. Multiple episodes of mild traumatic brain injury result in impaired cognitive performance in mice. *Academic Emergency Medicine*. 2004; 11(8): 809–819.

23. Kane MJ, Angoa–Perez M, Briggs DI, Viano DC, Kreipke CW, Kuhn DM. A mouse model of human repetitive mild traumatic brain injury. *Journal of Neuroscience Methods*. 2012; 203(1): 41–49.

24. Shitaka Y, Tran HT, Bennett RE et al. Repetitive closed-skull traumatic brain injury in mice causes persistent multifocal axonal injury and microglial reactivity. *Journal of Neuropathology and Experimental neurology*. 2011; 70(7): 551–567.

25. Mannix R, Berglass J, Berkner J et al. Chronic gliosis and behavioral deficits in mice following repetitive mild traumatic brain injury. *Journal of Neurosurgery*. 2014; 121(6): 1342–1350.

26. Aungst SL, Kabadi SV, Thompson SM, Stoica BA, Faden AI. Repeated mild traumatic brain injury causes chronic neuro-inflammation, changes in hippocampal synaptic plasticity, and associated cognitive deficits. *Journal of Cerebral Blood Flow and Metabolism*. 2014; 34(7): 1223–1232.

27. Xu L, Nguyen JV, Lehar M et al. Repetitive mild traumatic brain injury with impact acceleration in the mouse: Multifocal axonopathy, neuroinflammation, and neurodegeneration in the visual system. *Experimental Neurology*. 2014.

28. Goddeyne C, Nichols J, Wu C, Anderson T. Repetitive mild traumatic brain injury induces ventriculomegaly and cortical thinning in juvenile rats. *Journal of Neurophysiology*. 2015; 113(9): 3268–3280.

29. Bolton AN, Saatman KE. Regional neurodegeneration and gliosis are amplified by mild traumatic brain injury repeated at 24-hour intervals. *Journal of Neuropathology and Experimental Neurology*. 2014; 73(10): 933–947.

30. Laurer HL, Bareyre FM, Lee VM et al. Mild head injury increasing the brain's vulnerability to a second concussive impact. *Journal of Neurosurgery*. 2001; 95(5): 859–870.

31. Longhi L, Saatman KE, Fujimoto S et al. Temporal window of vulnerability to repetitive experimental concussive brain injury. *Neurosurgery*. 2005; 56(2): 364–374.

32. Friess SH, Ichord RN, Ralston J et al. Repeated traumatic brain injury affects composite cognitive function in piglets. *Journal of Neurotrauma*. 2009; 26(7): 1111–1121.

33. Raghupathi R, Mehr MF, Helfaer MA, Margulies SS. Traumatic axonal injury is exacerbated following repetitive closed head injury in the neonatal pig. *Journal of Neurotrauma*. 2004; 21(3): 307–316.

34. Petraglia AL, Plog BA, Dayawansa S et al. The pathophysiology underlying repetitive mild traumatic brain injury in a novel mouse model of chronic traumatic encephalopathy. *Surgical Neurology International*. 2014; 5: 184.

35. Mannix R, Meehan WP, Mandeville J et al. Clinical correlates in an experimental model of repetitive mild brain injury. *Annals of Neurology*. 2013; 74(1): 65–75.

36. Donovan V, Kim C, Anugerah AK et al. Repeated mild traumatic brain injury results in long-term white-matter disruption. *Journal of Cerebral Blood Flow Metabolism*. 2014; 34(4): 715–723.

37. Mouzon BC, Bachmeier C, Ferro A et al. Chronic neuropathological and neurobehavioral changes in a repetitive mild traumatic brain injury model. *Annals of Neurology*. 2014; 75(2): 241–254.

38. Huang L, Coats JS, Mohd-Yusof A et al. Tissue vulnerability is increased following repetitive mild traumatic brain injury in the rat. *Brain Research*. 2013; 1499: 109–120.

39. Weber JT. Experimental models of repetitive brain injuries. *Progress in Brain Research*. 2007; 161: 253–261.

40. Mayers LB. Outcomes of sport-related concussion among college athletes. *The Journal of Neuropsychiatry and Clinical Neurosciences*. 2013; 25(2): 115–119.

41. Lovell MR, Collins MW, Iverson GL et al. Recovery from mild concussion in high school athletes. *Journal of Neurosurgery*. 2003; 98(2): 296–301.

42. McCrory P, Meeuwisse W, Aubry M et al. Consensus statement on Concussion in Sport - The 4th International Conference on Concussion in Sport held in Zurich, November 2012. *Physical Therapy in Sport*. 2013; 14(2): e1–e13.

43. Coughlin JM, Wang Y, Munro CA et al. Neuroinflammation and brain atrophy in former NFL players: An in vivo multimodal imaging pilot study. *Neurobiology of Disease*. 2015; 74: 58–65.

44. Meier TB, Bellgowan PS, Bergamino M, Ling JM, Mayer AR. Thinner cortex in collegiate football players with, but not without, a self-reported history of concussion. *Journal of Neurotrauma*. 2015.

45. Strain JF, Womack KB, Didehbani N et al. Imaging correlates of memory and concussion history in retired national football league athletes. *The Journal of the American Medical Association Neurology*. 2015; 72(7): 773–780.

46. Singh R, Meier TB, Kuplicki R et al. Relationship of collegiate football experience and concussion with hippocampal volume and cognitive outcomes. *The Journal of the American Medical Association.* 2014; 311(18): 1883–1888.

47. Goswami R, Dufort P, Tartaglia MC et al. Frontotemporal correlates of impulsivity and machine learning in retired professional athletes with a history of multiple concussions. *Brain Structure & Function.* 2015.

48. Albaugh MD, Orr C, Nickerson JP et al. Postconcussion symptoms are associated with cerebral cortical thickness in healthy collegiate and preparatory school ice hockey players. *Journal of Pediatric.* 2015; 166(2): 394–400.e391.

49. Tysvaer AT, Sortland O, Storli OV, Lochen EA. [Head and neck injuries among Norwegian soccer players. A neurological, electroencephalographic, radiologic and neuropsychological evaluation]. *Tidsskrift for Den Norske Laegeforening.* 1992; 112(10): 1268–1271.

50. Ford JH, Giovanello KS, Guskiewicz KM. Episodic memory in former professional football players with a history of concussion: an event-related functional neuroimaging study. *Journal of Neurotrauma.* 2013; 30(20): 1683–1701.

51. Tremblay S, De Beaumont L, Henry LC et al. Sports concussions and aging: a neuroimaging investigation. *Cerebral Cortex.* 2013; 23(5): 1159–1166.

52. Johnson B, Neuberger T, Gay M, Hallett M, Slobounov S. Effects of subconcussive head trauma on the default mode network of the brain. *Journal of Neurotrauma.* 2014; 31(23): 1907–1913.

53. Gronwall D, Wrightson P. Cumulative effect of concussion. *Lancet (London, England).* 1975; 2(7943): 995–997.

54. Iverson GL, Gaetz M, Lovell MR, Collins MW. Cumulative effects of concussion in amateur athletes. *Brain Injury.* 2004; 18(5): 433–443.

55. Matser EJ, Kessels AG, Lezak MD, Jordan BD, Troost J. Neuropsychological impairment in amateur soccer players. *The Journal of the American Medical Association.* 1999; 282(10): 971–973.

56. Breedlove EL, Robinson M, Talavage TM et al. Biomechanical correlates of symptomatic and asymptomatic neurophysiological impairment in high school football. *Journal of Biomechanics.* 2012; 45(7): 1265–1272.

57. Randolph C, Karantzoulis S, Guskiewicz K. Prevalence and characterization of mild cognitive impairment in retired national football league players. *Journal of the International Neurophysocological Society.* 2013; 19(8): 873–880.

58. Guskiewicz KM, Marshall SW, Bailes J et al. Association between recurrent concussion and late-life cognitive impairment in retired professional football players. *Neurosurgery.* 2005; 57(4): 719–726.

59. Guskiewicz KM, Marshall SW, Bailes J et al. Recurrent concussion and risk of depression in retired professional football players. *Medicine and Science in Sports and Exercise.* 2007; 39(6): 903–909.

60. De Beaumont L, Tremblay S, Henry LC, Poirier J, Lassonde M, Theoret H. Motor system alterations in retired former athletes: the role of aging and concussion history. *BMC Neurology.* 2013; 13: 109.

61. Bazarian JJ, Zhu T, Zhong J et al. Persistent, long-term cerebral white matter changes after sports-related repetitive head impacts. *PLoS One.* 2014; 9(4): e94734.

62. Davenport EM, Whitlow CT, Urban JE et al. Abnormal white matter integrity related to head impact exposure in a season of high school varsity football. *Journal of Neurotrauma.* 2014; 31(19): 1617–1624.

63. McAllister TW, Ford JC, Flashman LA et al. Effect of head impacts on diffusivity measures in a cohort of collegiate contact sport athletes. *Neurology.* 2014; 82(1): 63–69.

64. Koerte IK, Ertl-Wagner B, Reiser M, Zafonte R Shenton ME. White matter integrity in the brains of professional soccer players without a symptomatic concussion. *The Journal of the American Medical Association.* 2012; 308(18): 1859–1861.

65. Lipton ML, Kim N, Zimmerman ME et al. Soccer heading is associated with white matter microstructural and cognitive abnormalities. *Radiology.* 2013; 268(3): 850–857.

66. Bazarian JJ, Zhu T, Blyth B, Borrino A, Zhong J. Subject-specific changes in brain white matter on diffusion tensor imaging after sports-related concussion. *Magnetic Resonance Imaging.* 2012; 30(2): 171–180.

67. Lin AP, Ramadan S, Stern RA et al. Changes in the neurochemistry of athletes with repetitive brain trauma: preliminary results using localized correlated spectroscopy. *Alzheimer's Research & Therapy.* 2015; 7(1): 13.

68. Koerte IK, Lin AP, Muehlmann M et al. Altered Neurochemistry in former professional soccer players without a history of concussion. *Journal of Neurotrauma.* 2015; 32(17): 1287–1293.

69. Abbas K, Shenk TE, Poole VN et al. Alteration of default mode network in high school football athletes due to repetitive subconcussive mild traumatic brain injury: a resting-state functional magnetic resonance imaging study. *Brain Connectivity.* 2015; 5(2): 91–101.

70. Talavage TM, Nauman EA, Breedlove EL et al. Functionally-detected cognitive impairment in high school football players without clinically-diagnosed concussion. *Journal of Neurotrauma.* 2014; 31(4): 327–338.

71. Courville CB. Punch drunk. Its pathogenesis and pathology on the basis of a verified case. *Bulletin of the Los Angeles Neurological Society.* 1962; 27: 160–168.

72. Hollnagel P. ["Punch-drunk" syndrome. Reports of 3 cases of chronic encephalopathy in young boxers]. *Ugeskrift for Laeger.* 1974; 136(51): 2871–2874.

73. Montenigro PH, Corp DT, Stein TD, Cantu RC, Stern RA. Chronic traumatic encephalopathy: historical origins and current perspective. *Annual Review of Clinical Psychology.* 2015; 11: 309–330.

74. Millspaugh J. Dementia Pugilistica. *United States Naval Medical Bulletin.* 1937; 35: 297–303.

75. Tokuda T, Ikeda S, Yanagisawa N, Ihara Y, Glenner GG. Re-examination of ex-boxers' brains using immunohistochemistry with antibodies to amyloid beta-protein and tau protein. *Acta Neuropathologica.* 1991; 82(4): 280–285.

76. Critchley M. Medical aspects of boxing, particularly from a neurological standpoint. *British Medical Journal.* 1957; 1: 357–362.

77. Petraglia AL, Bailes J, Day AL. *Handbook of Neurological Sports Medicine.* Human Kinetics; 2015.

78. Omalu BI, DeKosky ST, Hamilton RL et al. Chronic traumatic encephalopathy in a national football league player: part II. *Neurosurgery.* 2006; 59(5): 1086–1092.

79. Omalu BI, Hamilton RL, Kamboh MI, DeKosky ST, Bailes J. Chronic traumatic encephalopathy (CTE) in a National Football League Player: Case report and emerging medicolegal practice questions. *Journal of Forensic Nursing.* 2010; 6(1): 40–46.

80. Maroon JC, Winkelman R, Bost J, Amos A, Mathyssek C, Miele V. Correction: chronic traumatic encephalopathy in contact sports: a systematic review of all reported pathological cases. *PLoS One.* 2015; 10(6): e0130507.

81. Stein TD, Alvarez VE, McKee AC. concussion in chronic traumatic encephalopathy. *Current Pain and Headache Reports.* 2015; 19(10): 47.

82. Geddes JF, Vowles GH, Nicoll JA, Revesz T. Neuronal cytoskeletal changes are an early consequence of repetitive head injury. *Acta Neuropathologica.* 1999; 98(2): 171–178.

83. Lepreux S, Auriacombe S, Vital C, Dubois B, Vital A. Dementia pugilistica: a severe tribute to a career. *Clinical Neuropathology*. 2015; 34(4): 193–198.

84. Omalu B, Hammers JL Bailes J et al. Chronic traumatic encephalopathy in an Iraqi war veteran with posttraumatic stress disorder who committed suicide. *Neurosurgical Focus*. 2011; 31(5): E3.

85. Omalu BI, Bailes J, Hammers JL, Fitzsimmons RP. Chronic traumatic encephalopathy, suicides and parasuicides in professional American athletes: the role of the forensic pathologist. *The American Journal of Forensic Medicine and Pathology*. 2010; 31(2): 130–132.

86. Omalu BI, Fitzsimmons RP, Hammers J, Bailes J. Chronic traumatic encephalopathy in a professional American wrestler. *Journal of Forensic Nursing*. 2010; 6(3): 130–136.

87. Aotsuka A, Kojima S, Furumoto H, Hattori T, Hirayama K. Punch drunk syndrome due to repeated karate kicks and punches. *Clinical Neurology*. 1990; 30(11): 1243–1246.

88. Baugh CM, Stamm JM, Riley DO et al. Chronic traumatic encephalopathy: neurodegeneration following repetitive concussive and subconcussive brain trauma. *Brain Imaging and Behavior*. 2012; 6(2): 244–254.

89. Roberts GW, Allsop D, Bruton C. The occult aftermath of boxing. *Journal of Neurology, Neurosurgery, and Psychiatry*. 1990; 53(5): 373–378.

90. Roberts GW, Whitwell HL, Acland PR, Bruton CJ. Dementia in a punch-drunk wife. *Lancet (London, England)*. 1990; 335(8694): 918–919.

91. Gavett BE, Stern RA, McKee AC. Chronic traumatic encephalopathy: a potential late effect of sport-related concussive and subconcussive head trauma. *Clinics in Sports Medicine*. 2011; 30(1): 179–188, xi.

92. Gavett BE, Cantu RC, Shenton M et al. Clinical appraisal of chronic traumatic encephalopathy: current perspectives and future directions. *Current Opinion in Neurology*. 2011; 24(6): 525–531.

93. Saigal R, Berger MS. The long-term effects of repetitive mild head injuries in sports. *Neurosurgery*. 2014; 75 Suppl 4: S149–155.

94. Clinton J, Ambler MW, Roberts GW. Post-traumatic Alzheimer's disease: preponderance of a single plaque type. *Neuropathology and Applied Neurobiology*. 1991; 17(1): 69–74.

95. McKee AC, Cantu RC, Nowinski CJ et al. Chronic traumatic encephalopathy in athletes: progressive tauopathy after repetitive head injury. *Journal of Neuropathology and Experimental Neurology*. 2009; 68(7): 709–735.

96. Mez J, Stern RA, McKee AC. Chronic traumatic encephalopathy: where are we and where are we going? *Current Neurology and Neuroscience Reports*. 2013; 13(12): 407.

97. Tartaglia MC, Hazrati LN, Davis KD et al. Chronic traumatic encephalopathy and other neurodegenerative proteinopathies. *Frontiers in Human Neuroscience*. 2014; 8: 30.

98. McKee AC, Cairns NJ, Dickson DW et al. The first NINDS/NIBIB consensus meeting to define neuropathological criteria for the diagnosis of chronic traumatic encephalopathy. *Acta Neuropathologica*. 2016; 131(1): 75–86.

99. Blumbergs PC, Scott G, Manavis J, Wainwright H, Simpson DA, McLean AJ. Staining of amyloid precursor protein to study axonal damage in mild head injury. *Lancet (London, England)*. 1994; 344(8929): 1055–1056.

100. Oppenheimer DR. Microscopic lesions in the brain following head injury. *Journal of Neurology, Neurosurgery, and Psychiatry*. 1968; 31(4): 299–306.

101. Breunig JJ, Guillot-Sestier MV, Town T. Brain injury, neuroinflammation and Alzheimer's disease. *Frontiers in Aging Neuroscience*. 2013; 5: 26.

102. Sivanandam TM, Thakur MK. Traumatic brain injury: a risk factor for Alzheimer's disease. *Neuroscience and Biobehavioral Reviews*. 2012; 36(5): 1376–1381.

103. Kahlson MA, Colodner KJ. Glial Tau pathology in tauopathies: functional consequences. *Journal of Experimental Neuroscience*. 2015; 9(Suppl 2): 43–50.

104. Lucke-Wold BP, Turner RC, Logsdon AF, Bailes JE, Huber JD, Rosen CL. Linking traumatic brain injury to chronic traumatic encephalopathy: identification of potential mechanisms leading to neurofibrillary tangle development. *Journal of Neurotrauma*. 2014; 31(13): 1129–1138.

105. Sendek A, Fuller HR, Hayre NR, Singh RR, Cox DL. Simulated cytoskeletal collapse via tau degradation. *PLoS One*. 2014; 9(8): e104965.

106. Omalu B. Chronic traumatic encephalopathy. *Progress in Neurological Surgery*. 2014; 28: 38–49.

107. McKee AC, Daneshvar DH. The neuropathology of traumatic brain injury. *Handbook Clinical Neurology*. 2015; 127: 45–66.

108. McKee AC, Daneshvar DH, Alvarez VE, Stein TD. The neuropathology of sport. *Acta Neuropathologica*. 2014; 127(1): 29–51.

109. Montenigro PH, Bernick C, Cantu RC. Clinical features of repetitive traumatic brain injury and chronic traumatic encephalopathy. *Brain Pathology (Zurich, Switzerland)*. 2015; 25(3): 304–317.

110. Hyman BT, Phelps CH, Beach TG et al. National Institute on Aging-Alzheimer's Association guidelines for the neuropathologic assessment of Alzheimer's disease. *Alzheimer's & Dementia*. 2012; 8(1): 1–13.

111. Jellinger KA, Paulus W, Wrocklage C, Litvan I. Traumatic brain injury as a risk factor for Alzheimer disease. Comparison of two retrospective autopsy cohorts with evaluation of ApoE genotype. *BMC Neurology*. 2001; 1: 3.

112. Montine TJ, Phelps CH, Beach TG et al. National Institute on Aging-Alzheimer's Association guidelines for the neuropathologic assessment of Alzheimer's disease: a practical approach. *Acta Neuropathologica*. 2012; 123(1): 1–11.

113. Stein TD, Montenigro PH, Alvarez VE et al. Beta-amyloid deposition in chronic traumatic encephalopathy. *Acta Neuropathologica*. 2015; 130(1): 21–34.

114. Geddes JF, Vowles GH, Robinson SF, Sutcliffe JC. Neurofibrillary tangles, but not Alzheimer-type pathology, in a young boxer. *Neuropathology and Applied Neurobiology*. 1996; 22(1): 12–16.

115. Djordjevic J, Sabbir MG, Albensi BC. Traumatic brain injury as a risk factor for Alzheimer's disease: Is inflammatory signaling a key player? *Current Alzheimer Research*. 2016.

116. Roberts GW. Immunocytochemistry of neurofibrillary tangles in dementia pugilistica and Alzheimer's disease: evidence for common genesis. *Lancet (London, England)*. 1988; 2(8626–8627): 1456–1458.

117. Tajiri N, Kellogg SL, Shimizu T, Arendash GW, Borlongan CV. Traumatic brain injury precipitates cognitive impairment and extracellular Abeta aggregation in Alzheimer's disease transgenic mice. *PLoS One*. 2013; 8(11): e78851.

118. Daneshvar DH, Goldstein LE, Kiernan PT, Stein TD, McKee AC. Post-traumatic neurodegeneration and chronic traumatic encephalopathy. *Molecular and Cellular Neurosciences*. 2015; 66(Pt B): 81–90.

119. Nordstrom P, Michaelsson K, Gustafson Y, Nordstrom A. Traumatic brain injury and young onset dementia: a nationwide cohort study. *Annals of Neurology*. 2014; 75(3): 374–381.

120. Fleminger S, Oliver DL, Lovestone S, Rabe-Hesketh S, Giora A. Head injury as a risk factor for Alzheimer's disease: the evidence 10 years on; a partial replication. *Journal of Neurology, Neurosurgery, and Psychiatry*. 2003; 74(7): 857–862.

121. Lehman EJ, Hein MJ, Baron SL, Gersic CM. Neurodegenerative causes of death among retired National Football League players. *Neurology*. 2012; 79(19): 1970–1974.

122. Gardner RC, Burke JF, Nettiksimmons J, Kaup A, Barnes DE, Yaffe K. Dementia risk after traumatic brain injury vs nonbrain trauma: the role of age and severity. *The Journal of the American Medical Association Neurology*. 2014; 71(12): 1490–1497.

123. Allsop D, Haga S, Bruton C, Ishii T, Roberts GW. Neurofibrillary tangles in some cases of dementia pugilistica share antigens with amyloid beta-protein of Alzheimer's disease. *The American Journal of Pathology*. 1990; 136(2): 255–260.

124. Guo Z, Cupples LA, Kurz A et al. Head injury and the risk of AD in the MIRAGE study. *Neurology*. 2000; 54(6): 1316–1323.

125. Lye TC, Shores EA. Traumatic brain injury as a risk factor for Alzheimer's disease: a review. *Neuropsychology Review*. 2000; 10(2): 115–129.

126. Mortimer JA, van Duijn CM, Chandra V et al. Head trauma as a risk factor for Alzheimer's disease: a collaborative re-analysis of case-control studies. EURODEM Risk Factors Research Group. *International Journal of Epidemiology*. 1991; 20 Suppl 2: S28–35.

127. O'Meara ES, Kukull WA, Sheppard L et al. Head injury and risk of Alzheimer's disease by apolipoprotein E genotype. *American Journal of Epidemiology*. 1997; 146(5): 373–384.

128. Plassman BL, Havlik RJ, Steffens DC et al. Documented head injury in early adulthood and risk of Alzheimer's disease and other dementias. *Neurology*. 2000; 55(8): 1158–1166.

129. Salib E, Hillier V. Head injury and the risk of Alzheimer's disease: a case control study. *International Journal of Geriatric Psychiatry*. 1997; 12(3): 363–368.

130. Schofield PW, Tang M, Marder K et al. Alzheimer's disease after remote head injury: an incidence study. *Journal of Neurology, Neurosurgery, and Psychiatry*. 1997; 62(2): 119–124.

131. Kutner KC, Erlanger D, Tsai J, Jordan B, Relkin N. Lower cognitive performance of older football players possessing apolipoprotein E epsilon4. *Neurosurgery*. 2000; 47(3): 651–657.

132. Jordan BD, Relkin NR, Ravdin LD, Jacobs AR, Bennett A, Gandy S. Apolipoprotein E epsilon4 associated with chronic traumatic brain injury in boxing. *The Journal of the American Medical Association*. 1997; 278(2): 136–140.

133. Yang Z, Lin F, Robertson CS, Wang KK. Dual vulnerability of TDP-43 to calpain and caspase-3 proteolysis after neurotoxic conditions and traumatic brain injury. *Journal of Cerebral Blood Flow and Metabolism*. 2014; 34(9): 1444–1452.

134. Chen-Plotkin AS, Lee VM, Trojanowski JQ. TAR DNA-binding protein 43 in neurodegenerative disease. *Nature Reviews Neurology*. 2010; 6(4): 211–220.

135. McKee AC, Gavett BE, Stern RA et al. TDP-43 proteinopathy and motor neuron disease in chronic traumatic encephalopathy. *Journal of Neuropathology and Experimental Neurology*. 2010; 69(9): 918–929.

136. Chen H, Richard M, Sandler DP, Umbach DM, Kamel F. Head injury and amyotrophic lateral sclerosis. *American Journal of Epidemiology*. 2007; 166(7): 810–816.

137. Chio A, Benzi G, Dossena M, Mutani R, Mora G. Severely increased risk of amyotrophic lateral sclerosis among Italian professional football players. *Brain*. 2005; 128(Pt 3): 472–476.

138. Fournier CN, Gearing M, Upadhyayula SR, Klein M, Glass JD. Head injury does not alter disease progression or neuropathologic outcomes in ALS. *Neurology*. 2015; 84(17): 1788–1795.

139. Gardner RC, Burke JF, Nettiksimmons J, Goldman S, Tanner CM, Yaffe K. Traumatic brain injury in later life increases risk for Parkinson disease. *Annals of Neurology*. 2015; 77(6): 987–995.

140. Bower JH, Maraganore DM, Peterson BJ, McDonnell SK, Ahlskog JE, Rocca WA. Head trauma preceding PD: a case-control study. *Neurology*. 2003; 60(10): 1610–1615.

141. Baugh CM, Robbins CA, Stern RA, McKee AC. Current understanding of chronic traumatic encephalopathy. *Current Treatment Options in Neurology*. 2014; 16(9): 306.

142. Blaylock RL, Maroon J. Immunoexcitotoxicity as a central mechanism in chronic traumatic encephalopathy-A unifying hypothesis. *Surgical Neurology International*. 2011; 2: 107.

143. Ojo JO, Mouzon B, Greenberg MB, Bachmeier C, Mullan M, Crawford F. Repetitive mild traumatic brain injury augments tau pathology and glial activation in aged hTau mice. *Journal of Neuropathology and Experimental Neurology*. 2013; 72(2): 137–151.

144. Uryu K, Laurer H, McIntosh T et al. Repetitive mild brain trauma accelerates Abeta deposition, lipid peroxidation, and cognitive impairment in a transgenic mouse model of Alzheimer amyloidosis. *Journal of Neuroscience*. 2002; 22(2): 446–454.

145. Smith DH, Chen XH, Nonaka M et al. Accumulation of amyloid beta and tau and the formation of neurofilament inclusions following diffuse brain injury in the pig. *Journal of Neuropathology and Experimental Neurology*. 1999; 58(9): 982–992.

146. Hamberger A, Huang YL, Zhu H et al. Redistribution of neurofilaments and accumulation of beta-amyloid protein after brain injury by rotational acceleration of the head. *Journal of Neurotrauma*. 2003; 20(2): 169–178.

147. Roberts GW, Gentleman SM, Lynch A, Graham DI. beta A4 amyloid protein deposition in brain after head trauma. *Lancet (London, England)*. 1991; 338(8780): 1422–1423.

148. Smith DH, Johnson VE, Stewart W. Chronic neuropathologies of single and repetitive TBI: substrates of dementia? *Nature Reviews Neurology*. 2013; 9(4): 211–221.

149. Nisenbaum EJ, Novikov DS, Lui YW. The presence and role of iron in mild traumatic brain injury: an imaging perspective. *Journal of Neurotrauma*. 2014; 31(4): 301–307.

150. Smith C. Review: the long-term consequences of microglial activation following acute traumatic brain injury. *Neuropathology and Applied Neurobiology*. 2013; 39(1): 35–44.

151. Smith C, Gentleman SM, Leclercq PD et al. The neuroinflammatory response in humans after traumatic brain injury. *Neuropathology and Applied Neurobiology*. 2013; 39(6): 654–666.

152. Smith DH, Chen XH, Pierce JE et al. Progressive atrophy and neuron death for one year following brain trauma in the rat. *Journal of Neurotrauma*. 1997; 14(10): 715–727.

153. Dashnaw ML, Petraglia AL, Bailes JE. An overview of the basic science of concussion and subconcussion: where we are and where we are going. *Neurosurgical Focus*. 2012; 33(6): E5: 1–9.

154. Turner RC, Lucke-Wold BP, Robson MJ, Omalu BI, Petraglia AL, Bailes JE. Repetitive traumatic brain injury and development of chronic traumatic encephalopathy: a potential role for biomarkers in diagnosis, prognosis, and treatment? *Frontiers in Neurology*. 2012; 3: 186.

155. Faden AI, Loane DJ. Chronic neurodegeneration after traumatic brain injury: Alzheimer disease, chronic traumatic encephalopathy, or persistent neuroinflammation? *Neurotherapeutics*. 2015; 12(1): 143–150.

156. Shultz SR, Bao F, Weaver LC, Cain DP, Brown A. Treatment with an anti-CD11d integrin antibody reduces neuroinflammation and improves outcome in a rat model of repeated concussion. *Journal of Neuroinflammation.* 2013; 10: 26.

157. Clavaguera F, Bolmont T, Crowther RA et al. Transmission and spreading of tauopathy in transgenic mouse brain. *Nature Cell Biology.* 2009; 11(7): 909–913.

158. Eisele YS, Bolmont T, Heikenwalder M et al. Induction of cerebral beta-amyloidosis: intracerebral versus systemic Abeta inoculation. *Proceedings of the National Academy of Sciences in the United States of America.* 2009; 106(31): 12926–12931.

159. Guo JL, Lee VM. Seeding of normal Tau by pathological Tau conformers drives pathogenesis of Alzheimer-like tangles. *The Journal of Biological Chemistry.* 2011; 286(17): 15317–15331.

160. Kane MD, Lipinski WJ, Callahan MJ et al. Evidence for seeding of beta-amyloid by intracerebral infusion of Alzheimer brain extracts in beta-amyloid precursor protein-transgenic mice. *Journal of Neuroscience.* 2000; 20(10): 3606–3611.

161. Meyer-Luehmann M, Coomaraswamy J, Bolmont T et al. Exogenous induction of cerebral beta-amyloidogenesis is governed by agent and host. *Science (New York, NY).* 2006; 313(5794): 1781–1784.

162. Walker LC, Callahan MJ, Bian F, Durham RA, Roher AE, Lipinski WJ. Exogenous induction of cerebral beta-amyloidosis in beta-APP-transgenic mice. *Peptides.* 2002; 23(7): 1241–1247.

163. Stern RA, Riley DO, Daneshvar DH, Nowinski CJ, Cantu RC, McKee AC. Long-term consequences of repetitive brain trauma: chronic traumatic encephalopathy. *PM & R.* 2011; 3(10 Suppl 2): S460–467.

164. Kiernan PT, Montenigro PH, Solomon TM, McKee AC. Chronic traumatic encephalopathy: a neurodegenerative consequence of repetitive traumatic brain injury. *Seminar in Neurology.* 2015; 35(1): 20–28.

165. Stern RA, Daneshvar DH, Baugh CM et al. Clinical presentation of chronic traumatic encephalopathy. *Neurology.* 2013; 81(13): 1122–1129.

166. Xu J, Murphy S, Kochanek K, Bastian B. Deaths: Final Data for 2013. *National Vital Statistics Report.* 2013; 64(2): 119.

167. Gardner A, Iverson GL, McCrory P. Chronic traumatic encephalopathy in sport: a systematic review. *British Journal of Sports Medicine.* 2014; 48(2): 84–90.

168. Montenigro PH, Baugh CM, Daneshvar DH et al. Clinical subtypes of chronic traumatic encephalopathy: literature review and proposed research diagnostic criteria for traumatic encephalopathy syndrome. *Alzheimer's Research & Therapy.* 2014; 6(5): 68.

169. Barkhoudarian G, Hovda DA, Giza CC. The molecular pathophysiology of concussive brain injury. *Clinics in Sports Medicine.* 2011; 30(1): 33–48, vii–iii.

170. Shlosberg D, Benifla M, Kaufer D, Friedman A. Blood–brain barrier breakdown as a therapeutic target in traumatic brain injury. *Nature Reviews Neurology.* 2010; 6(7): 393–403.

171. Barnes DE, Kaup A, Kirby KA, Byers AL, Diaz-Arrastia R, Yaffe K. Traumatic brain injury and risk of dementia in older veterans. *Neurology.* 2014; 83(4): 312–319.

172. Shively S, Scher AI, Perl DP, Diaz-Arrastia R. Dementia resulting from traumatic brain injury: what is the pathology? *Archives of Neurology.* 2012; 69(10): 1245–1251.

173. Sayed N, Culver C, Dams-O'Connor K, Hammond F, Diaz-Arrastia R. Clinical phenotype of dementia after traumatic brain injury. *Journal of Neurotrauma.* 2013; 30(13): 1117–1122.

174. Godbolt AK, Cancelliere C, Hincapie CA et al. Systematic review of the risk of dementia and chronic cognitive impairment after mild traumatic brain injury: results of the International Collaboration on Mild Traumatic Brain Injury Prognosis. *Archives of Physical Medicine and Rehabilitation*. 2014; 95(3 Suppl): S245–256.

175. Solomon GS, Kuhn AW, Zuckerman SL et al. Participation in pre-high school football and neurological, neuroradiological, and neuropsychological findings in later life: a study of 45 retired national football league players. *The American Journal of Sports Medicine*. 2016; 44(5): 1106–1115.

176. Bryan CJ, Clemans TA. Repetitive traumatic brain injury, psychological symptoms, and suicide risk in a clinical sample of deployed military personnel. *The Journal of the American Medical Association. Psychiatry*. 2013; 70(7): 686–691.

177. Iverson GL. Chronic traumatic encephalopathy and risk of suicide in former athletes. *British Journal of Sports Medicine*. 2014; 48(2): 162–165.

178. Kerr ZY, Marshall SW, Harding HP, Jr., Guskiewicz KM. Nine-year risk of depression diagnosis increases with increasing self-reported concussions in retired professional football players. *The American Journal of Sports Medicine*. 2012; 40(10): 2206–2212.

179. Didehbani N, Munro Cullum C, Mansinghani S, Conover H, Hart J, Jr. Depressive symptoms and concussions in aging retired NFL players. *Archives of Clinical Neuropsychology*. 2013; 28(5): 418–424.

180. Strain J, Didehbani N, Cullum CM et al. Depressive symptoms and white matter dysfunction in retired NFL players with concussion history. *Neurology*. 2013; 81(1): 25–32.

181. Jordan BD. The clinical spectrum of sport-related traumatic brain injury. *Nature Reviews Neurology*. 2013; 9(4): 222–230.

182. Victoroff J. Traumatic encephalopathy: review and provisional research diagnostic criteria. *NeuroRehabilitation*. 2013; 32(2): 211–224.

183. Lenihan MW, Jordan BD. The clinical presentation of chronic traumatic encephalopathy. *Current Neurology and Neuroscience Reports*. 2015; 15(5): 23.

184. Love S, Solomon GS. Talking with parents of high school football players about chronic traumatic encephalopathy: a concise summary. *The American Journal of Sports Medicine*. 2015; 43(5): 1260–1264.

185. Gardner RC, Hess CP, Brus-Ramer M et al. Cavum septum pellucidum in retired american pro-football players. *Journal of Neurotrauma*. 2015.

186. Tator CH. Chronic traumatic encephalopathy: how serious a sports problem is it? *British Journal of Sports Medicine*. 2014; 48(2): 81–83.

187. Ho L, Zhao W, Dams-O'Connor K et al. Elevated plasma MCP-1 concentration following traumatic brain injury as a potential "predisposition" factor associated with an increased risk for subsequent development of Alzheimer's disease. *Journal of Alzheimers Disease*. 2012; 31(2): 301–313.

188. Mitsis EM, Riggio S, Kostakoglu L et al. Tauopathy PET and amyloid PET in the diagnosis of chronic traumatic encephalopathies: studies of a retired NFL player and of a man with FTD and a severe head injury. *Translational Psychiatry*. 2014; 4: e441.

189. Small GW, Kepe V, Siddarth P et al. PET scanning of brain tau in retired national football league players: preliminary findings. *The American Journal of Geriatric Psychiatry*. 2013; 21(2): 138–144.

190. Yang ST, Hsiao IT, Hsieh CJ et al. Accumulation of amyloid in cognitive impairment after mild traumatic brain injury. *Journal of the Neurological Sciences*. 2015; 349(1–2): 99–104.

191. Barrio JR, Small GW, Wong KP et al. In vivo characterization of chronic traumatic encephalopathy using [F-18]FDDNP PET brain imaging. *Proceedings of the National Academy of Sciences of the United States of America.* 2015; 112(16): E2039–2047.

192. McCrory P. Sports concussion and the risk of chronic neurological impairment. *Clinical Journal of Sport Medicine.* 2011; 21(1): 6–12.

193. Hazrati LN, Tartaglia MC, Diamandis P et al. Absence of chronic traumatic encephalopathy in retired football players with multiple concussions and neurological symptomatology. *Frontiers in Human Neuroscience.* 2013; 7: 222.

194. Lakis N, Corona RJ, Toshkezi G, Chin LS. Chronic traumatic encephalopathy—neuropathology in athletes and war veterans. *Neurological Research.* 2013; 35(3): 290–299.

195. Lehman EJ. Epidemiology of neurodegeneration in American-style professional football players. *Alzheimer's Research & Therapy.* 2013; 5(4): 34.

196. Antonius D, Mathew N, Picano J et al. Behavioral health symptoms associated with chronic traumatic encephalopathy: a critical review of the literature and recommendations for treatment and research. *The Journal of Neuropsychiatry and Clinical Neurosciences.* 2014; 26(4): 313–322.

197. Castellani RJ. Chronic traumatic encephalopathy: A paradigm in search of evidence? *Laboratory Investigation; a Journal of Technical Methods and Pathology.* 2015; 95(6): 576–584.

198. Karantzoulis S, Randolph C. Modern chronic traumatic encephalopathy in retired athletes: what is the evidence? *Neuropsychology Review.* 2013; 23(4): 350–360.

199. Randolph C. Is chronic traumatic encephalopathy a real disease? *Current Sports Medicine Reports.* 2014; 13(1): 33–37.

200. Solomon GS, Zuckerman SL. Chronic traumatic encephalopathy in professional sports: retrospective and prospective views. *Brain Injury.* 2015; 29(2): 164–170.

CHAPTER 10

Promising advances in concussion diagnosis and treatment

Introduction

A concussion is classically considered as a traumatically-induced functional rather than a structural injury; therefore, neurological function, through the use of sideline assessments, such as the SCAT, coupled with symptom assessments and other clinical modalities, including ocular and balance testing, is used to appropriately evaluate and determine if injury occurred. If the athlete did receive a concussion, he/she is immediately removed from play and prescribed a period of rest. Graded academic and physical return to activity is then undertaken when clinically appropriate. Once the athlete is able to participate at full exertion without symptom exacerbation, neuropsychological testing and other adjunctive measures are used to determine if the athlete is deemed ready to return to play. As summarized, diagnosis, assessment of recovery, and final determination of return to play is made solely on clinical or functional outcome measurements. Through advanced imaging techniques and even analysis of biomarkers released following injury, research has conceded that considering concussion as only a functional entity is an inappropriate underestimation. Even noncomplicated concussions, excluding those with intracranial hemorrhage, may have structural neuronal injury as a response to secondary injury progression through propagation of the neurometabolic and inflammatory cascade. Exploiting our understanding of the microstructural neuronal damage that may occur will allow for advances in both diagnosis and treatment of concussion, moving away from the classical subjective or even clinical modalities testing function.

In this final chapter, we will discuss how knowledge of the pathophysiology of concussion, has led to not only the development of various biomarkers for potential diagnostic and predictive clinical use, but also provided the impetus to try different pharmaceutical regiments and therapeutic modalities to treat concussion, supported by their mechanism of action and conceivable effect on the neurometabolic cascade.

Biomarkers of concussion

A biomarker is a "characteristic that is objectively measured and evaluated as an indicator of normal biological process, pathogenic process, or pharmacologic responses to a therapeutic intervention."[1] Following a concussion, if severe enough, the initial insult or secondary injury may result in cellular death and release of axonal, neuronal, and astrocytic proteins (Figure 10.1).[2] Once the specific solute is released, it travels via diffusion from the brain interstitium to the cerebrospinal fluid (CSF), referred to as the glymphatic pathway. Then, the peripheral lymphatic vessels carry the solute from the CSF space to the serum where it becomes degraded by proteasomes or excreted via hepatic or renal clearance creating an optimum window for serum detections[3–5] (Figure 10.2).[6]

Therefore, following injury, it is possible to sample either the CSF, serum, or urine to evaluate for elevated levels of a specific protein biomarker (Figure 10.3).[5] CSF sampling has the highest concentration of solute, but requires invasive access (lumbar puncture or ventricular drain), which is most likely not indicated in the typical concussed patient. Conversely, obtaining biomarkers through serum is less invasive, but requires a more sensitive assay due to lower concentration levels from dilution and degradation.[2]

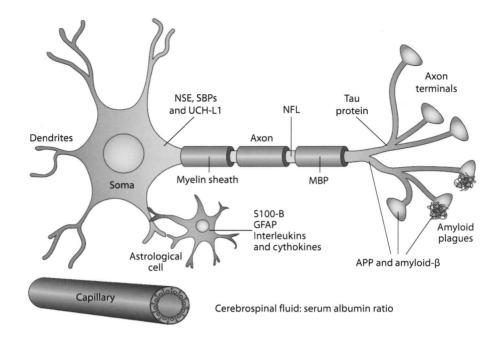

Figure 10.1 Biomarkers of concussion and location of origin. (From Zetterberg H et al. *Nat Rev Neurol.* Apr;9(4):201–10, 2013.)

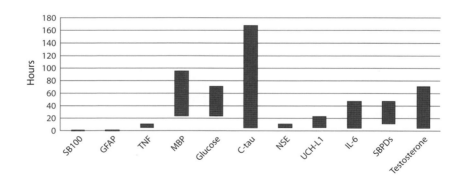

Figure 10.2 Optimum time for serum detection for various biomarkers of brain injury. (From Forde CT et al. *Br J Neurosurg.* Jan;28(1):8–15, 2014.)

Through a hypothesis driven approach, researchers have used our current understanding through preclinical models of the neurometabolic cascade to selectively screen for different markers following concussion in clinical models.[5] This methodology has identified numerous biomarkers of either neuronal, axonal, astroglial, and inflammatory mediator origin. We will discuss these in further detail but it is important to emphasize that their clinical utility and practical usage remains to be determined.

Neuronal biomarkers

Ubiquitin carboxy-terminal hydrolase isoenzyme L1

Ubiquitin carboxy-terminal hydrolase isoenzyme L1 (UCHL1) is an enzyme that is responsible for hydrolyzing ubiquitin (regulator of proteasome protein degradation) and is located in not only the cytoplasm of neurons but also the peripheral nervous system, neuroendocrine system, aortic endothelium, and smooth muscle cells.[5,7,8] UCHL1 has exhibited

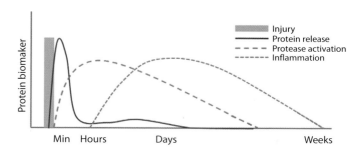

Figure 10.3 Following concussive injury, neuronal and astroglial protein components are released into the blood stream and subsequently degraded by proteasomes or renal/hepatic excretion. (From Mondello S et al. *Expert Rev Mol Diagn.* Jan;11(1):65–78, 2011.)

a capacity to acutely reflect extent of injury when obtained from serum less than 24 hours from injury and it correlates with the degree of the Glasgow Coma Scale Score (GCS).[9] In direct assessment of cohorts of milder brain injuries, Kou et al. obtained UCHL1 every 6 hours following injury for 24 hours in a cohort of nine mild TBI (mTBI) patients to find a 4.9 fold increase in UCHL1 acutely following injury.[10] However, elevation of UCHL1 among mTBI cohorts has not been universally appreciated and appears to be more consistently elevated in moderate to severe TBI.[9,11] Further, Puvenna et al. assessed the capability of UCHL1 to function as a biomarker for subconcussion by comparing healthy individuals, those that suffered a concussive injury, and players that participated in a competitive game without experiencing a concussion.[12] Unfortunately, UCHL1 was shown not to have a correlation with the number of exposed head contacts in the group that participated in the football game and therefore unable to be used as an objective measure of subconcussion.

Though UCHL1 has shown some evidence as a diagnostic biomarker, the outcome predictive value of UCHL1 elevation following injury has exhibited limited results. UCHL1 was not predictive of acute neurocognitive deficits (on standardized assessment of concussion), structural injury (diffusion tensor image findings on MRI), or long-term outcomes at 6 months in mild TBI patients.[7,10,11] One study did show a positive correlation with UCHL1 elevations following injury that predicted long-term Glasgow Outcome Scale scores, but was only seen in moderate to severe pediatric TBI patients.[13]

Interestingly, multiple studies have shown a predictive value of UCHL1 elevation in mTBI patients in those who also displayed an intracranial lesion on CT head imaging.[9,11,14] Papa et al. obtained serum UCHL1 values in 295 patients (10 with moderate TBI, 86 with mild TBI, and 199 negative controls) 4 hours after injury and demonstrated a statistically significant elevation in UCHL1 in those who had significant CT head findings (a mean of 1.618 ng/mL with a range of ±0.474 ng/mL vs. a mean of 0.620 ng/mL with a range of ±0.254 ng/mL, [$p < 0.001$]).[9] In a cohort of mild to moderate TBI patients, Welch et al. described a 100% sensitivity and 39% specificity for UCHL1 (over 0.04 ng/mL) for presence of intracranial lesions on imaging.[14] Since consistent significant results have only been seen in moderate and severe TBI, or those with intracranial hematomas, the use of UCHL1 as a predictor of concussive injury is still uncertain, but does appear to have a potential use as a screening tool for physicians to determine the need for obtaining cranial imaging, even in those with milder injuries. This futuristic application of a serum bioassay may reduce or limit the use of ionizing radiation.

Neuron specific enolase (NSE)

Neuron specific enolase (NSE) is an enzyme that is normally found in the cytoplasm of mature neurons, but also platelets, erythrocytes, neuroendocrine cells, and oligodendrocytes.[2,5,7,8] Following release into the serum, NSE has a half-life of roughly 24 hours, which is important to consider when determining when to test the athlete after injury.[15] Due to NSE's presence in multiple cells, hemolysis due to any reason, for example intracranial hemorrhage, extra-cranial trauma, or even serum sample lysis, can cause elevations in NSE levels.[5] As a result, NSE levels in patients who present with both intracranial and extracranial injuries are difficult to interpret. For example, Meric et al. was unable to show a statistically significant difference in NSE level elevation between those with mild TBI and those with noncranial head trauma.[16]

What makes NSE an interesting biomarker for head injury is that several studies have demonstrated elevations of NSE in mild, moderate, and severe TBI, in comparison to healthy controls, and importantly, a difference in prevalence of NSE elevation between severity of TBI.[16–21] As a diagnostic tool, Kruijk et al. showed that in their cohort of 104 mTBI patients, compared to 92 healthy controls, serum NSE levels obtained less than 6 hours from injury in the mTBI group had a mild elevation with an average 9.8 µg/L with a (10% to 90% range of 6.9 to 14.3 µg/L) while the healthy controls had an average NSE baseline level of 9.4 µg/L, (ranging from 6.3 to 13.3 µg/L).[20] Skogseid et al. obtained NSE levels a few hours after injury in 60 patients with mild to severe TBI and demonstrated that 88% of moderate to severe TBI and only 23% of minor head injury patients had an elevated serum NSE.[17] Others have demonstrated an even strikingly higher incidence of NSE elevation on admission in mTBI patients, ranging from 51% to 65%.[19,22] Instinctively, a higher severity of injury would cause greater neuronal injury and release of the intraneural biomarker, therefore increasing the likelihood to see elevations in more severe injuries.

Furthermore, elevation in NSE after injury has shown evidence of predicting outcomes, but solely in more severe TBI. Meric found that an elevation in NSE was 87% sensitive and 82% predictive of poor outcome (Glasgow outcome score) at one month in severe TBI, but had no association in mild TBI patients.[16] Other studies have shown conflicting results of correlation,[22] or lack of,[16,18,23] with NSE elevation and outcomes in mild TBI.

Interestingly, NSE elevation has also shown potential for predicating the presence of significant intracranial lesions on imaging. Due to its existence in both neurons and erythrocytes, a more significant cranial injury that leads to a hemorrhage would intuitively have greater elevation in NSE release. NSE elevation of more than 12.28 to 14.7 µg/L has been shown to have a 56% to 100% sensitivity and 6.9% to 77% specificity for the presence of intracranial lesions (subarachnoid, subdural, and intracerebral hemorrhage) on CT,

therefore is a potential screening test to determine the need for cranial imaging.[17,24,25] However due to its inconsistent specificity and sensitivity based on a narrow value to determine presence of intracranial hemorrhage, NSE currently is not realistic for clinical use at this time.

But what is NSE's role as a biomarker for subconcussion and concussive injury? Graham et al. was able to demonstrate elevated NSE levels, following a competition, in karate athletes subjected to head contacts, but not in those who received only body contacts (11.8 ng/mL, with a range of ±4.1 ng/mL vs. 20.2 ng/mL, with a range of ±9.1 ng/mL; $p < 0.05$).[26] But, NSE elevation a potential biomaker for concussion has been refuted by others due to lack of significant finding. Shahim et al. did not see elevations in NSE at 1, 12, 36, or 144 hours following concussive injury in their cohort of 35 professional hockey players.[27] Therefore, NSE's inconsistent results seen at more minor head injuries preclude its use as a sole biomarker for concussive injury.

Spectrin breakdown products (SBDPs)

Following a traumatic brain injury, calcium rushes into the neuron and activates a specific type of protease called calpains.[7] This leads to the degradation of cytoskeletal proteins of the neuron into spectrin.[5] In a preclinical study, two different types of spectrin breakdown products (SBDPs) were found to be elevated at 2, 6, and 24 hours following a controlled cortical impact in the rat model, which also correlated with the severity of injury and lesion size.[28] These findings have led to clinical studies showing the use of SBDP as an acute biomarker in severe TBI that has also been predictive of outcomes months after injury.[13,29]

More importantly, subsequent studies have focused on the strength in use of serum SBDP elevation in mTBI and concussive injuries. Siman et al. first studied a cohort of 38 patients with mTBI and negative CT head imaging, to demonstrate that a specific type of SBDP called N-terminal αII spectrin fragment (SNTF) was elevated in those with mTBI and, importantly, also correlated with white matter injury seen on DTI and persistent cognitive deficits at 3 months.[30] Following up with this finding, Siman et al. studied a cohort of professional ice hockey players to show that SNTF levels increased one hour after a concussion with decline to baseline levels by

6 days. Increased levels were predictive of delayed return to play (area under the curve = 0.87) and also not to be influenced by exercise.[31] Though data is limited, the current findings in these few studies express great promise of SBDP/SNTF for use as a biomarker of diagnosis and recovery for concussion, but further research is needed.

α-amino-3-hydroxy-5-methyl-4-isoxazolepropionic acid receptor peptide

An α-amino-3-hydroxy-5-methyl-4-isoxazolepropionic acid receptor (AMPAR) is a type of glutamate receptor located within neurons mostly located within the forebrain and subcortical areas.[32] Following neuronal injury and protease activation, AMPAR gets degraded and released into the CSF as smaller fragments/peptides. There is a huge scarcity in studies using AMPAR peptides as a biomarker and therefore characterization is limited. Dambinova et al. compared 33 athletes with a concussion (presenting within 1 to 2 weeks from injury), 51 athletes without a history of concussion, and 40 non-athletes.[32] All athletes received neurocognitive testing and serum AMPAR testing at the time of study inclusion. The researchers found a statistically significant increase of AMPAR values among those with concussion ($p < 0.0001$) that was 91% sensitive and 92% specific for concussion with a cut off value of 0.4 ng/mL, and that elevation was correlated with reduced scores on Impact testing.[32] Further clinical testing is required to determine the encouraging potential of AMPAR in concussion management.

Axonal biomarkers

Tau

Tau proteins are found within thin, non-myelinated axons and are responsible for microtubule stabilization.[2] Preclinical models have demonstrated that there exists a direct relationship between tau protein release and extent of traumatic injury,[7,33] but clinical studies have demonstrated conflicting results. Bulut et al. reviewed 60 adult patients with mTBI, who presented to the emergency department (ED), against 20 healthy controls.[34] Serum tau levels were not statistically different when comparing all mTBI patients to the healthy controls ($p = 0.445$), but those with intracranial lesions on CT scan (n = 11) had a greater mean serum tau level than those with mTBI without hemorrhage (307 pg/mL with a range of ±246 pg/mL vs. 77 pg/mL with a range of ±61 pg/mL [0.001]). Following up and contradicting this study, Kavalci et al. noted that admission serum tau levels between mTBI patients with (n = 33) and without (n = 55) intracranial hemorrhage had no significant difference (mean of 18.39 pg/mL, ranging from 2.19 to 714.47 pg/mL, vs. a mean of 16.29 pg/mL, ranging from 2.12 to 215.97 pg/mL).[35] A final study by Guzel et al. evaluated admission serum tau levels in 60 pediatric patients who presented to the ED with mTBI to healthy controls.[36] There was a statistically significant difference in tau protein levels between the controls and mTBI group ($p < .001$); but again, there was no difference between the mTBI groups when comparing presence of intracranial hemorrhage. As one can see from the data presented, there is still insufficient evidence to determine the role of serum tau in distinguishing patients who present with more complex injuries specifically those head injured patients that have intracranial pathology.

The role of serum tau specifically for sports concussive-injury diagnosis has shown promising results in two clinical studies. Both studies were performed by Shahim et al. in cohorts of professional hockey players. The first study demonstrated a significant increase in total serum tau levels compared to preseason baseline levels following a concussive injury (10 pg/mL, ranging from 2 to 102 pg/mL vs. 4.5 pg/mL, ranging from 0.06 to 22.7 pg/mL, $p < 0.001$).[27] Following up with this study, Shahim et al. performed a multicenter prospective study in 288 Swedish professional hockey players in which 28 that received a concussion had serum tau levels drawn at 1, 12, 36, and 144 hours from injury. Not only was serum Tau-C levels elevated following injury, serum Tau-A levels at 1 and 12 hours from injury were predictive of early versus late return to play.[37] This study underscores the future use of analyzing specific tau isotypes and not just evaluating total tau release as a predictive test in concussion. The use of total tau and tau isoforms has not consistently demonstrated a predictive role in outcomes of concussion in other studies, specifically when evaluating postconcussive syndrome at 3 months, therefore, further work must be undertaken before clinical use may be considered.[38,39] In lieu of the mentioned studies, Tau, with its relation to neurodegeneration and CTE, is a fascinating and promising biomarker in concussion that warrants further research.

Neurofilaments

Neurofilaments are a structural protein found in large caliber myelinated axons that assist in maintaining their shape, size, and overall integrity. There exists three neurofilament subunits, light, medium, and heavy chain, and these all have been studied as a biomarker for brain injury.[2,7] First, neurofilament light protein (NFL) has been evaluated through lumbar puncture in professional boxers from 2 weeks to 4 months following concussive injury (inclusion criteria included LOC for at least 5 seconds). Though the athletes had prompt recovery of symptoms and remained asymptomatic during the clinical study, NFL remained elevated until 36 weeks after injury.[40] The second subunit, neurofilament medium polypeptide (NFM), was studied in a cohort of 68 mTBI patients compared to 47 healthy controls. Martinez et al. demonstrated that there was a significant elevation of NFM in 44% of patients with mTBI; but of concern, patients with polytrauma had a significantly higher elevation ($p = 0.01$).[41] Lastly, neurofilament heavy chain (NFH) was evaluated by Neselius et al. in a cohort of amateur boxers. CSF and serum was obtained 1 to 6 days and 14 days following a competition among 30 boxers who did not have a concussion. Compared with controls, there was a significant increase in NFH in 80% of the boxers following the match, therefore due to subconcussive injury, that was not resolved by 14 days.[42] A follow-up study did indicate that those with persistent elevation of NFL at 14 days showed reduced performance on neurocognitive testing (Trail Making A, $p = 0.04$) and simple reaction time ($p = 0.042$).[43] Though research is limited, there exists a potential use of one or more neurofilament subunits as a diagnostic and predictive tool for concussive injury.

Astroglial biomarkers

S-100

S-100 is a calcium binding protein that is found not only in astrocytes, but also oligodendrocytes and other peripheral sources like Schwann cells, chondrocytes, adipocytes, and endocrine cells.[2,5,7,8] S-100 has become the most widely studied biomarker for use in traumatic brain injury due to serum elevation seen in in-vitro studies following more significant head trauma, where there is a breakdown of the blood–brain barrier (BBB).[3,44,45]

Research has also revealed serum S-100's role as a biomarker for the clinical diagnosis of minor head injuries. First, de Kruijk saw an increase in serum S-100 less than 6 hours from injury in a cohort of 104 mTBI patients (0.25 mcg/L, with a range of 0.00–0.68 mcg/L vs. 0.02 mcg/L, with a range of 0.00–0.13 mcg/L).[20] Even more recently, Graham et al. demonstrated that serum S-100 levels were elevated in 24 karate athletes, following a match that involved kicks to the head, in comparison to athletes that only received blows to the torso (0.12 mcg/L, with a range of ±0.17 vs. 0.37 mcg/L, with a range of ±0.26 mcg/L, $p < 0.05$).[26] These results shed light on the potential use of S-100 in the diagnosis of concussive and even subconcussive injuries that is not influenced by extracranial trauma.

Studies have also demonstrated the predictive value of some long-term outcomes, but not others, and also the presence of intracranial findings on imaging. Elevations in S-100 have correlated with severity, were predictive of requiring further medical care one week following injury, and return to baseline during rehabilitation in concussion and mTBI cohorts.[12,22,27] However, further studies in both adult and pediatric populations have shown limited predictive efficacy of postconcussive syndrome at follow-up or time till return to activity.[7,38,46–48]

S-100 has also shown strong predictive value as a screening test for presence of intracranial hematoma and contusions to the extent that many have advocated for its use in clinical practice.[5,24,25,49,50] A prospective study of 787 mTBI patients compared with 467 controls found that a cutoff value of 0.060 μg/L was 98% sensitive to rule out abnormal cranial imaging, with the potential of eliminating 22.9% of CT scans if applied to clinical use.[51] Two studies have directly compared the predictive value of S-100 to NSE, and in a prospective study of 139 mTBI patients, NSE greater than 12.28 ng/mL was 100% sensitive and 6.9% specific while S-100 greater than 0.21 ng/mL was 100% sensitive and 50% specific to determine presence/absence of cranial lesions on CT.[24,25]

Like the other biomarkers discussed, S-100 does have limitations and therefore use as a cornerstone biomarker is likely not conceivable. Since S-100 is also found in peripheral cells, noncranial trauma and even exertion have been shown to cause elevations in serum S-100 levels[3,4,44,50]; but again, this has not been universally seen.[52] Interestingly, Puvenna et al. compared serum S-100 levels of diagnosed mTBI patients, who presented to the ED, to healthy controls and 15 collegiate football players before and after a game.[12] It was found that not only did S-100 correlate with mTBI severity and had the ability to rule out mTBI in those presenting to the ED, S-100 elevations were also found to correlate with the number of subconcussive blows experienced by the collegiate cohort. Puvenna et al. concluded that S-100 may have potential as a biomarker for subconcussion; but as noted, this is difficult to conclude due to confounding factors like exertion and noncranial head trauma that may also cause elevation of S-100.

Glial fibrillary astrocytic protein (GFAP)

GFAP is a structural intermediate filament that composes the cytoskeleton of astrocytes.[3,4,7] Previous preclinical in vitro and in vivo studies have demonstrated acute increases in GFAP following head injury that also correlate with the extent of neuronal damage.[45,53] Kou et al. measured serum GFAP in nine mTBI patients every 6 hours for 24 hours following presentation to the ED, verifying the clinical application of serum GFAP elevation in a mTBI cohort.[10] It was shown that acutely after injury, GFAP increased 10.6 fold and, although a small cohort, GFAP elevations were even greater in those with intracranial lesions. Interestingly Kou et al. found no correlation with GFAP and findings on diffusion tensor imaging or the standardized assessment of concussion. Though not predictive of imaging or acute assessment modalities in the study by Kou et al., Mannix et al. showed in a cohort of thirteen 11- to 21-year-old concussed athletes who presented to the ED, that there was an association between GFAP elevation at time of injury and increased symptoms at one month follow-up.[54]

GFAP is also an attractive concussion biomarker because it is not influenced by extracranial injuries[50]

and is more predictive of intracranial hematoma than S-100.[50,55,56] Okonkwo et al. revealed that in a cohort of 215 TBI patients (83% with mTBI) a GFAP cutoff of more than 0.68 ng/mL had a 21.6 odds ratio of having a significant finding on CT head imaging, which was predictive of worse outcomes at 6 months from injury.[56]

Biomarkers of inflammation

Researchers have also used our knowledge of the neurometabolic cascade in concussion resulting in a proinflammatory state and blood brain barrier breakdown (BBB) as a source for potential biomarkers of injury. A specific biomarker for BBB breakdown is established by comparing the ratio of albumin in the CSF to the serum albumin. Since albumin is naturally present in the serum and not the CSF, any breakdown of the BBB would cause release of albumin into the CSF, and increase the ratio of CSF to serum albumin. Studies have shown a role of this biomarker in more severe TBI but there is limited data for concussive injury.[2] Believed to affect BBB, matrix metalloproteinase 9 (MMP-9) has also been shown clinically to increase 3.6 times within 8 hours of injury.[8] Further concussion biomarkers like galectin 3, phosphatidylserine coated platelets, and soluble urokinase plasminogen activator receptor (suPAR) are indicative of a proinflammatory state and have shown biomarker potential due to their acute increase following mTBI.[8,57,58]

For a more thorough discussion with potential application to concussive injury, we invite the reader to consult the literature concerning many other less researched biomarkers studied in TBI such as: brain derived neurotrophic factor (BDNF),[59] D-dimer,[60] plasma cellular prion protein (PrPc),[61] occludin,[8] copeptin,[8] c-reactive protein, brain natriuretic peptic (BNP), creatine kinase (CK), heart type fatty acid binding protein (h-FABP), prolactin,[62] cortisol,[4] myelin basic protein,[5,63,64] lipid peroxidation, microRNAs, and proteomics.[5]

Limitations of biomarkers

There are many obvious limitations displayed during our review of the literature of TBI biomarkers. First, the great variability in experimental design makes direct comparison of studies difficult: analysis of CSF versus serum fluid, lumbar cistern CSF versus ventricular CSF, different initial and ending time points of fluid collection, poorly described time points ("at follow-up," "at presentation," "within 24 hours" compared with more defined period like "within four hours"), and differing study populations (pediatric vs. adult, sports concussion vs. mTBI). Inter-study relationships also demonstrate poor definition consistency for concussion and mTBI thereby creating a heterogeneous sample. This is likely the fault of an evolving definition of concussion over the past decade.

Secondly, there is a preference of studies on biomarkers for more moderate and severe injury and a paucity of work in mTBI, specifically sports concussion cohorts. This may be due to the lack of research or even possibly a publication bias. At this point, the continuum of physiology is not completely understood between concussion and more severe TBI and the factors that differentiate them as distinct properties. For this reason, it is difficult to contribute work that has been validated in more severe TBI to that of concussive injury. Lastly, the specific cutoff values for each test are based on specific cohort studies and cannot be universally used. To advance the potential clinical use of biomarkers, further validation must take place to determine clinically significant serum/CSF cutoff values for each biomarker.

Future role of biomarkers in concussion

At this time, there is no biomarker that is available for clinical practice in concussion management. Nevertheless, research has shown great promise for the potential future use of biomarkers in concussion.[65] Further work needs to be performed to determine the best window to test for each specific biomarker and to better understand what an elevated value means clinically. Current clinical management of concussion lacks validated measures for diagnosis, guiding return to play, predicting outcomes, or assisting in determining retirement from sport; however, the application of biomarkers may provide clinicians this objective tool in the near future.[66,67]

Fascinating work is underway in preclinical and clinical models where biomarkers have been used to develop a "symptophenotype," where biomarkers are correlated with specific symptom appearance.[66] In a preclinical study, Evans et al. used proteomics to evaluate various biomarkers

following injury and interestingly correlated elevations in myelin associated glycoprotein, spectrin, and neurofilament light expression with deficits of grip strength in the animal model.[68] Further, in a clinical study of 63 patients with mTBI, upregulation of serum BMX, a protein kinase, was associated with "dizziness" measured by the dizziness handicap inventory.[69] These studies provide a novel tactic in biomarker use through their approach at developing an athlete's symptophenotype following injury. Pending further work, this methodology could potentially provide immediate, individualized information to clinicians of what specific symptoms would benefit from early rehabilitation.

Due to the gambit of biomarkers and their individual strengths and weaknesses regarding predictive capacity in outcomes for brain injury, specifically concussion, the future use of those biomarkers will like include not just one sole test but actually an array of multiple biomarkers in an attempt to provide an individualize description of the injury and recovery process of the athlete.[63,66,70] For example, Wolf et al. demonstrated in their mTBI cohort that the use of both S-100 and NSE together improved the sensitivity for predicting lack of intracranial lesion on imaging.[25] Therefore, only through the use of multiple biomarkers and improvement in overall predictive value will biomarkers be thrust into clinical practice.

Concussion pharmacological agents and treatment remedies

Pharmacotherapy

As discussed in Chapter 2, a neurometabolic and inflammatory cascade of events ensues after injury leading to secondary neuronal damage. Researchers have used a mechanistic approach to finding treatment remedies for traumatic brain injury by researching either specific pathways or more globally within this cascade of events.[71] Unfortunately, various medications that have shown great promise in preclinical studies have failed to demonstrate clinical efficacy in randomized trials for more moderate to severe TBI. Lack of experimental success can possibly be attributed to the already poor outcome associated with severe TBI, small cohort sizes, great variability in mechanism of injury, and the multitude of confounding variables. Assuming that concussion and severe

Table 10.1 Preclinical and Clinical Pharmaceutical Agents for TBI/Concussion

Pharmaceutical Class	Agent	
Steroid		
	Methylprednisolone	• Corticosteroid Randomization after Significant Head Injury trial (CRASH): multicenter, randomized, placebo controlled study, n = 10,008 (GCS <14) • Study terminated due to increased mortality at 14 days post injury in those treated with steroid (21.1% vs. 17.9%, p <0.001)[72,73]
	Progesterone	• Progesterone for traumatic brain injury, experimental clinical treatment (PROTECT): initial safety trial followed by efficacy trial: multicenter, randomized, placebo control, n = 882 moderate-severe TBI • No benefit of progesterone over control[74–81]
Natural/Herbal Supplements		
	Fatty Acids	• Types of Omega-3 polyunsaturated fatty acids: Docosahexaenoic (DHA, most abundant in brain) and eicosapentaenoic acid (EPA) • Can increase through diet by ingesting fish and nuts • Structural and functional role in brain: forms lipid bilayer of cells, role in cell signaling, neuronal growth, antioxidative, anti-inflammatory, and improves mitochondrial functioning[77–81] • Studied for potential role in mood disorders, Parkinson's, Alzheimer's, Huntington's disease, stroke, subarachnoid hemorrhage, epilepsy, and dementia[82–91] • In preclinical TBI models: • Animals shown to have reduction in brain DHA as a response to injury, and that supplementation reduced oxidative damage, BBB breakdown, axonal[92] injury, and improved behavioral outcomes[92–102]
	Resveratrol	• Present in wines and juices containing grapes and berries like blueberries, bilberries, and cranberries • Studied for use in cancer, heart disease, stroke, spinal cord injury, and Alzheimer's disease due to its antioxidant and anti-inflammatory properties[111–118] • In preclinical TBI models: • Decreased microglial activation, cytokine release, lesion volume, neuronal loss, and deficits on behavior testing[119–122]
	Curcumin	• Provides yellow color of the Indian spice, turmeric • Anti-inflammatory and antioxidant effects proposed to help in neurodegenerative diseases, subarachnoid hemorrhage, and stroke[123–136] • In preclinical TBI models: • Reduction in cerebral edema and oxidative stress, improved mitochondrial functioning, membrane integrity, and behavior outcomes[137–141]
	Enzogenol	• Flavonoid rich extract from pine bark of Pinus Radiata • Randomized, placebo control, cross over study in 60 adults 3 to 12 months following mTBI with persistent cognitive deficits. • No change in postconcussive symptoms or memory tests. Patients did report reduced subjective cognitive failures[149]
	Branched chain amino acids (Leucine, Isoleucine, and Valine)	• Precursors to GABA and glutamate neurotransmitters[150] • In preclinical TBI model: • Supplementation improved sleep quality, wakefulness, and cognitive deficits[150,151]

(Continued)

Table 10.1 (Continued)   Preclinical and Clinical Pharmaceutical Agents for TBI/Concussion

Pharmaceutical Class	Agent	
	Cannabinoids	• Found to have both anti-inflammatory and neuroprotective effects[152] • Use of endocannabinoid enzyme blocker, reduced BBB breakdown, microglial activation, infarct size and improved behavior outcomes in preclinical TBI and cerebral ischemia models[153–155] • In preclinical TBI models: • Blunted glutamate induced excitotoxicity, reduced contusion volume, cytokine release, neuronal atrophy, amyloid aggregation, and endoplasmic reticulum stress[156–159]
	Caffeine	• Central nervous system stimulant that functions as a nonspecific adenosine antagonist[160] • Studied for use in Parkinson's, Alzheimer's disease, and cognitive decline[160–166] • In preclinical TBI model • Preinjury supplementation was neuroprotective through reduced inflammation and modulation of glutamate release[160,167]

	Vitamin D	• In preclinical TBI model
		  • Deficiency worsened outcomes following TBI and attenuated benefits of progesterone therapy[91,168]
		  • Recommend screening for deficiency and replacement in TBI patients[169]

	Vitamin E	• In preclinical TBI model • Preinjury supplementation improved behavior outcomes, reduced oxidative stress, and increased synaptic plasticity[91,170]
Glycemic Medications		
	Glucagon like peptide-1 (GLP-1) analogues	• GLP-1 receptor is present on pancreatic beta cells and controls blood glucose levels • Also found on neurons and found to have antiapoptotic properties[171] • In preclinical TBI studies • Reduced oxidative stress and improved behavior outcomes,[171,172] but results have not been consistent[173]
Anti-Inflammatory/ Antioxidant		
	N-acetyl cysteine	• Precursor to the antioxidant glutathione found to reduce inflammation and reduce reactive oxygen species • Shown to improve behavior outcomes in a preclinical TBI model[174]
	Erythropoietin analogue	• Reduced inflammatory reaction and improved behavior outcomes in a preclinical TBI model[175]
	Minocycline	• Derivative of tetracycline (antibiotic) • Reduced microglial activation by 59% and reduced brain lesion volume by 58% in preclinical TBI model[176]
	Cytokine Receptor Inhibitors	• IL-1, IL-6, and TNFα receptor blockade showed reduction of injury and improved behavior outcomes in preclinical rat model[177–179]
	Intracellular Adhesion Molecule (ICAM) Inhibitors	• Role in cell signaling and transmigration of inflammatory cells from blood vessel to tissue • Used in preclinical ischemia and TBI model. Shown to reduce inflammatory cascade, BBB breakdown, and production of reactive oxygen species[180–184]
	Cerebrolysin	• Purified porcine brain proteins • Believed to improve oxygen utilization and therefore reduce oxidative stress and lactic acid formation • Randomized, placebo controlled study in 32 mTBI patients with parenchymal contusions • Intravenous injection improved cognitive function at 3 months[185]

TBI are within a continuum, proposed mechanistic therapies in moderate to severe TBI may be efficacious in milder injuries, like concussion. For this reason, we will briefly review some clinical trials in moderate–severe TBI, but will focus on the many remedies recommended by preclinical work over the past decade that have exhibited effects on blunting the neurometabolic and inflammatory cascade of concussion (Table 10.1).

Hyperbaric oxygen

Hyperbaric oxygen therapy is a medical treatment that entails placing the patient into a chamber filled with 100% oxygen at an increased atmospheric pressure. These chambers are used to prevent and treat decompression sickness (when scuba divers ascend too quickly and develop air emboli in their blood) and carbon monoxide poisoning (Figure 10.4). This therapy has shown promising results in animal studies, but has had variable outcomes in clinical trials for concussive injuries. In TBI and ischemic animal models, the use of hyperbaric oxygen therapy following injury has shown to reduce neuronal injury, infarct area, inflammation, improve neurological outcomes, and promote angiogenesis within the contused areas.[186–188]

Due to the preclinical effects on secondary injury progression, the use of hyperbaric oxygen therapy was theorized to improve those suffering with postconcussive syndrome (PCS). The application of hyperbaric oxygen for PCS was first proposed by Stoller et al. in a publication of two case

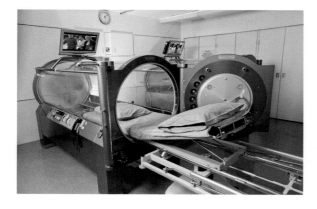

Figure 10.4 An example of a hyperbaric oxygen chamber.

studies of patients suffering from cognitive impairment.[189] One athlete was an ex-NFL player who was exposed to multiple concussions and, likely, years of subconcussions; the other athlete was a high school player who received multiple repetitive concussions during an acute time frame with persistent postconcussive symptoms. Remarkably, following 40 sessions of hyperbaric oxygen treatment, both athletes showed improvements on neuropsychological testing. Boussi et al. followed up with these findings in a randomized crossover controlled trial of 56 mTBI patients, 1 to 5 years after injury, who also had persistent postconcussive syndrome. Following the hyperbaric treatment regiment, athletes still exhibited improvements in cognitive functioning that also correlated with increased cerebral blood flow seen on single photon emission computed tomography (SPECT).[190]

Unfortunately, these positive findings have not been consistent in further randomized controlled trials, which could be contributed to the poor clinical design of the early studies (lack of blinding or placebo control)[191–195] Specifically, Walker et al. found no change in balance, fine motor skills, or neuropsychological testing between controls and those treated with 10 weeks of hyperbaric oxygen therapy in their cohort of 60 male military mTBI patients with persistent postconcussive syndrome lasting 3 to 36 months after injury.[191] Similarly, Miller et al. also demonstrated no benefit over controls in a multicenter sham, blinded, randomized control study in 72 military patients with persistent symptoms >4 months from mTBI.[79] Though hyperbaric treatment seems to be negated in the military mTBI population current literature still does not offer enough evidence to support or refute its role in sports concussion until stronger studies (randomized, placebo controlled) are performed.

Hypothermia

Preclinical and clinical studies have demonstrated the detrimental effect of hyperthermia on the injured brain.[196] For every one degree Celsius increase, the metabolic rate of the brain is increased by 7%![197] Following injury, the brain is in a state of mismatch where it is starving for energy, but is unable to efficiently produce it due to reduced blood flow and dysfunctional mitochondria. This lack of energy leads to byproduct formation of lactic acid and reactive oxygen/nitrogen species causing further secondary injury. Therefore, additional neuronal stress through hyperthermia and increased energy demand is critically undesirable. For these reasons, the inverse, mild hypothermia and reduced neuronal metabolism would theoretically protect the neuron from propagation of the neurometabolic cascade.[198]

When hypothermia was carried out following injury, animal models in single and repetitive TBI demonstrated astounding results in neuroprotection through blunting neurotransmitter release, calcium influx, BBB breakdown, the apoptosis pathway, APP accumulation, cytokine release, the inflammatory response, reduced contusion volume, preserved cerebral vascular reactivity, and improved brain glucose utilization, ultimately resulting in superior behavior and neurological outcomes.[197,199–205] However, the most recent randomized controlled studies for hypothermia in the pediatric and adult population have shown no improvement in long-term morbidity or mortality, possibly due to the negative systemic effects of hypothermia. [197,206,207]

The production of a scalp and neck-cooling device has been manufactured as a way to prevent the possible systemic detrimental effects

(increased intracranial pressure from shivering or reduced immune response) encountered with full body cooling. Wang et al. first demonstrated this novel idea in eight severe head injured or stroke patients, where the cooling device could be applied and monitored with invasive temperature devices. Through the use of warming blankets, they were able to maintain the patient's core temperature while isolating and raising the cerebral temperature by 1.84°C in one hour.[208,209] This therapy has been suggested for concussion and postconcussive syndrome but randomized clinical trial data is absent to prove efficacy (Figure 10.5).

Transcranial low level laser therapy

Transcranial low level laser therapy (LLLT), or "cold laser therapy, is a noninvasive treatment that involves the application of red and infrared light to the scalp[210–212] (Figure 10.6).[210–213] It is termed a "cold" laser because the intensity is not high enough to cause heat production or tissue injury.[212] Cadaveric studies have demonstrated that even through scalp application, the light penetrates beyond the skull and meninges to a depth of 40 mm into the cortical tissue.[214] It is believed that the LLLT has direct physiological effects on the mitochondria and has been proposed for use in inflammatory diseases, pain, stroke, TBI, neurodegenerative diseases, spinal cord injuries, and peripheral nerve disorders[215–220] (Figure 10.7).

A myriad of preclinical studies have demonstrated not only safety, but also efficacy in TBI

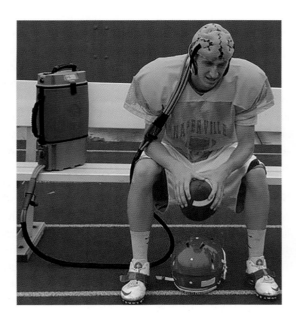

Figure 10.5 WElkins Sideline Cooling System.

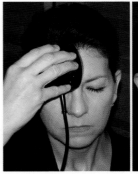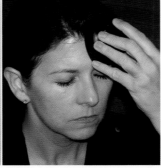

Figure 10.6 Transcranial Low Level Laser Therapy (LLLT). (From Huang YY et al. *J Biophotonics*. Nov;5(11–12): 827–37, 2012.)

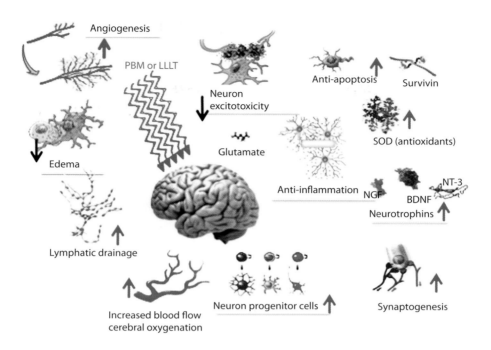

Figure 10.7 **Proposed mechanisms of LLLT.** (From Hamblin MR. *BBA Clin.* Oct 1;6:113–124, 2016.)

animal models. McCarthy et al. applied one to three treatments to rats and found no significant hematological, neoplastic, or histopathological changes one year after treatment.[221] Further work in TBI animal models has theorized that LLLT is absorbed by the mitochondria leading to improved energy production. This is tremendously important during the acute window period following injury where the neurons become further damaged due to their inability to provide the much needed energy necessary during this highly metabolic period. The application of LLLT, resulting in improved efficiency of the mitochondria, reduces production of reactive oxygen and nitrogen species, ultimately diminishing secondary neuronal death/apoptosis and improving outcomes.[210,222] Histologically, LLLT has also been shown to reduce edema, inflammation, cytokine release, infarct progression, and also stimulate release of neuronal and synaptic growth factors.[210,223–229] It is important to note that this is a complex and poorly understood technology where even the specific wavelength of light, dosing, and intensity is incredibly important in instigating the advantageous biochemical alterations within the neuron.[216,225,230–232]

To date, there is no randomized controlled clinical trial for the use of this therapy in concussion. Henderson et al. did publish a case study in which a patient with moderate TBI, who received 2 months of laser therapy, showed improvements in both cognitive and psychological symptoms (depression, anxiety, headaches, and insomnia).[233] Though supported by very limited clinical studies, the mitochondrial effects seen in preclinical models suggest great promise for use during the acute injury period following concussion, warranting further study.

Scalp light emitting diodes

Scalp light emitting diodes (LED) is a similar therapy to LLLT but uses a more inexpensive light source. Parallel to LLLT, LED has been demonstrated in cadaveric models to penetrate into cortical tissue, be absorbed by the mitochondria leading to improved energy production, and also have anti-inflammatory properties.[234,235] Also, LED has been shown clinically, in a vegetative state patient following severe TBI, to improve cerebral blood flow by 20% on SPECT imaging, as reported by Nawashiro et al.[236] It is currently unknown if there is any clinical advantage to LED over LLLT.[212]

Unlike LLLT, LED does provide slightly more clinical proof of its advantageous use in brain injured patients, but is still greatly limited. Naeser et al. first published a case report of the use of LED in two patients who suffered from cognitive disabilities following a mTBI. They revealed that the use of LED, even in the chronic postconcussive period, increased attention, improved sleep, reduced postconcussive symptoms, and improved neuropsychological testing.[237] Following up these intriguing results, Naeser et al. studied the use of LED in 11 chronic mTBI patients (10 months to 8 years following injury) who suffered with persistent cognitive deficits. After receiving a total of 18 outpatient treatments, the patients were also found to have improved neuropsychological testing, a reduction in post-traumatic stress symptoms, and improved social functioning.[234] But it is important to emphasize that neither of these studies included randomization of placebo-controls. Currently in recruitment, a clinical trial in mTBI patients who suffer from chronic (over 4 months) cognitive disabilities will be randomized to LED treatment versus placebo to determine its effect on neurocognitive testing.[238]

Transcranial magnetic stimulation

Transcranial magnetic stimulation (TMS) is a therapy that involves applying a brief magnetic pulse (1–4 tesla) over a specific cortical area to induce an electrical alteration to the neurons adjacent to the area on the skull that is being stimulated (Figure 10.8).[213,239] Depending on the type of pulse that is used and area of brain that is targeted, different responses can occur. For example, a single pulse over the primary motor cortex creates neuronal depolarization of the corticospinal neurons leading to muscle contraction, measured by percutaneous electrodes as a motor-evoked potential. Other repetitive or continuous pulses, like continuous theta burst stimulation, can be applied to neurons and thus the changes in electrical activity, either hypoexcitabilty or hyperexcitability, can be evaluated.[213] Though a noninvasive procedure, TMS does carry the risk of inducing seizures, which is concerning in patients that are already prone to developing them, especially in the case of severe TBI.[213]

The use of TMS has been applied to the different severities of TBI, as a potential diagnostic

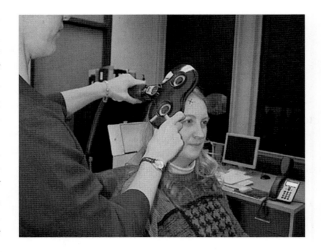

Figure 10.8 Transcranial Magnetic Stimulation (TMS). (From Pape TL et al. *J Head Trauma Rehabil.* Sep–Oct;21(5): 437–51, 2006.)

tool, and also as a therapeutic modality.[240,241] Application of TMS over the motor cortex has demonstrated neuronal inhibitory and excitatory alterations following a concussive injury. A specific measure, the cortical silent period, is the electrical silence occurring after muscle contraction and a TMS pulse. Following concussion, this period has been shown to be prolonged, presumably due to increased intracortical inhibition.[242] Multiple studies have evaluated this and other electrophysiological parameters through TMS to demonstrate distinct differences between patients with different severity of TBI,[243] acute injury versus healthy controls,[244–247] symptomatic versus asymptomatic patients in both the acute and chronic period following concussion,[241,244] and those exposed to repetitive concussions.[248,249] Interestingly, these changes also correlated with clinical outcomes and appear to have a prognostic value.[239,249] Pearce et al. studied 40 elite and amateur football players that suffered on average 3.2 concussions throughout their career.[249] In comparison to controls, the football cohort demonstrated intracortical inhibition through TMS that was also associated with reductions in performance on clinical tests (reaction time and fine motor control).

Further stimulating studies in TMS have demonstrated alterations within the acute (within

48 hours) interval with persistent changes weeks after injury.[245,246,250] Additionally, as demonstrated by Powers et al., athletes that were returned back to sport still displayed these functional differences of hypoexcitability through TMS.[241] TMS may have the potential to relay valuable information to the clinician regarding the functional neuronal changes that are persistent after a concussive injury, maybe precluding the individual from return to activity.

Not only has TMS shown potential for diagnosis and to measure injury evolution, there also is preliminary evidence that it may improve prolonged symptoms following brain injury. Koski et al. applied 20 sessions of TMS to 15 mTBI patients who had persistent postconcussive symptoms for greater than 3 months.[251] Not only did postconcussive syndrome scores decline by 14.6 points, these patients were also found to have an increase in cerebral activation during tasks on fMRI imaging. Though noteworthy, this study was not randomized and not placebo controlled. Leung et al. followed up this study with a cohort of mTBI patients who suffered from chronic daily headaches.[252] This randomized, sham controlled study did demonstrate a reduction in subjective headache intensity at 1 and 4 weeks in those treated with TMS compared to sham.

Conclusion

Though not all encompassing, this chapter reviewed the more recent experimental modalities being studied to improve concussion diagnosis, recovery monitoring, and treatment. Everything discussed within this chapter is considered investigational and not part of standard clinical practice. Further large prospective, randomized, placebo-controlled clinical studies need to be implemented for each modality to determine true clinical significance. Though dominated with preclinical animal and non-level 1 clinical studies, there are nevertheless encouraging outcomes to be noted. Only as research uncovers the pathophysiology of a concussive injury will further scientific advances occur in the objective measures of diagnosis and the monitoring of recovery following concussion.

References

1. Biomarkers Definitions Working G. Biomarkers and surrogate endpoints: preferred definitions and conceptual framework. *Clinical Pharmacology and Therapeutics.* 2001; 69(3): 89–95.

2. Zetterberg H, Smith DH, Blennow K. Biomarkers of mild traumatic brain injury in cerebrospinal fluid and blood. *Nature Reviews Neurology.* 2013; 9(4): 201–210.

3. Plog BA, Nedergaard M. Why have we not yet developed a simple blood test for TBI? *Expert Review of Neurotherapeutics.* 2015; 15(5): 465–468.

4. McCarthy MT, Kosofsky BE. Clinical features and biomarkers of concussion and mild traumatic brain injury in pediatric patients. *Annals of the New York Academy of Sciences.* 2015; 1345: 89–98.

5. Kulbe JR, Geddes JW. Current status of fluid biomarkers in mild traumatic brain injury. *Experimental Neurology.* 2015.

6. Forde CT, Karri SK, Young AM, Ogilvy CS. Predictive markers in traumatic brain injury: opportunities for a serum biosignature. *British Journal of Neurosurgery.* 2014; 28(1): 8–15.

7. Zetterberg H, Blennow K. Fluid markers of traumatic brain injury. *Molecular and Cellular Neurosciences.* 2015; 66(Pt B): 99–102.

8. Shan R, Szmydynger-Chodobska J, Warren OU, Mohammad F, Zink BJ, Chodobski A. A new panel of blood biomarkers for the diagnosis of mild traumatic brain injury/concussion in adults. *Journal of Neurotrauma.* 2015.

9. Papa L, Lewis LM, Silvestri S et al. Serum levels of ubiquitin C-terminal hydrolase distinguish mild traumatic brain injury from trauma controls and are elevated in mild and moderate traumatic brain injury patients with intracranial lesions and neurosurgical intervention. *The Journal of Trauma and Acute Care Surgery.* 2012; 72(5): 1335–1344.

10. Kou Z, Gattu R, Kobeissy F et al. Combining biochemical and imaging markers to improve diagnosis and characterization of mild traumatic brain injury in the acute setting: results from a pilot study. *PLoS One.* 2013; 8(11): e80296.

11. Diaz-Arrastia R, Wang KK, Papa L et al. Acute biomarkers of traumatic brain injury: relationship between plasma levels of ubiquitin C-terminal hydrolase-L1 and glial fibrillary acidic protein. *Journal of Neurotrauma.* 2014; 31(1): 19–25.

12. Puvenna V, Brennan C, Shaw G et al. Significance of ubiquitin carboxy-terminal hydrolase L1 elevations in athletes after subconcussive head hits. *PLoS One.* 2014; 9(5): e96296.

13. Berger RP, Hayes RL, Richichi R, Beers SR, Wang KK. Serum concentrations of ubiquitin C-terminal hydrolase-L1 and alphaII-spectrin breakdown product 145 kDa correlate with outcome after pediatric TBI. *Journal of Neurotrauma.* 2012; 29(1): 162–167.

14. Welch RD, Ayaz SI, Lewis LM et al. Ability of Serum Glial Fibrillary Acidic Protein, Ubiquitin C-Terminal Hydrolase-L1, and S100B to differentiate normal and abnormal head computed tomography findings in patients with suspected mild or moderate traumatic brain injury. *Journal of Neurotrauma.* 2015.

15. Berger RP, Adelson PD, Pierce MC, Dulani T, Cassidy LD, Kochanek PM. Serum neuron-specific enolase, S100B, and myelin basic protein concentrations after inflicted and noninflicted traumatic brain injury in children. *Journal of Neurosurgery.* 2005; 103(1 Suppl): 61–68.

16. Meric E, Gunduz A, Turedi S, Cakir E, Yandi M. The prognostic value of neuron-specific enolase in head trauma patients. *The Journal of Emergency Medicine.* 2010; 38(3): 297–301.

17. Skogseid IM, Nordby HK, Urdal P, Paus E, Lilleaas F. Increased serum creatine kinase BB and neuron specific enolase following head injury indicates brain damage. *Acta Neurochirurgica.* 1992; 115(3–4): 106–111.

18. Stalnacke BM, Bjornstig U, Karlsson K, Sojka P. One-year follow-up of mild traumatic brain injury: post-concussion symptoms, disabilities and life satisfaction in relation to serum levels of S-100B and neurone-specific enolase in acute phase. *Journal of Rehabilitation Medicine.* 2005; 37(5): 300–305.

19. Pelsers MM, Hanhoff T, Van der Voort D et al. Brain- and heart-type fatty acid-binding proteins in the brain: tissue distribution and clinical utility. *Clinical Chemistry.* 2004; 50(9): 1568–1575.

20. de Kruijk JR, Leffers P, Menheere PP, Meerhoff S, Twijnstra A. S-100B and neuron-specific enolase in serum of mild traumatic brain injury patients. A comparison with health controls. *Acta Neurologica Scandinavica.* 2001; 103(3): 175–179.

21. Pinelis VG, Sorokina EG, Semenova JB et al. Biomarkers in children with traumatic brain injury. *Zhurnal nevrologii i psikhiatrii imeni SS Korsakova/Ministerstvo zdravookhraneniia i meditsinskoi promyshlennosti Rossiiskoi Federatsii, Vserossiiskoe obshchestvo nevrologov [i] Vserossiiskoe obshchestvo psikhiat.* 2015; 115(8): 66–72.

22. Topolovec-Vranic J, Pollmann-Mudryj MA, Ouchterlony D et al. The value of serum biomarkers in prediction models of outcome after mild traumatic brain injury. *The Journal of Trauma.* 2011; 71(5 Suppl 1): S478–486.

23. De Kruijk JR, Leffers P, Menheere PP, Meerhoff S, Rutten J, Twijnstra A. Prediction of post-traumatic complaints after mild traumatic brain injury: early symptoms and biochemical markers. *Journal of Neurology, Neurosurgery, and Psychiatry.* 2002; 73(6): 727–732.

24. Mussack T, Biberthaler P, Kanz KG et al. Immediate S-100B and neuron-specific enolase plasma measurements for rapid evaluation of

primary brain damage in alcohol-intoxicated, minor head-injured patients. *Shock (Augusta, Ga)*. 2002; 18(5): 395–400.

25. Wolf H, Frantal S, Pajenda GS et al. Predictive value of neuromarkers supported by a set of clinical criteria in patients with mild traumatic brain injury: S100B protein and neuron-specific enolase on trial: clinical article. *Journal of Neurosurgery*. 2013; 118(6): 1298–1303.

26. Graham MR, Pates J, Davies B et al. Should an increase in cerebral neurochemicals following head kicks in full contact karate influence return to play? *International Journal of Immunopathology and Pharmacology*. 2015; 28(4): 539–546.

27. Shahim P, Tegner Y, Wilson DH et al. Blood biomarkers for brain injury in concussed professional ice hockey players. *The Journal of the American Medical Association Neurology*. 2014; 71(6): 684–692.

28. Ringger NC, O'Steen BE, Brabham JG et al. A novel marker for traumatic brain injury: CSF alphaII-spectrin breakdown product levels. *Journal of Neurotrauma*. 2004; 21(10): 1443–1456.

29. Mondello S, Robicsek SA, Gabrielli A et al. alphaII-spectrin breakdown products (SBDPs): diagnosis and outcome in severe traumatic brain injury patients. *Journal of Neurotrauma*. 2010; 27(7): 1203–1213.

30. Siman R, Giovannone N, Hanten G et al. Evidence that the blood biomarker sntf predicts brain imaging changes and persistent cognitive dysfunction in mild tbi patients. *Frontiers in Neurology*. 2013; 4: 190.

31. Siman R, Shahim P, Tegner Y, Blennow K, Zetterberg H, Smith DH. Serum sntf increases in concussed professional ice hockey players and relates to the severity of postconcussion symptoms. *Journal of Neurotrauma*. 2015; 32(17): 1294–1300.

32. Dambinova SA, Shikuev AV, Weissman JD, Mullins JD. AMPAR peptide values in blood of nonathletes and club sport athletes with concussions. *Military Medicine*. 2013; 178(3): 285–290.

33. Gabbita SP, Scheff SW, Menard RM, Roberts K, Fugaccia I, Zemlan FP. Cleaved-tau: a biomarker of neuronal damage after traumatic brain injury. *Journal of Neurotrauma*. 2005; 22(1): 83–94.

34. Bulut M, Koksal O, Dogan S et al. Tau protein as a serum marker of brain damage in mild traumatic brain injury: preliminary results. *Advances in Therapy*. 2006; 23(1): 12–22.

35. Kavalci C, Pekdemir M, Durukan P et al. The value of serum tau protein for the diagnosis of intracranial injury in minor head trauma. *The American Journal of Emergency Medicine*. 2007; 25(4): 391–395.

36. Guzel A, Karasalihoglu S, Aylanc H, Temizoz O, Hicdonmez T. Validity of serum tau protein levels in pediatric patients with minor head trauma. *The American Journal of Emergency Medicine*. 2010; 28(4): 399–403.

37. Shahim P, Linemann T, Inekci D et al. Serum tau fragments predict return to play in concussed professional ice hockey players. *Journal of Neurotrauma*. 2015.

38. Bazarian JJ, Zemlan FP, Mookerjee S, Stigbrand T. Serum S-100B and cleaved-tau are poor predictors of long-term outcome after mild traumatic brain injury. *Brain Injury*. 2006; 20(7): 759–765.

39. Ma M, Lindsell CJ, Rosenberry CM, Shaw GJ, Zemlan FP. Serum cleaved tau does not predict postconcussion syndrome after mild traumatic brain injury. *The American Journal of Emergency Medicine*. 2008; 26(7): 763–768.

40. Neselius S, Brisby H, Granholm F, Zetterberg H, Blennow K. Monitoring concussion in a knocked-out boxer by CSF biomarker analysis. *Knee Surgery, Sports Traumatology, Arthroscopy*. 2015; 23(9): 2536–2539.

41. Martinez-Morillo E, Childs C, Garcia BP et al. Neurofilament medium polypeptide (NFM) protein concentration is increased in CSF

and serum samples from patients with brain injury. *Clinical Chemistry and Laboratory Medicine*. 2015; 53(10): 1575–1584.

42. Neselius S, Zetterberg H, Blennow K, Marcusson J, Brisby H. Increased CSF levels of phosphorylated neurofilament heavy protein following bout in amateur boxers. *PLoS One*. 2013; 8(11): e81249.

43. Neselius S, Brisby H, Marcusson J, Zetterberg H, Blennow K, Karlsson T. Neurological assessment and its relationship to CSF biomarkers in amateur boxers. *PLoS One*. 2014; 9(6): e99870.

44. Schulte S, Podlog LW, Hamson-Utley JJ, Strathmann FG, Struder HK. A systematic review of the biomarker S100B: implications for sport-related concussion management. *Journal of Athletic Training*. 2014; 49(6): 830–850.

45. Di Pietro V, Amorini AM, Lazzarino G et al. S100B and glial fibrillary acidic protein as indexes to monitor damage severity in an in vitro model of traumatic brain injury. *Neurochemical Research*. 2015; 40(5): 991–999.

46. Babcock L, Byczkowski T, Wade SL, Ho M, Bazarian JJ. Inability of S100B to predict post-concussion syndrome in children who present to the emergency department with mild traumatic brain injury: a brief report. *Pediatric Emergency Care*. 2013; 29(4): 458–461.

47. BET 3: Can protein S100B add to current clinical guidelines in adult minor head injury? *EMJ*. 2013; 30(7): 597–599.

48. Ryb GE, Dischinger PC, Auman KM et al. S-100beta does not predict outcome after mild traumatic brain injury. *Brain Injury*. 2014; 28(11): 1430–1435.

49. Wolf H, Frantal S, Pajenda G, Leitgeb J, Sarahrudi K, Hajdu S. Analysis of S100 calcium binding protein B serum levels in different types of traumatic intracranial lesions. *Journal of Neurotrauma*. 2015; 32(1): 23–27.

50. Papa L, Silvestri S, Brophy GM et al. GFAP out-performs S100beta in detecting traumatic intracranial lesions on computed tomography in trauma patients with mild traumatic brain injury and those with extracranial lesions. *Journal of Neurotrauma*. 2014; 31(22): 1815–1822.

51. Bazarian JJ, Blyth BJ, He H et al. Classification accuracy of serum Apo A-I and S100B for the diagnosis of mild traumatic brain injury and prediction of abnormal initial head computed tomography scan. *Journal of Neurotrauma*. 2013; 30(20): 1747–1754.

52. Kiechle K, Bazarian JJ, Merchant-Borna K et al. Subject-specific increases in serum S-100B distinguish sports-related concussion from sports-related exertion. *PLoS One*. 2014; 9(1): e84977.

53. Yang SH, Gustafson J, Gangidine M et al. A murine model of mild traumatic brain injury exhibiting cognitive and motor deficits. *The Journal of Surgical Research*. 2013; 184(2): 981–988.

54. Mannix R, Eisenberg M, Berry M, Meehan WP, 3rd, Hayes RL. Serum biomarkers predict acute symptom burden in children after concussion: a preliminary study. *Journal of Neurotrauma*. 2014; 31(11): 1072–1075.

55. McMahon PJ, Panczykowski DM, Yue JK et al. Measurement of the glial fibrillary acidic protein and its breakdown products GFAP-BDP biomarker for the detection of traumatic brain injury compared to computed tomography and magnetic resonance imaging. *Journal of Neurotrauma*. 2015; 32(8): 527–533.

56. Okonkwo DO, Yue JK, Puccio AM et al. GFAP-BDP as an acute diagnostic marker in traumatic brain injury: results from the prospective transforming research and clinical knowledge in traumatic brain injury study. *Journal of Neurotrauma*. 2013; 30(17): 1490–1497.

57. Prodan CI, Vincent AS, Dale GL. Coated-platelet levels are persistently elevated in patients with mild traumatic brain injury.

The Journal of Head Trauma Rehabilitation. 2014; 29(6): 522–526.

58. Yu L, Wu X, Wang H, Long D, Yang J, Zhang Y. Diagnostic and prognostic significance of suPAR in traumatic brain injury. *Neurology India*. 2014; 62(5): 498–502.

59. Korley FK, Diaz-Arrastia R, Wu AH et al. Circulating brain-derived neurotrophic factor has diagnostic and prognostic value in traumatic brain injury. *Journal of Neurotrauma*. 2015.

60. Berger RP, Fromkin J, Rubin P, Snyder J, Richichi R, Kochanek P. Serum D-dimer concentrations are increased after pediatric traumatic brain injury. *Journal of Pediatrics*. 2015; 166(2): 383–388.

61. Pham N, Akonasu H, Shishkin R, Taghibiglou C. Plasma soluble prion protein, a potential biomarker for sport-related concussions: a pilot study. *PLoS One*. 2015; 10(2): e0117286.

62. La Fountaine MF, Toda M, Testa A, Bauman WA. Suppression of serum prolactin levels after sports concussion with prompt resolution upon independent clinical assessment to permit return-to-play. *Journal of Neurotrauma*. 2015.

63. Shen S, Loo RR, Wanner IB, Loo JA. Addressing the needs of traumatic brain injury with clinical proteomics. *Clinical Proteomics*. 2014; 11(1): 11.

64. Di Battista AP, Rhind SG, Baker AJ. Application of blood-based biomarkers in human mild traumatic brain injury. *Frontiers in Neurology*. 2013; 4: 44.

65. Papa L, Ramia MM, Edwards D, Johnson BD, Slobounov SM. Systematic review of clinical studies examining biomarkers of brain injury in athletes after sports-related concussion. *Journal of Neurotrauma*. 2015; 32(10): 661–673.

66. Jeter CB, Hergenroeder GW, Hylin MJ, Redell JB, Moore AN, Dash PK. Biomarkers for the diagnosis and prognosis of mild traumatic brain injury/concussion. *Journal of Neurotrauma*. 2013; 30(8): 657–670.

67. Mondello S, Schmid K, Berger RP et al. The challenge of mild traumatic brain injury: role of biochemical markers in diagnosis of brain damage. *Medicinal Research Reviews*. 2014; 34(3): 503–531.

68. Evans TM, Van Remmen H, Purkar A et al. Microwave & magnetic (m) proteomics of a mouse model of mild traumatic brain injury. *Translational Proteomics*. 2014; 3: 10–21.

69. Chen KY, Tsai TY, Chang CF et al. Worsening of dizziness impairment is associated with BMX level in patients after mild traumatic brain injury. *Journal of Neurotrauma*. 2015.

70. Buonora JE, Yarnell AM, Lazarus RC et al. Multivariate analysis of traumatic brain injury: development of an assessment score. *Frontiers in Neurology*. 2015; 6: 68.

71. Kochanek PM, Jackson TC, Ferguson NM et al. Emerging therapies in traumatic brain injury. *Seminars in Neurology*. 2015; 35(1): 83–100.

72. Roberts I, Yates D, Sandercock P et al. Effect of intravenous corticosteroids on death within 14 days in 10008 adults with clinically significant head injury (MRC CRASH trial): randomised placebo-controlled trial. *Lancet*. 2004; 364(9442): 1321–1328.

73. Beauchamp K, Mutlak H, Smith WR, Shohami E, Stahel PF. Pharmacology of traumatic brain injury: where is the "golden bullet"? *Molecular Medicine (Cambridge, Mass)*. 2008; 14(11–12): 731–740.

74. Wright DW, Kellermann AL, Hertzberg VS et al. ProTECT: a randomized clinical trial of progesterone for acute traumatic brain injury. *Annals of Emergency Medicine*. 2007; 49(4): 391–402, 402.e391–392.

75. Ma J, Huang S, Qin S, You C. Progesterone for acute traumatic brain injury. *The Cochrane Database of Systematic Reviews*. 2012; 10: Cd008409.

76. Wright DW, Yeatts SD, Silbergleit R et al. Very early administration of progesterone for acute traumatic brain injury. *The New*

England Journal of Medicine. 2014; 371(26): 2457–2466.

77. Barrett EC, McBurney MI, Ciappio ED. omega-3 fatty acid supplementation as a potential therapeutic aid for the recovery from mild traumatic brain injury/concussion. *Advances in Nutrition (Bethesda, Md).* 2014; 5(3): 268–277.

78. Bailes JE, Patel V. The potential for DHA to mitigate mild traumatic brain injury. *Military Medicine.* 2014; 179(11 Suppl): 112–116.

79. Robson LG, Dyall S, Sidloff D, Michael-Titus AT. Omega-3 polyunsaturated fatty acids increase the neurite outgrowth of rat sensory neurones throughout development and in aged animals. *Neurobiology of Aging.* 2010; 31(4): 678–687.

80. Lu DY, Tsao YY, Leung YM, Su KP. Docosahexaenoic acid suppresses neuroinflammatory responses and induces heme oxygenase-1 expression in BV-2 microglia: implications of antidepressant effects for omega-3 fatty acids. *Neuropsychopharmacology.* 2010; 35(11): 2238–2248.

81. Songur A, Sarsilmaz M, Sogut S et al. Hypothalamic superoxide dismutase, xanthine oxidase, nitric oxide, and malondialdehyde in rats fed with fish omega-3 fatty acids. *Progress in Neuro-Psychopharmacology & Biological Psychiatry.* 2004; 28(4): 693–698.

82. Petraglia AL, Winkler EA, Bailes JE. Stuck at the bench: Potential natural neuroprotective compounds for concussion. *Surgical Neurology International.* 2011; 2: 146.

83. Dyall SC, Michael-Titus AT. Neurological benefits of omega-3 fatty acids. *Neuromolecular Medicine.* 2008; 10(4): 219–235.

84. Poppitt SD, Howe CA, Lithander FE et al. Effects of moderate-dose omega-3 fish oil on cardiovascular risk factors and mood after ischemic stroke: a randomized, controlled trial. *Stroke.* 2009; 40(11): 3485–3492.

85. Yoneda H, Shirao S, Kurokawa T, Fujisawa H, Kato S, Suzuki M. Does eicosapentaenoic acid (EPA) inhibit cerebral vasospasm in patients after aneurysmal subarachnoid hemorrhage? *Acta Neurologica Scandinavica.* 2008; 118(1): 54–59.

86. Yuen AW, Sander JW, Fluegel D et al. Omega-3 fatty acid supplementation in patients with chronic epilepsy: a randomized trial. *Epilepsy and Behavior.* 2005; 7(2): 253–258.

87. Puri BK, Koepp MJ, Holmes J, Hamilton G, Yuen AW. A 31-phosphorus neurospectroscopy study of omega-3 long-chain polyunsaturated fatty acid intervention with eicosapentaenoic acid and docosahexaenoic acid in patients with chronic refractory epilepsy. *Prostaglandins Leukot Essent Fatty Acids.* 2007; 77(2): 105–107.

88. Kotani S, Sakaguchi E, Warashina S et al. Dietary supplementation of arachidonic and docosahexaenoic acids improves cognitive dysfunction. *Neuroscience Research.* 2006; 56(2): 159–164.

89. Morley JE, Banks WA. Lipids and cognition. *Journal of Alzheimer's Disease.* 2010; 20(3): 737–747.

90. Quinn JF, Raman R, Thomas RG et al. Docosahexaenoic acid supplementation and cognitive decline in Alzheimer disease: a randomized trial. *The Journal of the American Medical Association.* 2010; 304(17): 1903–1911.

91. Lucke-Wold BP, Logsdon AF, Nguyen L et al. Supplements, nutrition, and alternative therapies for the treatment of traumatic brain injury. *Nutritional Neuroscience.* 2016: 1–13.

92. Bailes JE, Mills JD. Docosahexaenoic acid reduces traumatic axonal injury in a rodent head injury model. *Journal of Neurotrauma.* 2010; 27(9): 1617–1624.

93. Wu A, Ying Z, Gomez-Pinilla F. Dietary omega-3 fatty acids normalize BDNF levels, reduce oxidative damage, and counteract learning disability after traumatic brain injury in rats. *Journal of Neurotrauma.* 2004; 21(10): 1457–1467.

94. Wu A, Ying Z, Gomez-Pinilla F. Exercise facilitates the action of dietary DHA on functional recovery after brain trauma. *Neuroscience.* 2013; 248: 655–663.

95. Begum G, Yan HQ, Li L, Singh A, Dixon CE, Sun D. Docosahexaenoic acid reduces ER stress and abnormal protein accumulation and improves neuronal function following traumatic brain injury. *Journal of Neuroscience.* 2014; 34(10): 3743–3755.

96. Hasadsri L, Wang BH, Lee JV et al. Omega-3 fatty acids as a putative treatment for traumatic brain injury. *Journal of Neurotrauma.* 2013; 30(11): 897–906.

97. Michael-Titus AT, Priestley JV. Omega-3 fatty acids and traumatic neurological injury: from neuroprotection to neuroplasticity? *Trends in Neurosciences.* 2014; 37(1): 30–38.

98. Mills JD, Bailes JE, Sedney CL, Hutchins H, Sears B. Omega-3 fatty acid supplementation and reduction of traumatic axonal injury in a rodent head injury model. *Journal of Neurosurgery.* 2011; 114(1): 77–84.

99. Russell KL, Berman NE, Gregg PR, Levant B. Fish oil improves motor function, limits blood–brain barrier disruption, and reduces Mmp9 gene expression in a rat model of juvenile traumatic brain injury. *Prostaglandins Leukot Essent Fatty Acids.* 2014; 90(1): 5–11.

100. Wang T, Van KC, Gavitt BJ et al. Effect of fish oil supplementation in a rat model of multiple mild traumatic brain injuries. *Restorative Neurology and Neuroscience.* 2013; 31(5): 647–659.

101. Wu A, Ying Z, Gomez-Pinilla F. Omega-3 fatty acids supplementation restores mechanisms that maintain brain homeostasis in traumatic brain injury. *Journal of Neurotrauma.* 2007; 24(10): 1587–1595.

102. Wu A, Ying Z, Gomez-Pinilla F. The salutary effects of DHA dietary supplementation on cognition, neuroplasticity, and membrane homeostasis after brain trauma. *Journal of Neurotrauma.* 2011; 28(10): 2113–2122.

103. Zheng GQ, Cheng W, Wang Y et al. Ginseng total saponins enhance neurogenesis after focal cerebral ischemia. *Journal of Ethnopharmacology.* 2011; 133(2): 724–728.

104. Li Y, Tang J, Khatibi NH et al. Treatment with ginsenoside rb1, a component of panax ginseng, provides neuroprotection in rats subjected to subarachnoid hemorrhage-induced brain injury. *Acta Neurochirurgica Supplement.* 2011; 110(Pt 2): 75–79.

105. Wang Y, Liu J, Zhang Z, Bi P, Qi Z, Zhang C. Anti-neuroinflammation effect of ginsenoside Rbl in a rat model of Alzheimer disease. *Neuroscience Letters.* 2011; 487(1): 70–72.

106. Ye R, Kong X, Yang Q et al. Ginsenoside rd in experimental stroke: superior neuroprotective efficacy with a wide therapeutic window. *Neurotherapeutics.* 2011; 8(3): 515–525.

107. Ye R, Zhang X, Kong X et al. Ginsenoside Rd attenuates mitochondrial dysfunction and sequential apoptosis after transient focal ischemia. *Neuroscience.* 2011; 178: 169–180.

108. Luo FC, Wang SD, Qi L, Song JY, Lv T, Bai J. Protective effect of panaxatriol saponins extracted from Panax notoginseng against MPTP-induced neurotoxicity in vivo. *Journal of Ethnopharmacology.* 2011; 133(2): 448–453.

109. Geng J, Dong J, Ni H et al. Ginseng for cognition. *The Cochrane Database of Systematic Reviews.* 2010(12): Cd007769.

110. Liang W, Ge S, Yang L et al. Ginsenosides Rb1 and Rg1 promote proliferation and expression of neurotrophic factors in primary Schwann cell cultures. *Brain Research.* 2010; 1357: 19–25.

111. Richard T, Pawlus AD, Iglesias ML et al. Neuroprotective properties of resveratrol and derivatives. *Annals of the New York Academy of Sciences.* 2011; 1215: 103–108.

112. Baur JA, Sinclair DA. Therapeutic potential of resveratrol: the in vivo evidence. *Nature Reviews Drug Discovery.* 2006; 5(6): 493–506.

113. Raval AP, Dave KR, Perez-Pinzon MA. Resveratrol mimics ischemic preconditioning in the brain. *Journal of Cerebral Blood Flow and Metabolism*. 2006; 26(9): 1141–1147.

114. Li C, Yan Z, Yang J et al. Neuroprotective effects of resveratrol on ischemic injury mediated by modulating the release of neurotransmitter and neuromodulator in rats. *Neurochemistry International*. 2010; 56(3): 495–500.

115. Gao D, Zhang X, Jiang X et al. Resveratrol reduces the elevated level of MMP-9 induced by cerebral ischemia-reperfusion in mice. *Life Sciences*. 2006; 78(22): 2564–2570.

116. Della-Morte D, Dave KR, DeFazio RA, Bao YC, Raval AP, Perez-Pinzon MA. Resveratrol pretreatment protects rat brain from cerebral ischemic damage via a sirtuin 1-uncoupling protein 2 pathway. *Neuroscience*. 2009; 159(3): 993–1002.

117. Yang YB, Piao YJ. Effects of resveratrol on secondary damages after acute spinal cord injury in rats. *Acta Pharmacologica Sinica*. 2003; 24(7): 703–710.

118. Karuppagounder SS, Pinto JT, Xu H, Chen HL, Beal MF, Gibson GE. Dietary supplementation with resveratrol reduces plaque pathology in a transgenic model of Alzheimer's disease. *Neurochemistry International*. 2009; 54(2): 111–118.

119. Ates O, Cayli S, Altinoz E et al. Neuroprotection by resveratrol against traumatic brain injury in rats. *Molecular and Cellular Biochemistry*. 2007; 294(1–2): 137–144.

120. Gatson JW, Liu MM, Abdelfattah K et al. Resveratrol decreases inflammation in the brain of mice with mild traumatic brain injury. *The Journal of Trauma and Acute Care Surgery*. 2013; 74(2): 470–474.

121. Singleton RH, Yan HQ, Fellows-Mayle W, Dixon CE. Resveratrol attenuates behavioral impairments and reduces cortical and hippocampal loss in a rat controlled cortical impact model of traumatic brain injury. *Journal of Neurotrauma*. 2010; 27(6): 1091–1099.

122. Sonmez U, Sonmez A, Erbil G, Tekmen I, Baykara B. Neuroprotective effects of resveratrol against traumatic brain injury in immature rats. *Neuroscience Letters*. 2007; 420(2): 133–137.

123. Scapagnini G, Caruso C, Calabrese V. Therapeutic potential of dietary polyphenols against brain ageing and neurodegenerative disorders. *Advances in Experimental Medicine and Biology*. 2010; 698: 27–35.

124. Wakade C, King MD, Laird MD, Alleyne CH, Jr., Dhandapani KM. Curcumin attenuates vascular inflammation and cerebral vasospasm after subarachnoid hemorrhage in mice. *Antioxidants and Redox Signaling*. 2009; 11(1): 35–45.

125. Yang F, Lim GP, Begum AN et al. Curcumin inhibits formation of amyloid beta oligomers and fibrils, binds plaques, and reduces amyloid in vivo. *The Journal of Biological Chemistry*. 2005; 280(7): 5892–5901.

126. Ng TP, Chiam PC, Lee T, Chua HC, Lim L, Kua EH. Curry consumption and cognitive function in the elderly. *American Journal of Epidemiology*. 2006; 164(9): 898–906.

127. Dohare P, Garg P, Jain V, Nath C, Ray M. Dose dependence and therapeutic window for the neuroprotective effects of curcumin in thromboembolic model of rat. *Behavioural Brain Research*. 2008; 193(2): 289–297.

128 Shah FA, Park DJ, Gim SA, Koh PO. Curcumin treatment recovery the decrease of protein phosphatase 2A subunit B induced by focal cerebral ischemia in Sprague-Dawley rats. *Laboratory Animal Research*. 2015; 31(3): 134–138.

129. Wu J, Li Q, Wang X et al. Neuroprotection by curcumin in ischemic brain injury involves the Akt/Nrf2 pathway. *PLoS One*. 2013; 8(3): e59843.

130. Li Y, Li J, Li S et al. Curcumin attenuates glutamate neurotoxicity in the hippocampus by suppression of ER stress-associated TXNIP/NLRP3 inflammasome activation in a manner

dependent on AMPK. *Toxicology and Applied Pharmacology*. 2015; 286(1): 53–63.

131. Tu XK, Yang WZ, Chen JP et al. Curcumin inhibits TLR2/4-NF-kappaB signaling pathway and attenuates brain damage in permanent focal cerebral ischemia in rats. *Inflammation*. 2014; 37(5): 1544–1551.

132. Liu L, Zhang W, Wang L et al. Curcumin prevents cerebral ischemia reperfusion injury via increase of mitochondrial biogenesis. *Neurochemical Research*. 2014; 39(7): 1322–1331.

133. Awad AS. Effect of combined treatment with curcumin and candesartan on ischemic brain damage in mice. *Journal of Stroke and Cerebrovascular Diseases*. 2011; 20(6): 541–548.

134. Zhao J, Yu S, Zheng W et al. Curcumin improves outcomes and attenuates focal cerebral ischemic injury via antiapoptotic mechanisms in rats. *Neurochemical Research*. 2010; 35(3): 374–379.

135. Yang C, Zhang X, Fan H, Liu Y. Curcumin upregulates transcription factor Nrf2, HO-1 expression and protects rat brains against focal ischemia. *Brain Research*. 2009; 1282: 133–141.

136. Shukla PK, Khanna VK, Ali MM, Khan MY, Srimal RC. Anti-ischemic effect of curcumin in rat brain. *Neurochemical Research*. 2008; 33(6): 1036–1043.

137. Laird MD, Sukumari-Ramesh S, Swift AE, Meiler SE, Vender JR, Dhandapani KM. Curcumin attenuates cerebral edema following traumatic brain injury in mice: a possible role for aquaporin-4? *Journal of Neurochemistry*. 2010; 113(3): 637–648.

138. Wu A, Ying Z, Schubert D, Gomez-Pinilla F. Brain and spinal cord interaction: a dietary curcumin derivative counteracts locomotor and cognitive deficits after brain trauma. *Neurorehabilitation and Neural Repair*. 2011; 25(4): 332–342.

139. Wu A, Ying Z, Gomez-Pinilla F. Dietary curcumin counteracts the outcome of traumatic brain injury on oxidative stress, synaptic plasticity, and cognition. *Experimental Neurology*. 2006; 197(2): 309–317.

140. Sharma S, Zhuang Y, Ying Z, Wu A, Gomez-Pinilla F. Dietary curcumin supplementation counteracts reduction in levels of molecules involved in energy homeostasis after brain trauma. *Neuroscience*. 2009; 161(4): 1037–1044.

141. Sharma S, Ying Z, Gomez-Pinilla F. A pyrazole curcumin derivative restores membrane homeostasis disrupted after brain trauma. *Experimental Neurology*. 2010; 226(1): 191–199.

142. Jiang J, Wang W, Sun YJ, Hu M, Li F, Zhu DY. Neuroprotective effect of curcumin on focal cerebral ischemic rats by preventing blood–brain barrier damage. *European Journal of Pharmacology*. 2007; 561(1–3): 54–62.

143. Xu M, Chen X, Gu Y et al. Baicalin can scavenge peroxynitrite and ameliorate endogenous peroxynitrite-mediated neurotoxicity in cerebral ischemia-reperfusion injury. *Journal of Ethnopharmacology*. 2013; 150(1): 116–124.

144. Shang Y, Zhang H, Cheng J et al. Flavonoids from Scutellaria baicalensis Georgi are effective to treat cerebral ischemia/reperfusion. *Neural Regeneration Research*. 2013; 8(6): 514–522.

145. Xue X, Qu XJ, Yang Y et al. Baicalin attenuates focal cerebral ischemic reperfusion injury through inhibition of nuclear factor kappaB p65 activation. *Biochemical and Biophysical Research Communications*. 2010; 403(3–4): 398–404.

146. Shang YZ, Miao H, Cheng JJ, Qi JM. Effects of amelioration of total flavonoids from stems and leaves of Scutellaria baicalensis Georgi on cognitive deficits, neuronal damage and free radicals disorder induced by cerebral ischemia in rats. *Biological and Pharmaceutical Bulletin*. 2006; 29(4): 805–810.

147. Cao Y, Li G, Wang YF et al. Neuroprotective effect of baicalin on compression spinal cord injury in rats. *Brain Research*. 2010; 1357: 115–123.

148. Hwang YK, Jinhua M, Choi BR et al. Effects of Scutellaria baicalensis on chronic cerebral hypoperfusion-induced memory impairments and chronic lipopolysaccharide infusion-induced memory impairments. *Journal of Ethnopharmacology*. 2011; 137(1): 681–689.

149. Theadom A, Mahon S, Barker-Collo S et al. Enzogenol for cognitive functioning in traumatic brain injury: a pilot placebo-controlled RCT. *European Journal of Neurology*. 2013; 20(8): 1135–1144.

150. Elkind JA, Lim MM, Johnson BN et al. Efficacy, dosage, and duration of action of branched chain amino Acid therapy for traumatic brain injury. *Frontiers in Neurology*. 2015; 6: 73.

151. Lim MM, Elkind J, Xiong G et al. Dietary therapy mitigates persistent wake deficits caused by mild traumatic brain injury. *Science Translational Medicine*. 2013; 5(215): 215ra173.

152. Xu JY, Chen C. Endocannabinoids in synaptic plasticity and neuroprotection. *The Neuroscientist*. 2015; 21(2): 152–168.

153. Katz PS, Sulzer JK, Impastato RA, Teng SX, Rogers EK, Molina PE. Endocannabinoid degradation inhibition improves neurobehavioral function, blood–brain barrier integrity, and neuroinflammation following mild traumatic brain injury. *Journal of Neurotrauma*. 2015; 32(5): 297–306.

154. Hayakawa K, Mishima K, Irie K et al. Cannabidiol prevents a post-ischemic injury progressively induced by cerebral ischemia via a high-mobility group box1-inhibiting mechanism. *Neuropharmacology*. 2008; 55(8): 1280–1286.

155. He XL, Wang YH, Gao M, Li XX, Zhang TT, Du GH. Baicalein protects rat brain mitochondria against chronic cerebral hypoperfusion-induced oxidative damage. *Brain Research*. 2009; 1249: 212–221.

156. Yang J, Wu X, Yu H, Liao X, Teng L. NMDA receptor-mediated neuroprotective effect of the Scutellaria baicalensis Georgi extract on the excitotoxic neuronal cell death in primary rat cortical cell cultures. *The Scientific World Journal*. 2014; 2014: 459549.

157. Chen SF, Hsu CW, Huang WH, Wang JY. Post-injury baicalein improves histological and functional outcomes and reduces inflammatory cytokines after experimental traumatic brain injury. *British Journal of Pharmacology*. 2008; 155(8): 1279–1296.

158. Lu JH, Ardah MT, Durairajan SS et al. Baicalein inhibits formation of alpha-synuclein oligomers within living cells and prevents Abeta peptide fibrillation and oligomerisation. *ChemBioChem*. 2011; 12(4): 615–624.

159. Choi JH, Choi AY, Yoon H et al. Baicalein protects HT22 murine hippocampal neuronal cells against endoplasmic reticulum stress-induced apoptosis through inhibition of reactive oxygen species production and CHOP induction. *Experimental and Molecular Medicine*. 2010; 42(12): 811–822.

160. Kalda A, Yu L, Oztas E, Chen JF. Novel neuroprotection by caffeine and adenosine A(2A) receptor antagonists in animal models of Parkinson's disease. *Journal of the Neurological Sciences*. 2006; 248(1–2): 9–15.

161. Costa J, Lunet N, Santos C, Santos J, Vaz-Carneiro A. Caffeine exposure and the risk of Parkinson's disease: a systematic review and meta-analysis of observational studies. *Journal of Alzheimer's Disease*. 2010; 20 Suppl 1: S221–238.

162. Santos C, Lunet N, Azevedo A, de Mendonca A, Ritchie K, Barros H. Caffeine intake is associated with a lower risk of cognitive decline: a cohort study from Portugal. *Journal of Alzheimer's Disease*. 2010; 20 Suppl 1: S175–185.

163. Santos C, Costa J, Santos J, Vaz-Carneiro A, Lunet N. Caffeine intake and dementia: systematic review and meta-analysis. *Journal of Alzheimer's Disease*. 2010; 20 Suppl 1: S187–204.

164. Cao C, Cirrito JR, Lin X et al. Caffeine suppresses amyloid-beta levels in plasma and brain of Alzheimer's disease transgenic mice. *Journal of Alzheimer's Disease*. 2009; 17(3): 681–697.

165. Arendash GW, Mori T, Cao C et al. Caffeine reverses cognitive impairment and decreases brain amyloid-beta levels in aged Alzheimer's disease mice. *Journal of Alzheimer's Disease*. 2009; 17(3): 661–680.

166. Arendash GW, Schleif W, Rezai-Zadeh K et al. Caffeine protects Alzheimer's mice against cognitive impairment and reduces brain beta-amyloid production. *Neuroscience*. 2006; 142(4): 941–952.

167. Li W, Dai S, An J et al. Chronic but not acute treatment with caffeine attenuates traumatic brain injury in the mouse cortical impact model. *Neuroscience*. 2008; 151(4): 1198–1207.

168. Cekic M, Cutler SM, VanLandingham JW, Stein DG. Vitamin D deficiency reduces the benefits of progesterone treatment after brain injury in aged rats. *Neurobiology of Aging*. 2011; 32(5): 864–874.

169. Cekic M, Stein DG. Traumatic brain injury and aging: is a combination of progesterone and vitamin D hormone a simple solution to a complex problem? *Neurotherapeutics*. 2010; 7(1): 81–90.

170. Aiguo W, Zhe Y, Gomez-Pinilla F. Vitamin E protects against oxidative damage and learning disability after mild traumatic brain injury in rats. *Neurorehabilitation and Neural Repair*. 2010; 24(3): 290–298.

171. Greig NH, Tweedie D, Rachmany L et al. Incretin mimetics as pharmacologic tools to elucidate and as a new drug strategy to treat traumatic brain injury. *Alzheimer's and Dementia*. 2014; 10(1 Suppl): S62–75.

172. Rachmany L, Tweedie D, Li Y et al. Exendin-4 induced glucagon-like peptide-1 receptor activation reverses behavioral impairments of mild traumatic brain injury in mice. *Age (Dordrecht, Netherlands)*. 2013; 35(5): 1621–1636.

173. Tweedie D, Rachmany L, Rubovitch V et al. Exendin-4, a glucagon-like peptide-1 receptor agonist prevents mTBI-induced changes in hippocampus gene expression and memory deficits in mice. *Experimental Neurology*. 2013; 239: 170–182.

174. Eakin K, Baratz-Goldstein R, Pick CG et al. Efficacy of N-acetyl cysteine in traumatic brain injury. *PLoS One*. 2014; 9(4): e90617.

175. Robertson CS, Garcia R, Gaddam SS et al. Treatment of mild traumatic brain injury with an erythropoietin-mimetic peptide. *Journal of Neurotrauma*. 2013; 30(9): 765–774.

176. Homsi S, Piaggio T, Croci N et al. Blockade of acute microglial activation by minocycline promotes neuroprotection and reduces locomotor hyperactivity after closed head injury in mice: a twelve-week follow-up study. *Journal of Neurotrauma*. 2010; 27(5): 911–921.

177. Perez-Polo JR, Rea HC, Johnson KM et al. Inflammatory cytokine receptor blockade in a rodent model of mild traumatic brain injury. *Journal of Neuroscience Research*. 2016; 94(1): 27–38.

178. Baratz R, Tweedie D, Wang JY et al. Transiently lowering tumor necrosis factor-alpha synthesis ameliorates neuronal cell loss and cognitive impairments induced by minimal traumatic brain injury in mice. *Journal of Neuroinflammation*. 2015; 12: 45.

179. Yang SH, Gangidine M, Pritts TA, Goodman MD, Lentsch AB. Interleukin 6 mediates neuroinflammation and motor coordination deficits after mild traumatic brain injury and brief hypoxia in mice. *Shock (Augusta, Ga)*. 2013; 40(6): 471–475.

180. Tang C, Xue HL, Bai CL, Fu R. Regulation of adhesion molecules expression in TNF-alpha-stimulated brain microvascular endothelial cells by tanshinone IIA: involvement of NF-kappaB and ROS generation. *PTR*. 2011; 25(3): 376–380.

181. Tang C, Xue H, Bai C, Fu R, Wu A. The effects of Tanshinone IIA on blood–brain barrier and brain edema after transient middle cerebral artery occlusion in rats. *Phytomedicine*. 2010; 17(14): 1145–1149.

182. Zhang WJ, Feng J, Zhou R et al. Tanshinone IIA protects the human blood–brain barrier model from leukocyte-associated hypoxia-reoxygenation injury. *European Journal of Pharmacology*. 2010; 648(1–3): 146–152.

183. Feuerstein GZ, Wang X, Barone FC. The role of cytokines in the neuropathology of stroke and neurotrauma. *Neuroimmunomodulation*. 1998; 5(3–4): 143–159.

184. Tsai YD, Liliang PC, Cho CL et al. Delayed neurovascular inflammation after mild traumatic brain injury in rats. *Brain Injury*. 2013; 27(3): 361–365.

185. Chen CC, Wei ST, Tsaia SC, Chen XX, Cho DY. Cerebrolysin enhances cognitive recovery of mild traumatic brain injury patients: double-blind, placebo-controlled, randomized study. *British Journal of Neurosurgery*. 2013; 27(6): 803–807.

186. Yin D, Zhou C, Kusaka I et al. Inhibition of apoptosis by hyperbaric oxygen in a rat focal cerebral ischemic model. *Journal of Cerebral Blood Flow and Metabolism*. 2003; 23(7): 855-864.

187. Vlodavsky E, Palzur E, Soustiel JF. Hyperbaric oxygen therapy reduces neuroinflammation and expression of matrix metalloproteinase-9 in the rat model of traumatic brain injury. *Neuropathology and Applied Neurobiology*. 2006; 32(1): 40–50.

188. Harch PG, Kriedt C, Van Meter KW, Sutherland RJ. Hyperbaric oxygen therapy improves spatial learning and memory in a rat model of chronic traumatic brain injury. *Brain Research*. 2007; 1174: 120–129.

189. Stoller KP. Hyperbaric oxygen therapy (1.5 ATA) in treating sports related TBI/CTE: two case reports. *Medical Gas Research*. 2011; 1(1): 17.

190. Boussi-Gross R, Golan H, Fishlev G et al. Hyperbaric oxygen therapy can improve post concussion syndrome years after mild traumatic brain injury—randomized prospective trial. *PLoS One*. 2013; 8(11): e79995.

191. Walker WC, Franke LM, Cifu DX, Hart BB. Randomized, sham-controlled, feasibility trial of hyperbaric oxygen for service members with postconcussion syndrome: cognitive and psychomotor outcomes 1 week post-intervention. *Neurorehabilitation and Neural Repair*. 2013; 28(5): 420–432.

192. Bennett M. Hyperbaric oxygen therapy no better than sham in improving postconcussion symptoms following mild traumatic brain injury. *Diving and Hyperbaric Medicine*. 2013; 43(3): 173.

193. Miller RS, Weaver LK, Bahraini N et al. Effects of hyperbaric oxygen on symptoms and quality of life among service members with persistent postconcussion symptoms: a randomized clinical trial. *The Journal of the American Medical Association Internal Medicine*. 2015; 175(1): 43–52.

194. Cifu DX, Hoke KW, Wetzel PA, Wares JR, Gitchel G, Carne W. Effects of hyperbaric oxygen on eye tracking abnormalities in males after mild traumatic brain injury. *Journal of Rehabilitation Research and Development*. 2014; 51(7): 1047–1056.

195. Cifu DX, Hart BB, West SL, Walker W, Carne W. The effect of hyperbaric oxygen on persistent postconcussion symptoms. *The Journal of Head Tauma Rehabilitation*. 2014; 29(1): 11–20.

196. Kochanek PM, Jackson TC. It might be time to let cooler heads prevail after mild traumatic brain injury or concussion. *Experimental Neurology*. 2015; 267: 13–17.

197. Karnatovskaia LV, Wartenberg KE, Freeman WD. Therapeutic hypothermia for neuroprotection: history, mechanisms, risks, and clinical applications. *The Neurohospitalist*. 2014; 4(3): 153–163.

198. Li YH, Zhang CL, Zhang XY, Zhou HX, Meng LL. Effects of mild induced hypothermia on hippocampal connexin 43 and glutamate transporter 1 expression following traumatic brain injury in rats. *Molecular Medicine Reports*. 2015; 11(3): 1991–1996.

199. Miyauchi T, Wei EP, Povlishock JT. Therapeutic targeting of the axonal and microvascular change associated with repetitive mild traumatic brain injury. *Journal of Neurotrauma*. 2013; 30(19): 1664–1671.

200. Kim JY, Kim N, Yenari MA, Chang W. Hypothermia and pharmacological regimens that prevent overexpression and overactivity of the extracellular calcium-sensing receptor protect neurons against traumatic brain injury. *Journal of Neurotrauma*. 2013; 30(13): 1170–1176.

201. Cheng SX, Zhang S, Sun HT, Tu Y. Effects of mild hypothermia treatment on rat hippocampal beta-amyloid expression following traumatic brain injury. *Therapeutic Hypothermia and Temperature Management*. 2013; 3(3): 132–139.

202. Lee JH, Wei L, Gu X, Wei Z, Dix TA, Yu SP. Therapeutic effects of pharmacologically induced hypothermia against traumatic brain injury in mice. *Journal of Neurotrauma*. 2014; 31(16): 1417–1430.

203. Gu X, Wei ZZ, Espinera A et al. Pharmacologically induced hypothermia attenuates traumatic brain injury in neonatal rats. *Experimental Neurology*. 2015; 267: 135–142.

204. Yokobori S, Gajavelli S, Mondello S et al. Neuroprotective effect of preoperatively induced mild hypothermia as determined by biomarkers and histopathological estimation in a rat subdural hematoma decompression model. *Journal of Neurosurgery*. 2013; 118(2): 370–380.

205. Jia F, Mao Q, Liang YM, Jiang JY. The effect of hypothermia on the expression of TIMP-3 after traumatic brain injury in rats. *Journal of Neurotrauma*. 2014; 31(4): 387–394.

206. Hutchison JS, Ward RE, Lacroix J et al. Hypothermia therapy after traumatic brain injury in children. *The New England Journal of Medicine*. 2008; 358(23): 2447–2456.

207. Maekawa T, Yamashita S, Nagao S, Hayashi N, Ohashi Y. Prolonged mild therapeutic hypothermia versus fever control with tight hemodynamic monitoring and slow rewarming in patients with severe traumatic brain injury: a randomized controlled trial. *Journal of Neurotrauma*. 2015; 32(7): 422–429.

208. Wang H, Olivero W, Lanzino G et al. Rapid and selective cerebral hypothermia achieved using a cooling helmet. *Journal of Neurosurgery*. 2004; 100(2): 272–277.

209. Wang H, Wang B, Jackson K et al. A novel head-neck cooling device for concussion injury in contact sports. *Translational Neuroscience*. 2015; 6(1).

210. Huang YY, Gupta A, Vecchio D et al. Transcranial low level laser (light) therapy for traumatic brain injury. *Journal of Biophotonics*. 2012; 5(11–12): 827–837.

211. Morries LD, Cassano P, Henderson TA. Treatments for traumatic brain injury with emphasis on transcranial near-infrared laser phototherapy. *Neuropsychiatric Disease and Treatment*. 2015; 11: 2159–2175.

212. Chung H, Dai T, Sharma SK, Huang YY, Carroll JD, Hamblin MR. The nuts and bolts of low-level laser (light) therapy. *Annals of Biomedical Engineering*. 2012; 40(2): 516–533.

213. Demirtas-Tatlidede A, Vahabzadeh-Hagh AM, Bernabeu M, Tormos JM, Pascual-Leone A. Noninvasive brain stimulation in traumatic brain injury. *The Journal of Head Trauma Rehabilitation*. 2012; 27(4): 274–292.

214. Tedford CE, DeLapp S, Jacques S, Anders J. Quantitative analysis of transcranial and intraparenchymal light penetration in human cadaver brain tissue. *Lasers in Surgery and Medicine*. 2015; 47(4): 312–322.

215. Hashmi JT, Huang YY, Osmani BZ, Sharma SK, Naeser MA, Hamblin MR. Role of

low-level laser therapy in neurorehabilitation. *PM & R.* 2010; 2(12 Suppl 2): S292–305.

216. Wu Q, Xuan W, Ando T et al. Low-level laser therapy for closed-head traumatic brain injury in mice: effect of different wavelengths. *Lasers in Surgery and Medicine.* 2012; 44(3): 218–226.

217. Cotler HB, Chow RT, Hamblin MR, Carroll J. The use of low level laser therapy (lllt) for musculoskeletal pain. *MOJ Orthopedics and Rheumatology.* 2015; 2(5).

218. Lee HI, Park JH, Park MY et al. Preconditioning with transcranial low-level light therapy reduces neuroinflammation and protects blood–brain barrier after focal cerebral ischemia in mice. *Restorative Neurology and Neuroscience.* 2016; 34(2): 201–214.

219. Gomes LE, Dalmarco EM, Andre ES. The brain-derived neurotrophic factor, nerve growth factor, neurotrophin-3, and induced nitric oxide synthase expressions after low-level laser therapy in an axonotmesis experimental model. *Photomedicine and Laser Surgery.* 2012; 30(11): 642–647.

220. Dong T, Zhang Q, Hamblin MR, Wu MX. Low-level light in combination with metabolic modulators for effective therapy of injured brain. *Journal of Cerebral Blood Flow and Metabolism.* 2015; 35(9): 1435–1444.

221. McCarthy TJ, De Taboada L, Hildebrandt PK, Ziemer EL, Richieri SP, Streeter J. Long-term safety of single and multiple infrared transcranial laser treatments in Sprague-Dawley rats. *Photomedicine and Laser Surgery.* 2010; 28(5): 663–667.

222. Xuan W, Vatansever F, Huang L et al. Transcranial low-level laser therapy improves neurological performance in traumatic brain injury in mice: effect of treatment repetition regimen. *PLoS One.* 2013; 8(1): e53454.

223. Zhang Q, Zhou C, Hamblin MR, Wu MX. Low-level laser therapy effectively prevents secondary brain injury induced by immediate early responsive gene X-1 deficiency.

Journal of Cerebral Blood Flow and Metabolism. 2014; 34(8): 1391–1401.

224. Xuan W, Vatansever F, Huang L, Hamblin MR. Transcranial low-level laser therapy enhances learning, memory, and neuroprogenitor cells after traumatic brain injury in mice. *Journal of Biomedical Optics.* 2014; 19(10): 108003.

225. Xuan W, Huang L, Hamblin MR. Repeated transcranial low-level laser therapy for traumatic brain injury in mice: biphasic dose response and long-term treatment outcome. *Journal of Biophotonics.* 2016.

226. Xuan W, Agrawal T, Huang L, Gupta GK, Hamblin MR. Low-level laser therapy for traumatic brain injury in mice increases brain derived neurotrophic factor (BDNF) and synaptogenesis. *Journal of Biophotonics.* 2015; 8(6): 502–511.

227. Quirk BJ, Torbey M, Buchmann E, Verma S, Whelan HT. Near-infrared photobiomodulation in an animal model of traumatic brain injury: improvements at the behavioral and biochemical levels. *Photomedicine and Laser Surgery.* 2012; 30(9): 523–529.

228. Oron A, Oron U, Streeter J et al. Near infrared transcranial laser therapy applied at various modes to mice following traumatic brain injury significantly reduces long-term neurological deficits. *Journal of Neurotrauma.* 2012; 29(2): 401–407.

229. Oron A, Oron U, Streeter J et al. low-level laser therapy applied transcranially to mice following traumatic brain injury significantly reduces long-term neurological deficits. *Journal of Neurotrauma.* 2007; 24(4): 651–656.

230. Giacci MK, Wheeler L, Lovett S et al. Differential effects of 670 and 830 nm red near infrared irradiation therapy: a comparative study of optic nerve injury, retinal degeneration, traumatic brain and spinal cord injury. *PLoS One.* 2014; 9(8): e104565.

231. Ando T, Xuan W, Xu T et al. Comparison of therapeutic effects between pulsed and

continuous wave 810–nm wavelength laser irradiation for traumatic brain injury in mice. *PLoS One.* 2011; 6(10): e26212.

232. Khuman J, Zhang J, Park J, Carroll JD, Donahue C, Whalen MJ. Low-level laser light therapy improves cognitive deficits and inhibits microglial activation after controlled cortical impact in mice. *Journal of Neurotrauma.* 2012; 29(2): 408–417.

233. Henderson TA, Morries LD. SPECT Perfusion imaging demonstrates improvement of traumatic brain injury with transcranial near-infrared laser phototherapy. *Advances in Mind-Body Medicine.* 2015; 29(4): 27–33.

234. Naeser MA, Zafonte R, Krengel MH et al. Significant improvements in cognitive performance post-transcranial, red/near-infrared light-emitting diode treatments in chronic, mild traumatic brain injury: open-protocol study. *Journal of Neurotrauma.* 2014; 31(11): 1008–1017.

235. Lim W, Lee S, Kim I et al. The anti-inflammatory mechanism of 635 nm light-emitting-diode irradiation compared with existing COX inhibitors. *Lasers in Surgery and Medicine.* 2007; 39(7): 614–621.

236. Nawashiro H, Wada K, Nakai K, Sato S. Focal increase in cerebral blood flow after treatment with near-infrared light to the forehead in a patient in a persistent vegetative state. *Photomedicine and Laser Surgery.* 2012; 30(4): 231–233.

237. Naeser MA, Saltmarche A, Krengel MH, Hamblin MR, Knight JA. Improved cognitive function after transcranial, light-emitting diode treatments in chronic, traumatic brain injury: two case reports. *Photomedicine and Laser Surgery.* 2011; 29(5): 351–358.

238. Meehan Iii WP. LED Therapy for the Treatment of Concussive Brain Injury. *NCT02383472* 2016; https://clinicaltrials.gov/ct2/show/NCT02383472. Accessed Sept. 19, 2016.

239. Major BP, Rogers MA, Pearce AJ. Using transcranial magnetic stimulation to quantify electrophysiological changes following concussive brain injury: a systematic review. *Clinical and Experimental Pharmacology & Physiology.* 2015; 42(4): 394–405.

240. Herrold AA, Kletzel SL, Harton BC, Chambers RA, Jordan N, Pape TL. Transcranial magnetic stimulation: potential treatment for co–occurring alcohol, traumatic brain injury and posttraumatic stress disorders. *Neural Regeneration Research.* 2014; 9(19): 1712–1730.

241. Powers KC, Cinelli ME, Kalmar JM. Cortical hypoexcitability persists beyond the symptomatic phase of a concussion. *Brain Injury.* 2014; 28(4): 465–471.

242. Miller NR, Yasen AL, Maynard LF, Chou LS, Howell DR, Christie AD. Acute and longitudinal changes in motor cortex function following mild traumatic brain injury. *Brain Injury.* 2014; 28(10): 1270–1276.

243. Chistyakov AV, Soustiel JF, Hafner H, Trubnik M, Levy G, Feinsod M. Excitatory and inhibitory corticospinal responses to transcranial magnetic stimulation in patients with minor to moderate head injury. *Journal of Neurology, Neurosurgery, and Psychiatry.* 2001; 70(5): 580–587.

244. Tallus J, Lioumis P, Hamalainen H, Kahkonen S, Tenovuo O. Transcranial magnetic stimulation-electroencephalography responses in recovered and symptomatic mild traumatic brain injury. *Journal of Neurotrauma.* 2013; 30(14): 1270–1277.

245. Livingston SC, Saliba EN, Goodkin HP, Barth JT, Hertel JN, Ingersoll CD. A preliminary investigation of motor evoked potential abnormalities following sport-related concussion. *Brain Injury.* 2010; 24(6): 904–913.

246. Pearce AJ, Hoy K, Rogers MA et al. Acute motor, neurocognitive and neurophysiological change following concussion injury in Australian amateur football. A prospective multimodal investigation. *Journal of Science and Medicine in Sport.* 2015; 18(5): 500–506.

247. Tremblay S, de Beaumont L, Lassonde M, Theoret H. Evidence for the specificity of intracortical inhibitory dysfunction in asymptomatic concussed athletes. *Journal of Neurotrauma*. 2011; 28(4): 493–502.

248. De Beaumont L, Lassonde M, Leclerc S, Theoret H. Long-term and cumulative effects of sports concussion on motor cortex inhibition. *Neurosurgery*. 2007; 61(2): 329–336.

249. Pearce AJ, Hoy K, Rogers MA et al. The long-term effects of sports concussion on retired Australian football players: a study using transcranial magnetic stimulation. *Journal of Neurotrauma*. 2014; 31(13): 1139–1145.

250. Tremblay S, Vernet M, Bashir S, Pascual-Leone A, Theoret H. Theta burst stimulation to characterize changes in brain plasticity following mild traumatic brain injury: A proof-of-principle study. *Restorative Neurology and Neuroscience*. 2015; 33(5): 611–620.

251. Koski L, Kolivakis T, Yu C, Chen JK, Delaney S, Ptito A. Noninvasive brain stimulation for persistent postconcussion symptoms in mild traumatic brain injury. *Journal of Neurotrauma*. 2015; 32(1): 38–44.

252. Leung A, Shukla S, Fallah A et al. Repetitive transcranial magnetic stimulation in managing mild traumatic brain injury-related headaches. *Neuromodulation*. 2016; 19(2): 133–141.

Index